Molecular and
Cellular Networks
for Cancer Therapy

Molecular and Cellular Networks for Cancer Therapy

From the International Symposium on Molecular and Cellular Networks for Cancer Therapy, May 20, 1988, Osaka, Japan

Editors:

Yuichi Yamamura
Ichiro Azuma

 1989

Excerpta Medica, Amsterdam–Princeton–Hong Kong–Tokyo–Sydney

International Congress Series No. 857
ISBN 0 444 81076 5

Published by:
Elsevier Science Publishers B.V.
(Biomedical Division)
P.O. Box 211
1000 AE Amsterdam
The Netherlands

Sole distributors for the USA and Canada:
Elsevier Science Publishing Company Inc.
655 Avenue of the Americas
New York, NY 10010
USA

Printed in Japan

Contents

Preface

During the past 2 decades, many immunostimulants have been developed with the aim of using them clinically to stimulate the host defense against cancer, infectious diseases, and other immunodisorders. From studies on the mechanism of action of these immunostimulants, it was shown that endogenous cytokines induced by administration of immunostimulants could play an important role in the stimulation of the host defense mechanism. Recently, different cytokines such as interferons α, β, and γ, interleukins 1–6, tumor necrosis factor, and colony-stimulating factor, which have been prepared in bulk, following the development of genetic engineering technology, and supplied for experimental study and clinical application in cancer patients. The symposium on which this book is based summarized the experimental and clinical results accumulated in the past decade on the effect of immunostimulants and cytokines as cancer therapy.

Immediately following the IVth International Conference on Immunopharmacology in Osaka, May 15 to 19, 1988, an international symposium on "Molecular and Cellular Networks for Cancer Therapy" was held, organized by a scientific committee consisting of Drs Y. Yamamura, I. Azuma, T. Ogura, and F. Takaku. The symposium took place on May 20, 1988, at the Osaka Hilton International, with 250 delegates. Ten speakers, including 5 from overseas, reviewed their special areas of experience in immunostimulants and cytokines as cancer therapy.

This volume is not purely a proceedings of the meeting, but has been especially edited to reflect the discussions which took place, as well as the reviews presented. It is also intended to provide a better understanding of the knowledge obtained in recent years and future research prospects in this area. The volume divides approximately into 2 sections: first, the present state of cytokine and immunostimulant research and its application in cancer therapy; and second, experimental and clinical studies on the efficacy of immunostimulants, especially *Nocardia rubra* cell wall skeleton (N-CWS), as cancer treatment. The book contains 22 papers, including 9 reviews which were presented at the symposium.

It is our real pleasure to thank warmly all the contributors to this volume and the participants in the symposium. We are also very grateful to Drs T. Ogura and F. Takaku for their most valuable contribution to the organization of the symposium.

We are particularly indebted to Fujisawa Pharmaceutical Co., Ltd., for financial support of the symposium, and especially to Mr Y. Konishi, of Fujisawa Pharmaceutical Co., Ltd., for his assistance in arranging the symposium and the publication of this proceedings. The expert assistance of the staff of Excerpta Medica, Ltd., in producing this volume is also greatly appreciated.

Y. Yamamura
I. Azuma

Cytokines and their role
in cancer therapy

Pleiotropisms and pleiomorphisms of cytokines— Immunostimulated and endogenous ways of hematopoiesis?

Fritz Melchers

Basel Institute for Immunology, Basel, Switzerland

Introduction

Blood cells are formed by proliferation and differentiation in a complex series of steps, first during embryonic development, and then continuously throughout adult life to replace those which die, used or unused for their effector functions. These steps are controlled by specific cell-cell contacts and by soluble cytokines. Both can be seen as ligand-receptor interactions mediated and received by specific cells at particular points in their developments.

The hierarchies of cellular developments in the blood cell system are experimentally defined by cellular precursor-product relationships, in which one cell is recognized as the progenitor (P) or precursor (pre) of a set of differentiated cells in a clonal assay. Such clonal assays define the soluble and cell contact-mediated activities which influence proliferation and differentiation of a given stage in blood cell development. It is hoped that these controlling elements of proliferation and differentiation can be used not only to specify the stage of lineage differentiation and the molecular parameters of their controls, but also to influence the future development of a given cell in this hierarchy through exogenous interference with cell-specific ligands of cell-cell contacts and of soluble mediators.

Stem cells and progenitors

The hematopoietic cell system of erythroid, myeloid, and lymphoid cells is derived from single pluripotent stem cells ($S_{M/E/L}$, Fig 1). Their existence has long been implied from experiments in which early bone marrow cells with unique chromosome aberrations induced by radiation have given rise to marked cells in all lineages of blood (1–3). Furthermore, single cells of embryonic blood from a donor could be introduced into the circulation of an embryonic host to

F. Melchers

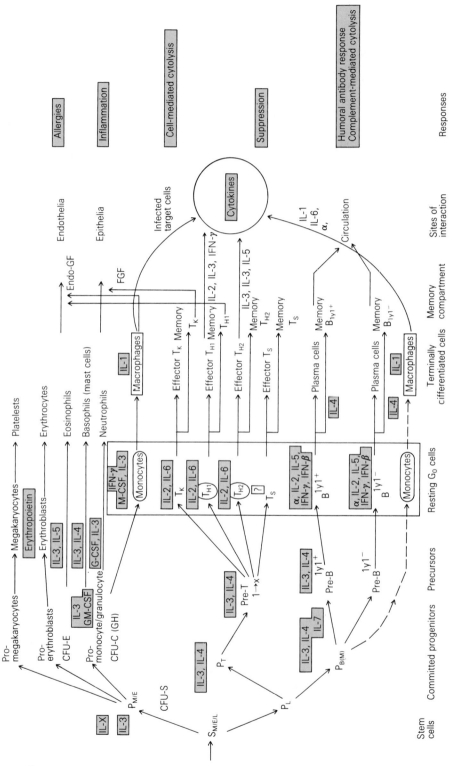

Fig 1 Hematopoiesis of blood cell lineages to their effector phases, and the role of cytokines in this development. The different stages are described in sequence by the bottom line.

4

repopulate all lineages (4). Recently, pluripotent stem cells from bone marrow (5) were infected in vitro with a retrovirus containing the neomycin-resistance gene. Upon transfer of these cells to a host the integrated virus and, therefore, the neomycin resistance has been detected in erythroid, myeloid, and lymphoid cells (6,7). So far, however, pluripotent stem cells cannot be detected by an in vitro colony assay.

The first cells detectable in vivo and in vitro as colony-forming, immature progenitors of the erythroid/myeloid parts of the blood system are the colony-forming units in spleen (8,9) (CFU-S, $P_{M/E}$ in Fig 1). A progenitor for all lymphoid cells (P_L) has not yet been discovered. From these early progenitors, more committed progenitors are derived. In the myeloid branch of blood cell differentiation they form colonies (CFU-C, CFU-GM) in which monocytes and granulocytes will differentiate (10). In the lymphoid branches progenitors committed to the various T cells (3,11) (P_T) and those committed to the ly 1^+ as well as ly 1^- B cell lineages are detectable in various in vivo and in vitro assays (for references see papers in ref 12).

All the early stages of blood cell differentiation are thought to depend on specialized, competent environments containing cooperating stromal cells. It is likely that contacts between progenitors and stromal cells control these stages of blood cell differentiation, although no structures forming these contacts have yet been specified by either genetic or biochemical evidence. For erythroid/myeloid differentiation and for B lymphocyte development this competent environment is provided by bone marrow, while T lymphocytes require the thymus for the expression of α and β chains of T cell receptors (TcRs) and for the CD4 and CD8 surface markers which are involved, respectively, in helper and cytolytic functions of T cells.

The resting state of the lymphoid compartment and its activation

Cells of the erythroid, megakaryocytic, basophilic, eosinophilic, and neutrophilic lineages, which are all thought to be derived from the myeloid/erythroid-committed progenitors ($P_{M/E}$) might never go through a resting, G_0 phase, from which they could be activated to their terminally differentiated effector phases. Lymphocytes, and maybe some of the monocytes, however, do (see box in Fig 1). I have speculated (13) that the insertion of an immunoglobulin (Ig) or a TcR molecule into the surface membrane of a pre-B or pre-T cell at the stage of transition to the mature B or T cell might signal the cell to go to rest. In this resting, G_0 state of the cell cycle, lymphocytes are refractory to the action of proliferation-inducing cytokines (14). Special signals have to be given to resting lymphocytes to render them susceptible to cytokines which stimulated proliferation and maturation to the terminally differentiated effector functions of T cell killing, help, and suppression, and of B cell Ig (antibody) secretion. These special signals are initiated by the binding of foreign materials, called antigens.

Immunostimulation

The response to antigen happens in the competent environment of the peripheral, secondary lymphoid organs, such as lymph nodes and spleen. They require the cooperation of several types of cells of the monocytic and lymphoid lineages. In the activation of primary B cells from their resting state, 2 types of cells have been identified to cooperate with B cells in 2 discernible steps (13–15). In the 1st step, antigen is taken up by accessory (A) cells, many of which belong to the monocyte–macrophage lineage. The antigen is then processed (in the case of proteins to peptides) (16,17), and the processed antigen is presented, in conjunction with membrane proteins encoded by genes of the major histocompatibility complex (MHC), on the surface of these A cells (Fig 2). This whole process is likely to activate a monocyte, if it was resting beforehand. The complex of processed antigen and MHC protein is then recognized by specific receptors on T cells, ie, by the antigen-specific, MHC-restricted TcR. This MHC-antigen/TcR-mediated contact between 2 types of cells (A and T) activates *both* cells.

Cytolytic T cells recognize processed antigen in conjunction with MHC class I molecules. They are helped in their contact to the A cells by the CD8 molecule (on the T cell) which establishes additional contact to the MHC class I molecules (on the A cell) (Fig 2, phase 1). Once activated, the cytolytic T cells will proliferate and mature to killer effector functions. They repeat the MHC-restricted, antigen-specific contacts when they kill the target cells (Fig 2, phase 2).

Helper T cells recognize processed antigen in conjunction with MHC class II molecules. They are helped in their contact to the A cells by the CD4 molecule, which makes additional contacts with MHC class II molecules. As a consequence of these contacts, T cells and A cells begin to produce and secrete cytokines.

In the 2nd step, resting B cells bind antigen by their antigen-specific Ig receptors, take up the antigen, process it and, finally, present the processed antigen in conjunction with MHC class II molecules on their surface. The same MHC-restricted, antigen-specific helper T cells now make contact with MHC-antigen via their MHC-restricted, antigen-specific TcR (Fig 2). Again, *both* types of cells are activated. B cells, as a consequence, become "excited," and become susceptible to the action of specific cytokines, to which they previously, ie, in their resting state, had been insensitive.

Cell-cycle control of lymphocytes

Once activated, lymphocytes will proceed through the cell cycle, ie, through G_1 phase, S phase, and G_2 phase, and complete the cycle with mitosis, provided that the appropriate signals are given (18). The cell cycle of primary B cells is controlled by multiple signals: signals of antigen via surface Ig; signals of helper T cells with their TcR via processed antigen in the context of MHC class II molecules; signals of complement-C3-like components, called α-factors, via the complement C3d receptor CR2 (19); and signals of interleukin 2 (IL-2) or IL-5 via receptors for IL-2 or IL-5 (Fig 3) (20,21; for further references see ref 13).

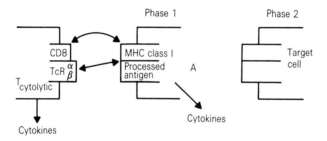

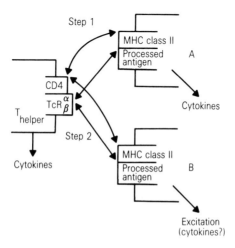

Fig 2 MHC-restricted, antigen-specific interactions of killer or helper T cells with accessory (A) cells and target cells, or accessory cells and B cells.

These multiple signals, initiated by the ligands binding to their corresponding receptors, control the cell cycle in a synergistic fashion, and at different restriction points within the cycle. Similarly, T cell growth appears to be synergistically controlled by binding of processed antigen plus MHC molecules on A cells to TcR on T cells, by IL-2 and by IL-6 (22,23).

The synergistic growth control of lymphocytes is a consequence of the cooperation of different cells both by cell-cell contacts as well as by interactions of receptors with specific soluble cytokines. The soluble cytokines themselves are produced as a consequence of cell-cell contacts, and all contacts require antigen to initiate these cascades of reactions of lymphocytes and A cells.

Clonal assays for important phases of normal lymphocyte growth are often not available, since both the activation and the cell-cycle progression phases are not only dependent on soluble cytokines but also on cell-cell contacts. Further-

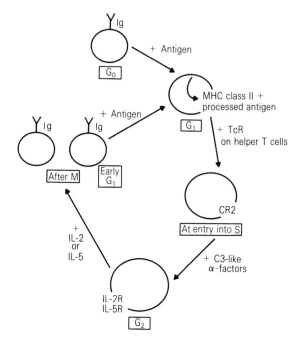

Fig 3 Different phases of the B cell cycle controlled by different ligands interacting with different surface-bound receptors (phase 1: binding of antigen to Ig; phase 2: binding of TcR on helper T cells to processed antigen in the context of MHC class II molecules; phase 3: binding of C3-like α-factors to the complement receptor CR2; phase 4: binding of either IL-2 or IL-5 to IL-2 or IL-5 receptors).

more, the efficiency of plating of lymphocytes in tissue culture drops to practically zero below cell concentrations of $1-5 \times 10^4$ cells/mL. Cultures of normal lymphocytes are never 100% pure, as a single cell would be. Consequently, actions of cells and cytokines on lymphocytes may be direct, or indirect via contaminating cells. In many instances, studies of lymphocyte activation do not really measure the completion of one or several cell cycles, but monitor early changes in surface marker expression, biochemical signaling reactions, or thymidine uptake, which might all occur without mitoses. All this often makes it impossible to assign unambiguously the activity of a given cytokine to a *direct* action on lymphocytes.

Cell-cell contacts and cytokines in the development of the blood cell lineages

Cells within the hierarchies of development of the different blood lineages begin to be well defined not only by their morphology, cell-surface marker, and gene-expression patterns (for references see ref 12) but also by their patterns of reactivities with other cells and with soluble cytokines (Fig 1). The recent advances in these fields have been made possible by several developments: by the isolation and structural identification of genes for many cytokines, and by the expression of those genes as single, pure proteins in large quantities; by the identification of receptors for these lymphokines; by the generation of monoclonal antibodies specific for cytokines and for their receptors; by the long-term growth of normal (or almost normal) cells of the hematopoietic system and of the cooperating stromal cells, often as clones of cells; by the development of serum-substituted tissue-culture systems; and by in situ detection of expressed genes and proteins in single cells (for contributions from our laboratory to these advances, see refs 24–26).

The picture that emerges is not simple. One cell does not react with only one other cell, but with more than one, and those cells are from different lineages and differentiation stages. The example already mentioned is the helper T cell- *and* accessory cell-dependent activation and cell-cycle propagation of B cells.

Whenever the response to the cell-cell contact is cytokine production, it is not one, but several lymphokines that are produced by one cell. Examples are: helper T cells of type T_{H1} (27), which produce IL-2, IL-3, and interferon-γ (IFN-γ); helper T cells of type T_{H2}, which produce IL-3, IL-4, IL-5, and IL-6; or macrophages which produce IL-1, IL-6, complement-like components, and other growth factors. It also becomes evident that one cytokine can be produced by more than one differentiated type of cell.

One cytokine can act on more than one type of differentiated cell of the hematopoietic cell system, and maybe even on cells outside it. IL-2 acts on the different functional subpopulations of T cells and on B cells. IL-5 acts on B cells and on eosinophils, and IFN-γ acts on lymphocytes, monocytes, macrophages, and even on glial cells (28) . The actions of IL-1 are very diverse indeed (29).

Finally, one cell does not react only to one cytokine but can alternatively use more than one in the induction to the same function. Examples are IL-3 and all the alternative cytokines of the myeloid differentiation lineages (shown in Fig 1), and IL-2 and IL-5 as alternative β-type growth factors of B cells (18,20,21).

Endogenously controlled and exogenously induced hematopoiesis

Particularly striking in the scheme of hematopoiesis (Fig 1) is the role of IL-3 as a panhematopoietic activity, acting throughout the granulocytic–monocytic pathway of differentiation and in early stages of lymphocyte progenitors and precursors (30,31). It is puzzling that IL-3 acts on early progenitors and precursors although it is produced by T_{H1} and T_{H2} helper cells which develop from IL-3-sensitive precursors. How can these progenitors and precursors grow in the absence of T_{H1} and T_{H2} cells, ie, in bone marrow, in fetal liver, or in congenitally athymic animals such as nu/nu mice, or when T_{H1} and T_{H2} cells are resting, are not stimulated by antigen, and, therefore, do not produce IL-3?

In the myeloid lineage of differentiation, alternative cytokines appear to exist in the forms of IL-X (32), GM-CSF, G-CSF, and M-CSF, which can stimulate the generation of granulocytes and monocytes. They are likely to allow the

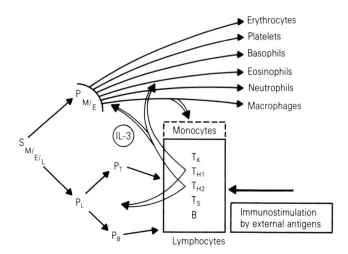

Fig 4 Exogenous control of hematopoiesis by IL-3 produced in T_{H1} and T_{H2} cells as a response to immunostimulation by antigen. The endogenous routes of hematopoietic differentiation (see also Fig 1) are expected to be controlled by different, endogenous cytokines.

development of these cell lineages in the absence of IL-3-producing T_H cells. The discovery of IL-7, acting on progenitor and precursor cells of the B lineage (33), might indicate that such alternative cytokines also exist for the lymphoid cell lineages. IL-7 is produced in stromal cells, consequently independently of T_H cells. There might, therefore, be two alternative ways to generate myeloid and lymphoid cells (Fig 4). One is *endogenous*, and the other is *induced* by exogenous stimuli. Immunostimulation by foreign antigens will exogenously induce T_{H1} and T_{H2} helper cells to produce, among other cytokines, IL-3—this will be in times of excessive need for cells to be generated in the acute defense against the foreign invader. In this view, the immune system has developed its own ways to mobilize hematopoiesis.

The physiological roles and importance of the multitude of cellular sites for cytokine production, of the multitude of cytokines produced at one site, and of the pleiomorphism and pleiotropism of the action of cytokines in the hematopoietic cell lineages all remain challenging problems for future research.

Acknowledgment

The Basel Institute for Immunology was founded and is supported by F. Hoffmann-La Roche & Co. Ltd, Basel, Switzerland.

References

1. Wu AM, Till JE, Siminovitch L, McCulloch EA. J Exp Med. 1968;127:458-63.
2. Wu AM. J Cell Physiol 1967;69:177-84.
3. Abramson S, Miller RC, Phillips RA. J Exp Med 1977;145:1567-79.
4. Fleischmann RA, Custer RP, Mintz B. Cell 1982;30:351-9.
5. Micklem HS, Ford CE, Evans EP, Gray J. Proc R Soc Lond Biol Sci 1966;165:78-102.
6. Keller G, Paige C, Gilboa E, Wagner EF. Nature 1985;318:149-54.
7. Dick JE, Magli MC, Auszar D, et al. Cell 1985;42:71-9.
8. Till JE, McCulloch EA. Radiat Res 1961;14:213-22.
9. Johnson GR, Metcalf D. Differentiation of normal and neoplastic hematopoietic cells. Cold Spring Harbor 1987:49-62.
10. Metcalf D. Recent Results Cancer Res 1977;61:1-227.
11. Kadish JL, Basch RS. J Exp Med 1976;143:1082-99.
12. Paige CJ, Gisler RH, eds. Curr Top Microbiol Immunol 1987;135:1-148.
13. Melchers F. In: Honjo T et al, eds. Immunoglobulin genes. New York: Academic Press; 1989:23-44.
14. Melchers F, Andersson J. Cell 1984;37:715-20.
15. Melchers F, Andersson J. Annu Rev Immunol 1986;4:13-36.
16. Buss S, Sette A, Colon SM, et al. Science 1876;235:1353-8.
17. Unanue ER, Allen PM. Science 1987;236:551-7.
18. Melchers F, Lernhardt W. Proc Natl Acad Sci USA 1985;82:7681-5.
19. Melchers F, Erdei A, Schulz T, Dierich MP. Nature 1985;317:1353-8.
20. Lernhardt W, Karasuyama H, Rolink A, Melchers F. Immunol Rev 1987;99:241-62.
21. Karasuyama H, Rolink A, Melchers F. J Exp Med 1988;18:97-104.
22. Hardt C, Nobuko S, Wagner H. Eur J Immunol 1987;17:209-18.
23. Uyttenhove C, Conlie PG, Van Snick J. J Exp Med 1988;167:1417-27.
24. Iscove NN, Melchers F. J Exp Med 1976;147:923-8.
25. Berger CN. EMBO (Eur Molec Biol Organ) J 1986;5:85-93.
26. Karasuyama H, Melchers F. Eur J Immunol 1988;18:97-104.
27. Coffman RL, Seymour BWP, Lebman DA, et al. Immunol Rev 1988;102:5-28.
28. Fontana A, Frei K, Bodmer S, Hofer E. Immunol Rev 1987;100:185-201.
29. Oppenheim JJ, Kovac EJ, Mitsushima K, Durum SK. Immunol Today 1986;7:45-56.
30. Schrader JW. Annu Rev Immunol 1986;4:205-30.
31. Palacios R, Hanson G, Steinmetz M, McKearn JP. Nature 1984;309:126-131.
32. Iscove NN, Fagg B, Keller G. Blood (in press).
33. Namen AE, Schmierer AE, March CJ, et al. J Exp Med 1988;167:988-1002.

Hemopoietic regulators in the treatment of cancer and myeloid leukemia

Donald Metcalf

Cancer Research Unit, The Walter and Eliza Hall Institute of Medical Research, Royal Melbourne Hospital, Melbourne, Victoria, Australia

Introduction

With the notable exception of a few types of less common tumor, the introduction of chemotherapy to the treatment of cancer has in general failed to achieve cures and, even when having a measurable effect, has usually achieved only temporary remissions. In many instances, the completion of what might otherwise have been a successful course of therapy is prevented by the development of severe drug-induced marrow damage. The use of chemotherapy alone in the treatment of cancer appears often to reach an impasse, with the maximum tolerated doses not able to destroy fully the tumor population.

In such a situation it is the view of many that the stimulation of host resistance, either via lymphoid cells or hemopoietic cells, might be an important adjunct to chemotherapy, thus allowing the complete suppression of some tumors. This is the reasoning behind the use of lymphokine-activated killer (LAK) cells and behind numerous in vitro studies that analyze the capacity of granulocytes and macrophages to exhibit significant tumoricidal effects. While it is clear that granulocytes and macrophages can be tumoricidal in vitro, it has to be admitted that the evidence is less compelling for a useful role of these cells in vivo in cancer subjects.

For nonhemopoietic cancers, stimulation of hemopoiesis, and in particular formation of granulocytes and macrophages, may be useful therapeutically in two ways. These are: a) in preventing or minimizing drug-induced marrow aplasia, thus allowing chemotherapy to be continued and preventing serious secondary infections; and b) in stimulating both the formation of more granulocytes and macrophages and their tumoricidal action, thereby killing more tumor cells.

Colony-stimulating factors

Of the various molecules that have now been identified as influencing the different stages and subsets of hemopoietic cells, those most likely to stimulate granulocyte and macrophage formation and function are the glycoprotein colony-stimulating factors (CSFs) (1). There is strong evidence that these molecules are the major regulators controlling the proliferation of committed precursors of granulocytes and macrophages to form mature progeny. Furthermore, the same CSFs have a strong capacity to stimulate the functions of mature granulocytes and macrophages, including phagocytosis, microbial killing, and cytotoxicity for model tumor target cell systems.

Four CSFs have been identified in mice and humans—GM-CSF, G-CSF, multi-CSF (IL-3), and M-CSF (CSF-1). Each has been purified and characterized; cDNA and genomic clones for each have been isolated, and recombinant CSF has been produced in bacteria, yeast, or mammalian cell expression systems. In vitro analysis has shown that the various recombinant CSFs exhibit the same range of functions as the corresponding native molecules and are therefore valid for use in vivo to establish the responses produced by the injection of CSF.

The CSFs exhibit some specialization in their action in vitro, with GM-CSF and multi-CSF being able to stimulate both granulocytic and macrophage formation, G-CSF being primarily a stimulus for granulocyte formation and M-CSF for monocyte–macrophage formation (2).

Studies on the responses of mice to injection with CSFs have demonstrated a corresponding selectivity in action, with G-CSF greatly increasing blood granulocyte levels and GM-CSF being more effective, when injected intraperitoneally, in increasing the number of peritoneal macrophages (2–4).

In the limited studies performed in primates and humans, both G-CSF and GM-CSF have been found capable of stimulating major rises in blood granulocyte levels, the rises being sustainable for as long as the CSF is injected. Interestingly, the injection of G-CSF has been observed to shorten the duration of the neutropenia that follows chemotherapy associated with marrow toxicity (5–7). In primate studies, use of G-CSF and GM-CSF in marrow-transplanted animals has also shortened the period of neutropenia that follows irradiation, and has accelerated the recovery of white cell levels (8–10). Similarly, in mice with cyclophosphamide-induced marrow damage, injection of G-CSF strongly enhanced resistance of the animals to lethal challenge with a variety of microorganisms (11).

These early studies have indicated that the CSFs may be valuable in treating cancer either by chemotherapy or by ablative therapy with bone marrow transplantation, by virtue of their capacity to minimize hemopoietic damage and to accelerate hemopoietic regeneration. These effects of the CSFs can reasonably be expected to reduce significantly the rise of serious infections in such patients, and to allow more aggressive chemotherapy to be used.

It is not yet known whether the stimulation of granulocyte and macrophage function in vivo, by the injection of CSFs, will increase the cancer cell killing by these cells in vivo. It may be useful to explore such a possibility in ovarian cancer with extensive local peritoneal metastases, where local infusion of an agent such as GM-CSF might result in significant macrophage-mediated killing.

For the present, at least, the CSFs are likely to be useful in the management of many cancers, if only by enhancing the patient's resistance to secondary infections.

CSFs and myeloid leukemia

The myeloid leukemias differ quite sharply from other cancers when we consider the role of hemopoietic regulators. The myeloid leukemias are neoplasms of granulocyte and monocyte populations, cells normally dependent on the CSFs for all proliferation. In vitro, the proliferation of leukemic cells from the majority of patients with acute myeloid leukemia (AML) and those from all patients with chronic myeloid leukemia depend absolutely on the addition of exogenous CSF (1). In the minority of cases where AML cells appear to proliferate autonomously, analysis has revealed autocrine production of CSF by the cells (12) so, again, the leukemic cells can be regarded as CSF dependent.

Furthermore, in mice, insertion of CSF genes into CSF-dependent hemopoietic cell lines has been found to transform such cells into fully leukemic cells (13,14). This indicates that the CSF genes are classifiable as protooncogenes. In addition, insertion of GM-CSF and multi-CSF cDNAs into normal hemopoietic stem cells, by using a retroviral vector, results in a cell population capable of unrestrained progressive proliferation in recipient animals, leading to death with pathological changes resembling myeloid leukemia in many aspects.

These observations indicate that the CSFs must be involved in the initiation and progressive expansion of myeloid leukemic populations. At face value there would be no conceivable therapeutic role for CSF administration in myeloid leukemia. An exception may arise where ablation therapy prior to marrow transplantation is believed to have eliminated all residual leukemic cells and where the CSFs are being used solely to enhance hemopoietic regeneration.

However, the role of CSFs in myeloid leukemia is more complex because of their ability to induce differentiation commitment in hemopoietic cells (1). In a leukemic population such an action can be monitored either by a reduction in leukemic stem-cell self-generation (clonogenicity) or by the induction of differentiation. These 2 processes are not necessarily linked.

As a consequence of this type of action, G-CSF has been found to be effective on cells of the murine myelomonocytic line WEHI-3B, both in suppressing clonogenicity and in inducing the development of maturing granulocytes and monocytes (15,16). Continued culture of WEHI-3B cells in the presence of G-CSF can eventually entirely suppress the leukemic population in vitro. Injection of G-CSF to mice with transplanted myeloid leukemic cells leads to prolonged survival with an apparent absence of leukemic cells (17). In this model system, GM-CSF has similar but weaker action while multi-CSF and M-CSF are inactive.

Parallel studies, using HL60 cells and human GM-CSF or G-CSF, indicated that both factors had some capacity to suppress self-generation of the clonogenic cells, the action of G-CSF being slightly stronger (18,19). In this human model, morphological maturation was not observed, but the cells did express membrane markers typical of differentiated granulocytes and monocytes (19).

In theory, it should be possible to test the actions of the various CSFs in primary cultures of human myeloid leukemic cells, to determine whether primary cells of the various AML subtypes exhibit some suppression similar to that observed with the model leukemic cell lines. The practical difficulties with such a study are that the colonies or clones usually grown from such myeloid leukemic populations exhibit no evidence of clonogenic cell self-renewal and thus, no easy method is available for the assessment of altered self-renewal. The reason for this is unclear. It may be that the clonogenic cells detected are too differentiated and have already lost their capacity for self-renewal. Alternatively, the CSF used to stimulate cell proliferation may, itself, suppress self-renewal. Since CSF addition is mandatory for most cultures, no CSF-free control cultures can be studied. It may be valuable to concentrate attention on those examples of AML where the cells appear capable of autonomous proliferation, but no analysis of CSF action on such cultures has yet been reported.

Thus a role for CSF administration, particularly of G-CSF, in the management of myeloid leukemia by enforcing differentiation is unassessable at present. Furthermore, in view of the known proliferative actions of the CSFs on myeloid leukemic cells, it would be irresponsible to inject CSF into myeloid leukemic patients known still to harbor leukemic cells until some in vitro method is devised for predicting in which particular patients differentiation induction will dominate over cell proliferation.

Leukemia inhibitory factor

In studying the in vitro behavior of murine M1 myeloid leukemic cells Ichikawa (20) observed that addition of various organ-conditioned media could induce differentiation in M1 colonies. Initial characterization of the active molecule in such media was confused somewhat by parallel work on the CSFs also produced by these same tissues. A defined molecule able to induce differentiation in M1 cells was purified from L cell-conditioned medium by Tomida et al (21) and was distinct from the known CSFs. A parallel human molecule able to induce differentiation in human myeloid leukemic cells was ultimately identified as tumor necrosis factor (22).

A better resolution of the active murine molecules that induce differentiation in M1 cells was obtained by purifying the active factors from Krebs II ascites tumor-conditioned media (23). Three molecules able to induce differentiation in M1 or WEHI-3B cells were identified—G-CSF, GM-CSF, and an additional molecule named leukemia inhibitory factor (LIF). It is likely that LIF is identical to the D-factor purified by Tomida et al (21) and to MGI-2 as characterized by Lipton and Sachs (24). LIF is a glycoprotein of M_r 58 000 which in clonal cultures of M1 cells induces differentiation in colony cells and, at slightly higher concentrations (10^{-9} M), completely inhibits colony formation. Evidence suggests that this inhibitory action, causing death of initiating clones, is in part the consequence of induction of CSF dependency in the cells and is preventable by addition of M-CSF but not other CSFs (25).

LIF has no colony-stimulating activity, and appears not to be a proliferative stimulus for normal hemopoietic cells. Its normal function remains obscure, but monocytes and macrophages exhibit membrane receptors for the molecule and it may well play a role in regulating macrophage function.

Sequencing of a cDNA for murine LIF indicated no sequence homology with any CSF or other hemopoietic regulator and no sequence homology with tumor necrosis factor (26). Furthermore, antisera against tumor necrosis factor did not block the action of LIF on M1 cells.

Sequencing of a genomic clone for human LIF indicated a high degree (approximately 80%) of homology with the murine analogue and both native and recombinant human LIF are fully active on murine M1 leukemic cells (27).

While there is no structural similarity between G-CSF and LIF, some functional interrelationships may exist: 1) addition of G-CSF potentiates the action of LIF on M1 leukemic cells; 2) the genes for both murine G-CSF and LIF are on chromosome 11; and 3) combination of human LIF with GM-CSF or G-CSF appears to enhance the action of LIF on HL60 or U937 cells.

The therapeutic potential of LIF is not really assessable until more is known of the distribution of its receptors on human leukemic cells and of the biological effects of LIF in cultures of primary leukemic cells. A favorable aspect of its properties is the lack of proliferative effects—the disadvantage possessed by G-CSF.

Studies using the murine M1 myeloid leukemia model have identified a large number of chemical substances or biological factors able to induce these cells to differentiate (28). Biologically active agents range from cortisone to tumor necrosis factor, IL-6, interferon-γ, G-CSF, and LIF. The biological significance, if any, of this multiplicity of apparently active agents is difficult to assess purely from in vitro studies. In theory, many of these agents might constitute a network of interacting regulatory molecules able to influence significantly the behavior of such leukemic cells in vivo. On the other hand, many of these in vitro observations may be irrelevant in vivo, either because the required concentration of the agent is nonphysiological or because the factor might not exist in adequate concentrations in vivo.

An interesting and complex biological control system exists that has the potential to influence profoundly the behavior of myeloid leukemic populations in vivo. This may well explain the unusual behavior of AML populations where prolonged remissions can be obtained without absolute elimination of all leukemic cells. Much more investigation is required, however, before such a network can be advanced as a serious possibility.

References

1. Metcalf D. The molecular control of normal and leukemic blood cells. Boston: Har-

vard University Press; 1988.

2. Metcalf D. The molecular control of normal and leukemic granulocytes and macrophages. Proc R Soc Lond B Biol Sci 1987;230:389–423.

3. Metcalf D, Begley CG, Williamson DJ, et al. Hemopoietic responses in mice injected with purified recombinant murine GM-CSF. Exp Hematol 1987;15:1–9.

4. Metcalf D, Begley CG, Johnson GR, et al. Effects of purified bacterially-synthesized murine Multi-CSF (IL-3) on hemopoiesis in adult mice. Blood 1986;68:46–57.

5. Morstyn G, Souza LM, Keech J, et al. Effect of granulocyte colony stimulating factor on neutropenia induced by cytotoxic chemotherapy. Lancet 1988;i:667–72.

6. Bronchud MH, Scarffe JH, Thatcher N, et al. Phase I/II study of recombinant human granulocyte colony-stimulating factor in patients receiving intensive chemotherapy for small cell lung cancer. Br J Cancer 1987;56:809–13.

7. Gabrilove J, Jakubowski A, Grous J, et al. Initial results of a study of recombinant human granulocyte colony stimulating factor (rhG-CSF) in cancer patients. Exp Hematol 1987;815:461.

8. Donahue RE, Wang EA, Stone D, et al. Stimulation of haematopoiesis in primates by continuous infusion of recombinant human GM-CSF. Nature 1986;321:872–5.

9. McVittie TJ, D'Alesandro MA, Monroy RL, et al. Recombinant human granulocyte-macrophage stimulating factor (RHG-CSF): Effects of in vivo infusion in primates on hemopoiesis and activation of circulating neutrophils. Exp Hematol 1987;15:460.

10. Welte K, Bonilla MA, Gillio AP, et al. Recombinant human granulocyte colony-stimulating factor. Effects on hematopoiesis in normal and cyclophosphamide-treated primates. J Exp Med 1987;165:941–8.

11. Matsumoto M, Matsubara S, Matsuno T, et al. Protective effect of human granulocyte colony-stimulating factor on microbial infection in neutropenic mice. Infect Immun 1987;55:2715–20.

12. Young DC, Griffin JD. Autocrine secretion of GM-CSF in acute myeloblastic leukemia. Blood 1986;68:1178–81.

13. Lang RA, Metcalf D, Gough NM, et al. Expression of a hematopoietic growth factor cDNA in a factor-dependent cell line results in autonomous growth and tumorigenicity. Cell 1985;43:531–42.

14. Hapel AJ, Vande Woude GV, Campbell HD, et al. Generation of an autocrine leukaemia using a retroviral expression vector carrying the interleukin-3 gene. Lymphokine Res 1986;5:249–54.

15. Metcalf D, Nicola NA. Autoinduction of differentiation in WEHI-3B leukemia cells. Int J Cancer 1982;30:773–80.

16. Metcalf D. Regulator-induced suppression of myelomonocytic leukemia cells: Clonal analysis of early cellular events. Int J Cancer 1982;30:203–10.

17. Tamura M, Nomura H, Hata S, et al. Prolongation of the survival time of leukemic mice by the administration of recombinant human granulocyte colony stimulating factor. Exp Hematol 1987;15:558.

18. Metcalf D. Clonal analysis of the response of HL60 human myeloid leukemia cells to biological regulators. Leuk Res 1983;7:117–32.

19. Begley CG, Metcalf D, Nicola NA. Purified colony stimulating factors (G-CSF and GM-CSF) induce differentiation in human HL60 leukemic cells with suppression of clonogenicity. Int J Cancer 1987;39:99–105.

20. Ichikawa Y. Further studies on the differentiation of a cell line of myeloid leukemia. J Cell Physiol 1970;76:175–84.

21. Tomida M, Yamamoto-Yamaguchi Y, Hozumi M. Purification of a factor inducing

differentiation of mouse myeloid leukemic M1 cells from conditioned medium of mouse fibroblast L929 cells. J Biol Chem 1984;279:10978–82.

22. Takada K, Iwamoto S, Sugimoto H, et al. Identity of differentiation inducing factor and tumor necrosis factor. Nature 1986;323:338–40.
23. Hilton DJ, Nicola NA, Gough NM, Metcalf D. Resolution and purification of three distinct factors produced by Krebs ascites cells which have differentiation-inducing activity on murine myeloid leukemic cell lines. J Biol Chem 1988;263:9238–43.
24. Lipton JH, Sachs L. Characterization of macrophage- and granulocyte-inducing proteins for normal and leukemic myeloid cells produced by the Krebs ascites tumor. Biochim Biophys Acta 1981;673:552–69.
25. Metcalf D, Hilton DJ, Nicola NA. Clonal analysis of the actions of the murine leukemia inhibitory factor (LIF) on leukemic and normal hemopoietic cells. Leukemia 1988;2:216–21.
26. Gearing DP, Gough NM, King JA, et al. Molecular cloning and expression of cDNA encoding a murine leukemia inhibitory factor (LIF). EMBO (Eur Mol Biol Organ) J 1987;6:3995–4002.
27. Gough NM, Gearing DP, King JA, et al. Molecular cloning and expression of the human gene homologous to murine myeloid leukemia inhibitory factor (LIF). Proc Natl Acad Sci USA 1988;85:2623–7.
28. Hozumi M. Fundamentals of chemotherapy of myeloid leukemia by induction of leukemia cell differentiation. Adv Cancer Res 1983;38:121–69.

Effectiveness of cytokines in cancer therapy

Fumimaro Takaku

Faculty of Medicine, University of Tokyo, Tokyo, Japan

In this review, results of Japanese clinical studies will be compared with studies from other countries. Of the various cytokines, only the interferons (IFNs), interleukin 2 (IL-2), and granulocyte colony-stimulating factor (G-CSF) have been clinically tested in Japan for their usefulness in cancer treatment, and therefore this article will be restricted to results obtained with these cytokines.

Interferons

The clinical effectiveness of various IFNs has been extensively studied in Japan (1–7). Nineteen Japanese companies started to prepare recombinant IFN-α, IFN-β, or IFN-γ, either independently or in collaboration with foreign companies. Some of these companies have now discontinued the development of some products. Currently, 2 groups are marketing natural IFN-α and IFN-β and another 12 companies either have submitted the necessary data to the Ministry of Health and Welfare to obtain permission for marketing, or are still conducting clinical trials. Many data have accumulated from clinical trials in Japan, and they will be compared here with results from other countries.

Effectiveness of interferons on solid tumors

The solid tumor most extensively studied for the effectiveness of IFNs has been renal cell carcinoma (1–10). Five kinds of natural or recombinant IFN-α have been used to treat a total of 313 cases of renal cell carcinoma in several studies, with results in effectiveness ranging from 6% to 23% (mean 17%). Natural or recombinant IFN-β was given to 62 patients, with a response rate ranging from 4% to 20% (mean 8%). Recombinant IFN-γ, given to 108 patients, was not as effective as IFN-α or IFN-β, with a response rate of only 0–6% (mean 4%), however, the number of units of IFN-γ given to each patient was lower than that for IFN-α or IFN-β, and when a high dose of IFN-γ (40×10^6 units/m^2 per day) was given to 30 patients with renal cell carcinoma, 6 (20%) responded (10). IFNs are useful for treating patients with relapsed or metastatic renal cell carcinoma because no effective chemotherapy for this disease is available.

Brain tumor was the first malignancy reported to respond to IFNs in Japan (1–7,11–13). Administration of natural IFN-β to 57 patients with various brain tumors induced remission in 13% to 17% (mean 14%). Natural and recombinant IFN-α was given to 121 patients, with a response rate of 4% to 20% (mean 14%). Again, IFN-γ given to 43 patients with brain tumors was less effective than other IFNs, with a mean response rate of less than 5%, although the number of units of IFN-γ given to the patients was lower than those of IFN-α or IFN-β. Medulloblastoma showed the highest response rate (44%), followed by glioblastoma and malignant astrocytoma (17% and 14%, respectively). In 65 brain tumor patients, IFNs were given locally via an Ommaya reservoir. The mean reponse rate was 14% and there was no significant difference in response to the different IFNs.

IFNs were ineffective on other kinds of solid tumors, including those of the breast, head and neck, and others, with the highest response rate being only 3%.

Effectiveness of IFNs on hematologic malignancies

Many cases of multiple myeloma have been treated with IFNs during phase II studies. The progress of multiple myeloma is usually very slow. It is ethically possible, therefore, to give IFNs to patients as an initial treatment. Five study groups treated a total of 181 patients with either natural or recombinant IFN-α (1–7,14). The response rate (complete plus partial response) was 0–30% (mean 18%). This value was not significantly different from that reported in other countries (15–19). In 50 cases treated with natural or recombinant IFN-β, a response rate of 4–25% (mean 14%) was observed and when IFN-γ was given to 45 patients a mean response rate of less than 3% was seen. The number of units of IFN-γ was lower than those of IFN-α or IFN-β. The response rate depended to some extent on the dose of IFN-α; patients who showed a partial response were all treated with a mean daily dose of 16×10^6 units, while those who showed weak or no response were treated with $7–8 \times 10^6$ units/day. IFNs were effective in patients who became resistant to conventional chemotherapeutic agents. In 126 patients who had previously been treated by chemotherapeutic agents and in 45 new patients, mean response rates to IFN-α of 22% and 20%, respectively, were observed. There was no significant difference in response rate among the immunoglobulin subtypes of multiple myeloma. The IgG, IgA, and B-J types of multiple myeloma responded to IFN-α with rates of 17%, 22%, and 7%, respectively.

Malignant lymphoma had been reported to respond to IFNs (1–7). Sixty-one cases of non-Hodgkin's lymphoma responded to natural or recombinant IFN-α with a response rate of 0–28% (mean 13%). One case had a complete response, with total regression of the cancer. Natural IFN-β given to 38 non-Hodgkin's lymphoma patients was effective in 0–29% (mean 16%). Two cases showed a complete response. No cases of non-Hodgkin's lymphoma responded to IFN-γ therapy, although only 8 patients were studied, and the number of units of IFN-γ given to each patient was lower than those of IFN-α or IFN-β. Two patients with mycosis fungoides, however, responded to the systemic administration of IFN-γ, showing a complete response (7).

Response rates in Japan of malignant lymphoma to IFNs are lower than those reported in the USA or in European countries (26–28). Most patients with non-Hodgkin's lymphoma in Japan were treated with 3–10 × 10⁶ units per day. However, this dose was lower than that used in the USA or Europe, where patients received 10–50 × 10⁶ units/m² per day. The difference in response rates could therefore be due to the different dose of IFNs used. Furthermore, the Japanese studies were on non-Hodgkin's lymphoma, while those from other countries included cases of Hodgkin's disease. The difference in the response rate may, therefore, be accounted for by the different types of malignant lymphoma included in the different studies. Racial differences in the clinical course of the patients with malignant lymphoma could be another explanation for the differences observed in response rate to IFNs in this disorder.

A similar difference was observed in the reponse of hairy cell leukemia to IFN-α. It is well known that in this disease IFN-α should be given as initial treatment. A high response rate of 78.3% has been reported in the USA and Europe (29–36). However, only 6 of our 15 patients responded to IFN-α, with a partial response (Table 1) (37). The hematologic features of the hairy cell leukemia observed in many Japanese patients are somewhat different from those in other countries (38) and often do not show leukocytopenia. Japanese patients with hairy cell leukemia who had hematologic profiles identical to those in patients in other countries responded to IFN-α with a similar high response rate and patients with atypical blood profiles did not. Thus, the observed differences in response to IFN-α in patients with hairy cell leukemia could be due to racial differences in the types of the disease or due to the inclusion of atypical cases in our study.

Talpaz et al and others have shown that IFN-α could also be given as initial treatment in chronic myelogenous leukemia (CML) (39–44). The disappearance of a Philadelphia chromosome (Ph¹)-positive clone after treatment with IFN-α has been reported by several groups. The results of a Japanese phase II study of IFNs in CML showed an overall response rate of 39%, however the patients were not treated long enough for the disappearance of the Ph¹-positive clone to be observed. Long-term treatment of CML patients with IFN-α in our depart-

Table 1 Effectiveness of IFN-α on hairy cell leukemia.

Area of study	No. of patients	Dose (× 10⁶ units/d)	Complete response no. (%)	Partial response no. (%)	Response rate (%)‡
USA and Europe*	563	2–12	50 (8.9)	391 (69.4)	78.3
Japan†	15	3	1 (6.7)	5 (33.3)	40.0

*Natural and recombinant IFN-α; †natural IFN-α; ‡sum of % complete response and % partial response.

ment revealed a decrease in the percentage of Ph^1-positive cells, as shown in Table 2 (45). However, the decrease was not as marked as that reported by other researchers.

Adult T cell leukemia (ATL) is a regional disease observed mainly in certain districts in Japan. It is resistant to various antileukemic agents and has a rapid course and a poor prognosis. Some cases, however, remain "smouldering." Nineteen patients were treated with recombinant IFN-α and 14 with recombinant IFN-γ. The response rate in both groups was 21% (46). No difference was observed between the 2 groups.

Other hematologic malignancies treated with IFNs in Japan include acute leukemia and chronic lymphocytic leukemia (CLL). Among 33 cases of acute leukemia treated with IFNs, only 2 cases (6%) showed a partial response, while the response of CLL patients to IFNs was, however, fairly good. Among 37 cases treated by various IFNs, 10 patients (27%) showed a response. No differences in effectiveness between IFN-α, IFN-β, or IFN-γ were observed in CLL patients.

Effectiveness of local injection of IFNs into skin malignancies

Clinical trials of IFNs in Japan, involving many types of skin malignancies, were conducted by local injection of IFNs in phase II studies. Treatment of 465 patients with various skin malignancies has been carried out by local injection of natural or recombinant IFN-α, IFN-β, or IFN-γ by many groups (47–50). A complete response was observed in 4–33% (mean 20%) of patients and the response rate was 33–72% (mean 49%). The criteria for complete or partial response of skin tumors to IFNs were defined by dermatologists for local administration of chemotherapeutic agents. Skin lymphomas, including mycosis fungoides, showed the highest mean response rate of 66%. The complete response rate of patients with skin lymphoma was 43%. Malignant melanoma also responded to local administration of IFNs, with a mean reponse rate of 43% and a complete response rate of 7%. Spindle-cell carcinoma of the skin also responded to treatment with a rate of 28%. The differences in effectiveness of IFN-α, IFN-β, and IFN-γ, which were observed after systemic administration of the IFNs, were not apparent when local administration was used; IFN-γ given locally was as effective as the other IFNs given locally.

Table 2 Effect of IFN-α administration on Ph^1 cells in CML patients.

Patient	% Ph^1 cells before IFN-α	3 months	% Ph^1 cells after IFN-α		
			6 months	9 months	12 months
1	100	—	75	100	100
2	100	100	—	75	—
3	100	100	92*	85*	—

*With additional chromosomal change.

Interleukin 2

Table 3 shows the results of our study on the effectiveness of systemically administered interleukin 2 (IL-2) on various kinds of malignancies. Doses of 1–3 $\times$ 10^6 units per day were given intravenously and the responses observed in patients with renal cell carcinoma, bladder carcinoma, mycosis fungoides, and malignant hemangioendothelioma. Of the 60 renal cell carcinoma patients that could be evaluated after treatment with IL-2, 3 showed a total regression of all cancer (complete response), 6 had more than a 50% tumor reduction (partial response), 1 had a 25% to 50% tumor reduction (minor response), while 23 had stable disease and 27 had more than a 25% tumor increase (progressive disease) (51). The incidence of objective response was therefore 15%. Both Rosenberg et al (52) and West et al (53) have reported a complete response of renal cell carcinoma to IL-2 administration. Administration of IL-2 alone, or in combination with IFNs, may therefore be an effective treatment for relapsed or metastatic renal cell carcinoma. Another group using IL-2 in Japan reported a complete response in 2 patients with cutaneous lymphoma and 1 patient with oral cavity tumors (54). A partial response was observed in 1 patient each with gastric cancer, hepatoma, skin lymphoma, or atypical leukemia. Three patients with head and neck tumor also had a partial response to to IL-2.

Administration of IL-2 directly into the pleural or peritoneal cavity to treat patients with carcinomatous pleuritis or peritonitis has been reported to be very

Table 3 Effectiveness of IL-2 on various malignancies (systemic administration).

Type of cancer	No. of evaluable cases	CR	PR	MR	NC	PD	Response rate (%)*
Hepatoma	14	0	0	0	6	8	
Colorectal	6			1	3	2	
Lung	65	1					
Renal cell	60	3	6	1	23	27	15.0
Bladder	2		1		1		50.0
Oral cavity	5				3	2	
Nasopharyngeal	3			1	1	1	
Malignant melanoma	7				4	3	
Mycosis fungoides	2		1	1			50.0
Malignant hemangioendothelioma	1		1				100.0
Others	14				8	6	
Total	120	3	9	4	54	50	

CR, complete response (total regression); PR, partial response (>50% tumor reduction) MR, minor response (25–50% tumor reduction); NC, no change (stable disease); PD, progressive disease (>25% tumor increase).

effective (55). Local injection of IL-2 into malignant hemangioendothelioma induced a complete disappearance of the tumor (56). However, further studies are needed to confirm these findings.

Malignant tumors have also been treated in Japan by infusions of lymphokine-activated killer (LAK) cells, by several study groups. Since the collection and incubation of the large numbers of mononuclear cells, as originally described by Rosenberg (57) and his group, is costly and time consuming, we tried to reduce the number of such incubated cells by infusing the LAK cells into the artery supplying blood to the tumor tissue via an indwelling catheter. In this way we treated patients with hepatoma in whom treatment by transartery embolization was not indicated because of the presence of tumor cell emboli in the portal vein or because of diffuse infiltration of hepatoma cells. Usually 1×10^9 LAK cells are infused into the hepatic artery in each treatment through an indwelling catheter. Results of our adoptive immunotherapy using LAK cells are shown in Table 4 (58–60).

As shown in Table 4, 1 case of advanced hepatoma in a 63-year-old male showed diffuse infiltration of tumor cells into the liver, but nevertheless showed a marked response to adoptive immunotherapy; serum levels of tumor markers, including α-fetoprotein, returned to normal. An arteriogram of the hepatic artery showed the disappearance of the tumor stain. This patient remains alive, more than 3 years after the start of the therapy with IL-2 plus LAK cells. Another case of advanced hepatoma, in a 21-year-old female, also responded to a LAK cell infusion through the hepatic artery, showing an apparent reduction of tumor size and a marked decrease in serum tumor marker levels. The other 7 cases of hepatoma also responded to this adoptive immunotherapy to some extent. Since our first report, the effectiveness of local administration of LAK cells for the

Table 4 Results of adoptive immunotherapy with LAK cells and IL-2 via hepatic artery for hepatocellular carcinoma (December 1987).

Patient	Age (y)	Sex	Extension*	LAK cells (total number)	rIL-2 (total units)	Effect
1	63	M	E$_4$	$7.7 \times 10^{10\dagger}$	3.8×10^8	Partial response
2	21	F	E$_4$	$9.7 \times 10^{10\dagger}$	1.9×10^8	Partial response + decreased serum AFP
3	68	M	E$_4$	$7.5 \times 10^{9\ddagger}$	2.3×10^7	
4	52	M	E$_1$	$6.6 \times 10^{9\ddagger}$	3.8×10^7	
5	50	M	E$_2$	$3.1 \times 10^{9\ddagger}$	2.3×10^7	
6	57	M	E$_1$	$5.3 \times 10^{9\ddagger}$	1.8×10^7	Decreased serum AFP
7	67	F	E$_1$	$2.1 \times 10^{9\ddagger}$	1.8×10^7	Decreased serum AFP
8	62	M	E$_1$	$2.2 \times 10^{9\ddagger}$	6.8×10^6	Tumor necrosis
9	54	M	E$_1$	$6.0 \times 10^{9\ddagger}$	8.5×10^6	Decreased serum AFP

*Extension of the tumor (E): E$_1$, <10%; E$_2$, 20–40%; E$_3$, 40–60%; E$_4$, >60%. †Long-term treatment. ‡Short-term treatment. AFP, alphafetoprotein.

treatment of hepatoma, as described here, has been tested by several groups in Japan (61,62). They have all confirmed our results.

Local administration of LAK cells has also been tried in Japan in the treatment of brain tumors (63). The method used to inject IFNs locally was applied to the local infusion of LAK cells. Although the number of brain tumor patients treated by this method is still low, the authors of the report of this treatment claimed that this method is effective. One patient with carcinomatous peritonitis was treated in our hospital by intraperitoneal administration of IL-2 and LAK cells which were induced by incubating mononuclear cells collected from the patient's ascites with IL-2. He responded to this treatment, with no further accumulation of ascites.

Induction of allogenic LAK cells or of LAK cells from surgically removed spleen or from the tumor itself has been tried by several groups in Japan. Except for the infusion of allogenic LAK cells, the trials are still at the experimental stage.

Granulocyte colony-stimulating factor

Granulocyte-macrophage (GM-) and granulocyte (G-) colony-stimulating factors (CSFs) were initially identified as hematopoietic factors stimulating the in vitro formation of granulocyte-macrophage and granulocyte colonies. Success in cloning the CSF genes and in producing recombinant CSFs using bacteria or cultured animal cells has made it possible to study the effects of CSFs in vivo.

In vivo administration of GM-CSF and G-CSF induced a marked increase in peripheral blood white cell counts in humans, as well as in experimental animals if they were given the CSFs effective for their species (64). Peripheral white blood cell counts reached $5-6 \times 10^4/mm^3$ if the CSFs were given daily for several days. Only neutrophils were increased in response to G-CSF, while the administration of GM-CSF caused an increase of neutrophils, monocytes, and eosinophils. Side effects of G-CSF were minimal, with only transient medullary bone pain in some patients who were given large doses (65). GM-CSF, on the other hand, was associated with many side effects, such as myalgia, fever, queasiness, headache, and occasionally hypotension, in addition to medullary bone pain (66,67).

In Japan, 2 kinds of recombinant G-CSF, one produced from Chinese hamster ovary (CHO) cells and the other from *Escherichia coli*, have been used in a phase II study to observe the effectiveness of G-CSF in neutropenic patients after anticancer chemotherapy or after bone marrow transplantation. Since only G-CSF is available in Japan and is considered to be superior to GM-CSF in the treatment of neutropenia, owing to its specificity to neutrophils and its fewer side effects, only clinical results on G-CSF will be described in this paper.

Effectiveness of G-CSF on neutropenia induced by anticancer drugs

Multicenter clinical trials of the effectiveness of G-CSF in neutropenia following treatment with anticancer drugs are currently in progress in Japan. We are studying patients with malignant lymphoma and small cell lung cancer. To eliminate individual differences in bone marrow suppression after anticancer chemotherapy and in responses to G-CSF, each patient receives 2 courses of the same chemotherapy. After the 1st course, the patients are treated with G-CSF 100–200 $\mu g/m^2$ daily for 2–3 weeks. After the 2nd course, the same patients receive a placebo. Changes in peripheral white blood cell and neutrophil counts after chemotherapy are compared between the 2 courses. Although we are now accumulating patients thus treated for a crossover study, results obtained so far clearly show that G-CSF accelerates recovery from neutropenia after chemotherapy and shortens the duration of neutropenia. In some patients, neutrophil counts at the nadir were higher during the G-CSF treatment than during the control course. Results from a typical patient with lung cancer, who showed a remarkable acceleration in recovery from neutropenia following G-CSF therapy, are shown in Fig 1. So far, about 80 cases of malignant lymphoma and 20 cases of small cell lung cancer have been entered into this study. They have all shown a favorable response to G-CSF produced in both CHO cells and *E. coli.*

Effectiveness of G-CSF on neutropenia after bone marrow transplantation

Neutropenia is a consequence of autologous as well as allogenic bone marrow transplantation. To accelerate recovery from neutropenia, 100–200 $\mu g/m^2$ of G-

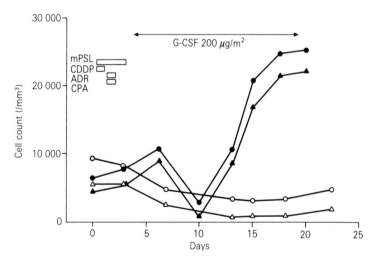

Fig 1 Effect of G-CSF 200 $\mu g/m^2$ for 2 weeks on the granulocytopenia after chemotherapy in a patient with lung adenocarcinoma. After the 2nd course, the same patient received placebo. ● WBC and ▲ granulocyte counts while receiving G-CSF injection; ○ WBC and △ granulocyte counts during control period; mPSL, methyl prednisolone; CDDP, cisplatin; ADR, Adriamycin (doxorubicin); CPA, cyclophosphamide. Patient was a 56-year-old female.

CSF was given daily, starting from the 3rd day after transplantation until the peripheral blood leukocyte levels returned to normal. So far, about 30 patients undergoing bone marrow transplantion have been treated with G-CSF in this way.

The mean period between allogenic bone marrow transplantation and recovery of peripheral blood neutrophil counts up to 500/mm^3 has been 28.5 ± 9.1 days, for 37 patients with leukemia (T. Masaoka, personal communication). In almost all cases treated with G-CSF, peripheral blood granulocytes returned to 500/mm^3 or more 10–14 days after transplantation. Hematologic changes in a typical patient who received G-CSF after bone marrow transplantation are shown in Fig 2. We believe that G-CSF will become a most useful supportive drug in bone marrow transplantation.

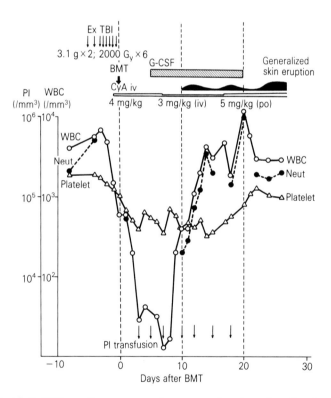

Fig 2 Effect of G-CSF on the recovery from granulocytopenia after bone marrow transplantation in a 16-year-old female patient with acute lymphoblastic leukemia. From 5 days after bone marrow transplantation (BMT), the patient started to receive iv injection of rG-CSF 200 μg/m^2. ○ White blood cell counts; ● neutrophil counts; △ platelet (Pl) counts; CyA, cyclosporin A. Data from T. Masaoka, The Center for Adult Disease, Osaka, Japan.

Effectiveness of G-CSF on myelodysplastic syndrome and acute leukemia

Myelodysplastic syndrome (MDS) is a preleukemic state often associated with neutropenia and dysfunction of mature granulocytes, which renders the patient susceptible to infections. Since both GM-CSF and G-CSF increase the number as well as the activity of neutrophils, administration of these CSFs has been expected to be of clinical value in MDS. Increased activity of neutrophils from MDS patients, after in vitro incubation of the neutrophils with G-CSF, has been reported recently by Yuo et al (68). We therefore gave G-CSF daily to patients with MDS and so far we have observed a significant increase in neutrophil count in all the patients studied (Table 5). There was no significant difference between CHO and *E. coli* recombinant G-CSF in their granulopoietic effects on MDS patients.

G-CSF induced varying hematologic changes in patients with acute leukemia. In some patients, the numbers of both leukemic blasts and mature granulocytes were increased in peripheral blood and the leukemic blast cells returned to their basal levels soon after cessation of G-CSF administration. In other cases, however, only the mature granulocytes were increased, while a decrease in leukemic blast cells was observed. Since both GM-CSF and G-CSF increased the number of leukemic colonies, the hematologic changes after administration of G-CSF should be carefully monitored in more patients with acute leukemia.

Acknowledgment

The author acknowledges Dr T. Masaoka at The Center for Adult Disease, Osaka, Japan for supplying data on the patient (Fig 2) who had received bone marrow transplantation and G-CSF injection.

Table 5 Effects of G-CSF on MDS and acute leukemia.

Patient	Age (y)	Sex	Diagnosis	Dose of rhG-CSF (μg/m$_2$ × d)	Responses ANC (/mm^3)
1	61	M	MDS, RA	400 × 6 iv	860 → 3000
2	22	F	MDS, RA	400 × 6 iv	1300* → 4000*
3	50	M	MDS, RAEB	100 × 7 iv	400 → 3500
4	63	M	MDS, RA	100 × 7 iv	7400 → 8100
5	42	M	MDS, RA	0.8 × 5 sc	1000 → 3100
6	56	M	AML (M2)	400−1600 × 9 iv	60 → 400
7	17	M	ALL (L2)	0.8 × 20 iv	0 → 1360
8	49	M	AML (M3)	5.0 × 4 sc	500 → 7350
9	24	M	ALL (L1)	5.0** × 14 iv	0 → 1100

*WBC. RA, refractory anemia; RAEB, refractory anemia with excess blasts; ANC, absolute neutrophil counts.

References

1. Kimura K. Cooperative study group of HLBI. A cooperative phase I and II study of HLBI in patients with malignant tumors. Jpn J Cancer Chemother 1984;11:1324. (In Japanese)

2. Takaku F. Phase II study of interferon α-2 (Sch 30,500) for hematopoietic tumors. Rinsho Iyaku 1985;1:59. (In Japanese)

3. Kimura K. Cooperative study group of Ro 22-8181. Phase II study of recombinant leukocyte A interferon (Ro 22-8181) in hematological malignancies. Jpn J Cancer Chemother 1985;12:928. (In Japanese)

4. Furue H. Phase II clinical study on interferon-α produced from human lymphoblast (Interferol α) for malignant tumor. Rinsho Iyaku 1985;1:1103. (In Japanese)

5. Ohno R. Clinical studies of interferon on cancer in Japan. Jpn J Cancer Chemother 1985;14:1194. (In Japanese)

6. Tsubura H. Phase I and II studies of human lymphoblast IFN (MOR-22) on malignant tumors. Jpn J Cancer Chemother 1986;21:1049. (In Japanese)

7. Takaku F. IFN-γ study group. Treatment of various malignancies with recombinant IFN-γ (S6810). Jpn J Cancer Chemother 1987;14:645. (In Japanese)

8. Niijima T. Clinical evaluation of recombinant IFN A (rIFN-αA) on urological malignancies. Jpn J Cancer Chemother 1985;12:921. (In Japanese)

9. Niijima M. Clinical effect of human lymphoblast interferon (MOR-22) on renal cell carcinoma. J Jpn Soc Cancer Ther 1986;21:1277.

10. Koiso K. Recombinant human interferon gamma (S-6810) research group on renal cell carcinoma. Phase II study of recombinant human interferon gamma (S-6810) on renal cell carcinoma. Cancer 1987;60:929.

11. Kitamura K. Phase II study of interferon α-2 (Sch. 30500) on brain tumor. Rinsho Igaku 1986;21:1068. (In Japanese)

12. Hirakawa K. Phase II study of human lymphoblast interferon (MOR-22) on brain tumor. J Jpn Soc Cancer Ther 1986;21:1068. (In Japanese)

13. Takakura K. Phase II study on the effectiveness of human interferon αA (rIFN-αA, Ro 22-8181) on malignant brain tumor. Jpn J Cancer Chemother 1987;12:913. (In Japanese)

14. Ohno R, Kimura K, Amaki I, et al. Treatment of multiple myeloma with recombinant human leukocyte A interferon. Cancer Treat Rep 1985;69:14343.

15. Mellstedt H, Bjorkholm M, Johansson B, et al. Interferon therapy in myelomatosis. Lancet 1979;i:245.

16. Alexanian R, Gutterman JU, Levy H. Interferon treatment in multiple myeloma. Clin Hematol 1982;2:211.

17. Costanzi JJ, Cooper MR, Scarffe JH, et al. Phase II study of recombinant alpha-2 interferon in resistant multiple myeloma. J Clin Oncol 1985;3:654.

18. Wagstaff J, Loynds P, Scarffe JH. Phase III study of rDNA human alpha-2 interferon in multiple myeloma. Cancer Treat Rep 1985;69:495.

19. Quesada JR, Alexanian R, Hawkins M, et al. Treatment of multiple myeloma with recombinant α-interferon. Blood 1986;67:275.

20. Merigan T, Sikora K, Breeden JH, et al. Preliminary observations on the effect of human leukocyte interferon in non-Hodgkin's lymphoma. N Engl J Med 1978;299:1449.

21. Gutterman JU, Blumenschein G, Alexanian R, et al. Leukocyte interferon-induced tumor regression in human metastatic breast cancer, multiple myeloma, and malig-

nant lymphoma. Ann Intern Med 1980;93:399.

22. Bunn PA, Foon XA, Ihde DC, et al. Recombinant leukocyte A interferon: an active agent in advanced cutaneous T-cell lymphomas. Ann Intern Med 1984;101:484.

23. Louie AC, Gallagher JG, Sikora K, et al. Follow-up observations on the effect of human leukocyte interferon in non-Hodgkin's lymphoma. Blood 1981;58:712.

24. Foon KA, Sherwin SA, Abrams PG, et al. Treatment of advanced non-Hodgkin's lymphoma with recombinant leukocyte A interferon. N Engl J Med 1984;311:1148.

25. Bottino GC, Schoenberger CS, Zefferen J, et al. Treatment of advanced non-Hodgkin's lymphoma with recombinant leukocyte A interferon. N Engl J Med 1984;311:1148.

26. Quesada JR, Hawkins M, Horning S, et al. Leukocyte interferon (Clone A) in metastatic breast cancer, malignant lymphoma, and multiple myeloma. Am J Med 1984;77:427.

27. Foon KA, Bottino GC, Abrams PG, et al. Phase II trial of recombinant leukocyte A interferon in patients with advanced chronic lymphocytic leukemia. Am J Med 1985;78:216.

28. O'Connel MJ, Colgan JP, Oken MM, et al. Clinical trial of recombinant leukocyte A interferon as initial therapy for favorable histology non-Hodgkin's lymphomas and chronic lymphocytic leukemia. An Eastern Cooperative Oncology Group Pilot Study. J Clin Oncol 1986;4:128.

29. Quesada JR, Reuben J, Manning JT, et al. Alpha interferon for induction of remission in hairy-cell leukemia. N Engl J Med 1984;310:15.

30. Thompson JA, Brady J, Kidd P, Fefer A. Recombinant alpha-2 interferon in the treatment of hairy cell leukemia. Cancer Treat Rep 1985;93:399.

31. Jacobs AD, Champlin RE, Golde DW. Recombinant alpha-2-interferon for hairy cell leukemia. Blood 1985;65:107.

32. Worman CP, Catovsky D, Bevan PC, et al. Interferon is effective in hairy cell leukaemia. Br J Haematol 1985;60:759.

33. Ratain MJ, Golomb HM, Vardiman JW, et al. Treatment of hairy cell leukemia with recombinant alpha$_2$ interferon.Blood 1985;65:644.

34. Quesada JR, Hersh EM, Gutterman JU. Treatment of hairy cell leukemia with recombinant DNA-derived interferon alpha: a phase II study. Blood 1986;68:493.

35. Catovsky D, Quesada JR, Golomb HM. Guidelines for the treatment of hairy cell leukemia. Leukemia 1987;1:405–6.

36. Cheson BD, Martin A. Clinical trials in hairy cell leukemia. Current status and future directions. Ann Intern Med 1987;106:871.

37. Kitani T, Tokumine S. Immunotherapy. In: Takaku F, ed., Leukemia and lymphoma. Tokyo: Nankodo; 1988:85. (In Japanese)

38. Machii T, Inoue R, Kitani T. Hairy cell leukemia. Pathophysiology and clinical findings in Japanese cases. Naika 1987;60:1281. (In Japanese)

39. Talpaz M, McCredie KB, Mavligit GM, Gutterman JU. Leukocyte interferon-induced myeloid cytoreduction in chronic myelogenous leukemia. Blood 1983;62:689.

40. Talpaz M, Kantarijian HM, McCredie KB, et al. Chronic myelogenous leukemia: Hematologic remissions and cytogeneic improvements induced by recombinant alpha A interferon. N Engl J Med 1986;314:1065.

41. Talpaz M, Kantarjian HM, McCredie KB, et al. Clinical investigation of human alpha interferon in chronic myelogenous leukemia. Blood 1987;69:1280.

42. Talpaz M, McCredie K, Kantarjian H, et al. Chronic myelogenous leukemia: Hematologic remissions with alpha interferon. Br J Haematol 1986;64:87.

43. Yoffe G, Blich M, Katarjian H, et al. Molecular analysis of interferon-induced sup-

pression of Philadelphia chromosome in patients with chronic myeloid leukemia. Blood 1987;69:961.

44. Talpaz M, Kantarjian HM, McCredie KB, et al. Clinical investigation of human leukocyte interferon in chronic myelogenous leukemia. Blood 1987;69:1280.

45. Ogura H, Shirafuji N, Kumakawa T, et al. Two cases of chronic myeloid leukemia showing favorable clinical course after treatment with interferon α. Clin Hematol 1987;28:1599. (In Japanese)

46. Tamura K, Makino S, Araki Y, et al. Recombinant interferon beta and gamma in the treatment of adult T-cell leukemia. Cancer 1987;59:1059–62

47. Ishihara K. Clinical study on the effectiveness of local injection of human fibroblastoid interferon (Hu IFN-β) in cutaneous malignant tumors. J Jpn Soc Cancer Chemother 1983;18:41. (In Japanese)

48. Ishihara K. Clinical study of human lymphoblast interferon α on cutaneous malignant tumors. Rinsho Iyaku 1985;1:1123. (In Japanese)

49. Ikeda S. Phase II study of human recombinant leukocyte interferon A (rIFN-αA, Ro 22-8181) on cutaneous malignant tumors. Jpn J Cancer Chemother 1985;12:936. (In Japanese)

50. Mishima Y. Phase II study of interferon-α (Mor-22) on cutaneous malignant tumors. Jpn J Cancer Chemother 1986;21:1059. (In Japanese)

51. Aso Y, Tazaki H, Umeda T, et al. Treatment of renal cell carcinoma with systemic administration of intermediate doses of recombinant human interleukin 2 alone. International symposium on therapeutic progress in urological cancer, Paris: 1988. (Abstract)

52. Rosenberg SA, Lotze MT, Muul LM, et al. A progress report on the treatment of 157 patients with advanced cancer using lymphokine-activated killer cells and interleukin 2 or high-dose interleukin 2 alone. N Engl J Med 1987;316:889–97.

53. West WH, Tauer KW, Yannelli JR, et al. Constant-infusion recombinant interleukin 2 in adoptive immunotherapy of advanced cancer. N Engl J Med 1987;316:898.

54. Taguchi T, Kimoto Y. Clinical application of biological response modifiers: Interleukin 2. Saishin Igaku 1987;42:325. (In Japanese)

55. Yasumoto K, Miyazaki K, Nagashima A, et al. Induction of lymphokine-activated killer cells by intrapleural instillations of recombinant interleukin 2 in patients with malignant pleurisy due to lung cancer. Cancer Res 1987;47:2184.

56. Masuzawa M, Higashi K, Nishioka K, Nishiyama S. Successful immunotherapy for malignant hemangioendothelioma using recombinant interleukin 2. Jpn J Dermatol 1988;98:367. (In Japanese)

57. Rosenberg SA, Lotze MT, Muul LM, et al. Observations on the systemic administration of autologous lymphokine-activated killer cells and recombinant interleukin-2 to patients with metastatic cancer. N Engl J Med 1985;313:1485.

58. Imawari M, Moriyama T, Ishikawa T, et al. LAK therapy. Kan Tan Sui 1987; 15:583. (In Japanese)

59. Moriyama T, Matsuhashi N, Nakamura I, et al. Adoptive immunotherapy of hepatocellular carcinoma with autologous lymphokine-activated killer cells and recombinant interleukin 2. Submitted for publication.

60. Ishikawa T, Imawari M, Moriyama T, et al. Immunotherapy of hepatocellular carcinoma with autologous lymphokine-activated killer cells and/or recombinant interleukin-2. J Cancer Res Clin Oncol 1988;114:283.

61. Komatsu T, Yamauchi K, Hasegawa K, et al. Effect of infusion of lymphokine-activated killer (LAK) cells and interleukin 2 (IL-2) into hepatic artery on 2 cases of

hematoma. Acta Hepatol Jpn 1987;27:477. (In Japanese)

62. Sakeda K, Nishihara T, Matsuura Y, et al. A case of hepatoma which responded to adoptive immunotherapy by lymphokine activated killer cells with a marked decrease of serum α-fetoprotein level. Acta Hepatol Jpn 1987;28:606.

63. Nakamura H, Shitara N, Wada T, et al. Basic and clinical studies on the adoptive immunotherapy for malignant brain tumor. Biotherapy 1987;1:307.

64. Azuma T, Takaku F. Phase I study of human recombinant granulocyte colony stimulating factor. Submitted for publication.

65. Gabrillove JL, Jakubowski A, Scher H, et al. Effect of granulocyte colony-stimulating factor on neutropenia and associated morbidity due to chemotherapy for transitional-cell carcinoma of the urothelium. N Engl J Med 1988;318:1414.

66. Vadhan-Raj S, Keating M, LeMaistre A, et al. Effect of recombinant human granulocyte macrophage colony-stimulating factor in patients with myelodysplastic syndrome. N Engl J Med 1987;317:1545.

67. Brandt SJ, Peters WP, Atwater SK, et al. Effect of recombinant human granulocyte-macrophage colony-stimulating factor on hematopoietic reconstitution after high-dose chemotherapy and autologous bone marrow transplantation. N Engl J Med 1983;318:869.

68. Yuo A, Kitagawa S, Okabe T, et al. Recombinant human granulocyte colony-stimulating factor repairs the abnormalities of neutrophils in patients with myelodysplastic syndrome and chronic myelogenous leukemia. Blood 1987;70:404.

Regulation of immune and inflammatory responses by T cell-derived lymphokines

Kiyohiko Hatake, Atsushi Miyajima, Ken-ichi Arai

Department of Molecular Biology, DNAX Research Institute of Molecular and Cellular Biology, Palo Alto, California, USA

T cell activation and production of lymphokines

T cells have been classified as helper, cytotoxic, and suppressor cells. Helper T cells are activated to initiate an immune response following recognition of an antigen presented in the context of the major histocompatibility complex on macrophages or B cells. Activated T cells produce a variety of lymphokines such as the interleukins (ILs) 2, 3, 4, 5, and 6, granulocyte-macrophage colony-stimulating factors (GM-CSF), interferon-γ (IFN-γ), tumor necrosis factor α (TNF-α), and lymphotoxin. These lymphokines amplify and modify the physiologic responses after antigenic stimulation by regulating proliferation and differentiation of a variety of lymphoid and hemopoietic cells. Initially, lymphokines were named after their activities on a unique target cell. However, molecular cloning of the lymphokine genes and characterization of the biological properties of the recombinant products have revealed that many lymphokines have more than one function and can interact with more than 1 type of cell. Likewise, different lymphokines can evoke similar biological responses by interacting with the same target cell, for example, both IL-2 and IL-4 have T cell growth factor (TCGF) activity. Over the past few years, several lymphokines, performing more than one function by interacting with multiple cell types, have been renamed subsequent to the establishment of the primary structure of the protein or the nucleotide sequence of the gene. Of the 4 major CSFs, IL-3 (multi-CSF), and GM-CSF are produced by activated T cells and stimulate early progenitor cells to produce hemopoietic cells of multiple lineages. A number of molecules, including IL-2, IL-4, IL-5, and B cell-stimulating factor 2 (BSF-2 or IL-6) (1–7) stimulate B cells. IL-4, which has been called BSF-1 on the basis of its activity on B cells, also stimulates T cells (TCGFII), mast cells (MCGFII), macrophages, and myeloid cells. IL-5, which has also been named T cell-replacing factor I (TRFI) and BCGFII, based on its activity on B cells, also stimulates eosinophils (Eo-CSF). BSF-2, which has been considered to be a B cell tropic lymphokine (8), is identical to the hepatocyte-stimulating factor (HSF) which mediates the acute phase reaction (9). This discovery, plus molecular cloning and elucidation of the roles of the lymphokines now permit us to examine the functional link between the different cellular compartments such as lymphocytes and hemopoietic cells in an immune response. Here we describe the structure of T cell-derived lymphokine genes, regulation of their expression, biological properties, and the role in the immune response and hemopoiesis.

Isolation of lymphokine genes using a cDNA expression vector

Since all known lymphokines are composed of a single polypeptide chain, their coding sequences can be isolated by functional expression in appropriate host cells using cDNA expression-cloning vectors, as originally designed by Okayama and Berg. We have used the pcD vector which carries the SV40 early promoter and a replication origin that permits replication of the pcD plasmid in COS7 monkcy cells (10,11). Culture supernatants of transiently transfected COS7 cells were assayed for several lymphokine activities. Results using this system show that full-length cDNAs for many lymphokines can be isolated entirely by functional expression in appropriate host cells. Recombinant lymphokines produced in COS7 cells by transient transfection of cDNA clones have been useful for characterization of lymphokine biological activities. Larger amounts of recombinant lymphokines have been produced by use of heterologous host vector systems such as *E. coli*, yeast (12), mammalian stable transformants, and silkworm baculovirus (13).

Molecular cloning of lymphokine cDNAs has revealed that each lymphokine is composed of a single polypeptide containing a hydrophobic signal sequence at the N-terminus characteristic of secretable proteins. Sequences of lymphokines are well conserved between mouse and human, except for IL-3 and, generally, homology at the nucleotide level is about 70% and that at the amino acid level 50%. Most lymphokines show no obvious homology with other growth factors or oncogenes and no significant homology is found between lymphokines either at the nucleotide sequence or amino acid sequence level. However, lymphotoxin and TNF-α, which interact with the same receptor on target cells, share extensive amino acid sequence homology (14). Similarly, BSF-2 (IL-6) and G-CSF share homology at the amino acid sequence level (7,15), although they do not share receptors on target cells.

Structure of lymphokine genes and regulation of their expression

Many lymphokine genes exist as a single copy gene in the haploid genome and GM-CSF, IL-3, IL-4, IL-5, M-CSF, and M-CSF receptor (c-fms) genes are located on human chromosome 5 (16). TNF-α and lymphotoxin genes are located close together on human chromosome 6. Loss of the whole or the long arm of chromosome 5 has been observed in malignant cells in patients with acute nonlymphocytic leukemia (ANLL). A family of genes encoding hemopoietic growth factors and their receptors may be clustered within limited region(s) of a chromosome and thereby coordinately regulate hemopoiesis.

Lymphokine genes are coordinately expressed during T cell activation. Similar to other eukaryotic genes, the 5′ flanking sequences play an important role for regulated expression of lymphokine genes. For example, insertion of a retrovirus long terminal repeat (LTR) at the 5′ flanking region of the mouse IL-3 gene resulted in constitutive expression (17) and 5′ flanking regions have been highly conserved between mouse and human lymphokine genes. There is approximately 85% homology in the 5′ flanking regions extending around 330 bp or 500 bp upstream of TATA boxes of human and mouse GM-CSF (18) or IL-4 genes (19–21). In contrast, there is no obvious homology among different lymphokine genes except for about a 10 bp consensus sequence which is present in the 5′ flanking region of several lymphokine genes (16). The importance of the 5′ flanking regions of lymphokine genes for antigen-induced expression was confirmed by transfection experiments using chloramphenicol acetyltransferase as a reporter gene. Regulatory regions of IL-2, GM-CSF, IL-3, and IL-4 have been located within a few hundred bp from the transcription initiation site (16).

Two types of helper T cell clones have been recognized in the mouse on the basis of a differential pattern of lymphokine production (21). Although both types produce IL-3 and GM-CSF, IL-2 and INF-γ are produced by T_H1 cells but not by T_H2 cells. In contrast, IL-4 and IL-5 are produced by T_H2 but not by T_H1 (Fig 1). However, the expression of T_H1-specific and T_H2-specific lymphokines is not always mutually exclusive. Somatic cell hybrids generated by fusion of T_H1

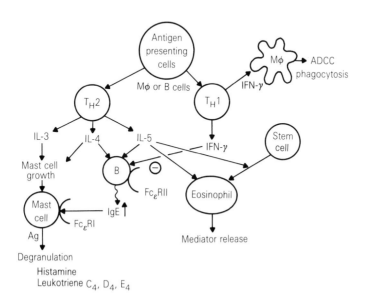

Fig 1 Regulatory circuit for IgE-mediated allergic response formed by T cell-derived lymphokines. ADCC, antibody-dependent cell-mediated cytotoxicity.

and T_H2 cells produce both IL-2 and IL-4 (22) indicating that the expression of these lymphokines is codominant. T_H1 cells mediate delayed-type hypersensitivity and cell-mediated and complement-mediated cytotoxity (23). T_H2, on the other hand, mediates IgE-dependent allergic response (23). Unlike the mouse system, most CD4$^+$ human T cell clones produce IL-2, IL-4, and IFN-γ. There is no clear separation of human clones into two subsets and different modes of activation such as antigen, lectin, or anti-CD2 stimulation can result in both qualitative and quantitative differences in lymphokine production (19).

Activation of lymphokine genes initiated by antigen or lectin stimulation is temporal and is regulated at the transcriptional level. Lymphokine-specific mRNA reaches a maximum level of 0.01–1.0% of total mRNA, 5 to 8 h after stimulation and transcription ceases thereafter (24). The production of lymphokine is also regulated at the posttranscriptional level; the AU-rich motif within the 3′ noncoding region, found in c-fos and lymphokine mRNAs, affects mRNA stability (25).

IL-3 and GM-CSF: Lymphokines that stimulate hemopoietic progenitor cells

Activated T cells produce 2 potent CSFs that stimulate early hemopoietic progenitor cells. IL-3, initially defined as a factor which induced 20-α-steroid dehydrogenase in thymus-deficient mice, has numerous biological activities including MCGF, Thy1 antigen induction, and multi-CSF activities which support colony formation composed of various cell lineages (26). The murine IL-3 cDNA encodes a polypeptide of 166 amino acids including a signal sequence (27). Almost all activities of natural IL-3 including multi-CSF have been confirmed using recombinant IL-3 (16) (Table 1). In contrast to other lymphokines, the IL-3

Table 1 Biological activities of murine IL-3 and GM-CSF.

IL-3	GM-CSF
1. Multi-CSF*	1. GM colony formation*
2. Burst promoting activity*	2. Burst promoting activity*
3. CFU-S stimulation	3. Eosinophil colony formation*
4. 20α SDH induction	4. Growth factor for hemopoietic cell lines*
5. Thy1 induction	5. Blast cell colony formation*
6. MCGF	6. Histamine release activity
7. Growth factor for hemopoietic cell lines*	
8. P cell stimulating factor	
9. Histamine producing cell stimulating factor	
10. Histamine release activity	

*Activity confirmed in human.

sequence diverged extensively during evolution. Only 54% homology was observed at the nucleotide level even between mouse and rat and the existence of a human homologue of murine IL-3 was only recently confirmed. Gibbon IL-3 cDNA, isolated by its ability to support growth of human circulating blast cells of chronic myelogenous leukemia patients, has 43% homology at the nucleotide level and only 29% homology at the amino acid level with murine IL-3 (28). Human IL-3 cDNA isolated from activated T cells is almost identical to gibbon IL-3 and encodes a protein 152 amino acid residues long which has multi-CSF activity (29) and stimulates basophil growth (30). However, it is not clear at presenty whether human IL-3 stimulates the growth of mast cells.

GM-CSF stimulates the formation of colonies composed of neutrophil, macrophage, and eosinophil lineages. Murine and human GM-CSF are glycoproteins of 141 and 144 amino acids, respectively, including a signal sequence (16, 18). Although they share about 50% homology at the amino acid level, the action of GM-CSF is species specific, like that of IL-3. Human GM-CSF also supports the growth of leukemic cells from patients and interacts with early progenitors and supports the proliferation of erythroid progenitors in the presence of erythropoietin. Mouse GM-CSF supports colony formation of blast cells that differentiate into various lineages. Administration of recombinant human GM-CSF into normal monkeys induced a marked leukocytosis (31) and when given to neutropenic patients resulted in a dose-dependent increase in white blood cell count (32). GM-CSF is also produced by cells other than T cells such as stroma, macrophage, and endothelial cells and its production is stimulated by IL-1 (33). For clinical trials, human GM-CSF has been introduced to neutropenic patients with serious conditions such as acquired immune deficiency syndrome (AIDS), aplastic anemia, and myelodysplastic syndrome (32). GM-CSF was especially effective in these patients. In myelodysplastic syndrome, human GM-CSF acts as a differentiation inducer on leukemic cells. Human IL-3 and/or GM-CSF may be a powerful tool for stem cell reserve or stem cell propagation for bone marrow transplantation.

IL-4 and IL-5: Lymphokines that stimulate lymphocytes and hemopoietic cells

Activation of resting B cells into antibody-producing plasma cells requires interaction with antigen, as well as with soluble factors produced by activated T cells or macrophages. Characterization of multiple biological activities in supernatants of mouse T cell clones indicated that T_H2 clones produce at least 4 activities not found in T_H1 cells. These are a TCGF activity distinct from IL-2 (TCGFII), an MCGF activity distinct from IL-3 (MCGFII) (19,23), the ability to induce Ia antigen on resting B cells (19,23), and IgE-inducing activity with lipopolysaccharide (LPS)-treated B cells (19,23). Recent studies have shown that all of these activities are properties of BSF-1 (19,23) and molecular cloning and expression studies have established that a single protein encoded by a cDNA clone termed IL-4 has all of these activities (1,2).

T_H2 cells also produce two other activities not found in T_H1 cells, ie, IgA-enhancing factor (IgA-EF) activity in cultures of LPS-stimulated mouse B cells (33) and Eo-CSF activity in cultures of human bone marrow cells. Molecular cloning and expression studies established that these 2 activities are mediated by a single cDNA clone which is identical to the IL-5 cDNA clone that encodes T cell replacing factor I (TRFI)/BCGFII activities (6). Association of Eo-CSF activity with mouse IL-5 is consistent with the observation that BCGFII is identical to eosinophil differentiation factor (19,23). Human IL-4 and IL-5 cDNA clones were isolated from activated human T cell clones based on nucleotide sequence homology with their mouse counterparts (3,6).

Mature murine IL-4 and human IL-4 are glycoproteins, 120 and 129 amino acid residues long, respectively. Studies with recombinant molecules revealed that human IL-4 has activities similar to mouse IL-4 (19) on B cells, as well as the ability to induce expression of the low affinity receptor for IgE (FcεRII/CD23) on B cells (19,23) (Table 2). Actions of IL-4 on B cells to enhance IgE production and induce FcεRII are inhibited by IFN-γ (19,23). Murine IL-4 stimulates the proliferation of immature thymocytes in the presence of the phorbol ester, PMA (19,23). Therefore, IL-4 may play a role in T cell ontogeny. IL-4 acts as a macrophage activation factor (MAF) by enhancing the antigen-presenting ability of certain macrophages (19,23) and stimulates the fusion of bone marrow and alveolar macrophages to form giant multinucleated cells (34). The latter activity is known as macrophage fusion factor (MFF) or macrophage inhibition factor (MIF) and may play a role in cell-mediated immune responses. In chronic granulomatous disease, such as Crohn's disease, tuberculosis, and sarcoidosis, giant multinucleated cells have been found in the center of these lesions. Human IL-4 may play an important role in forming such giant multinucleated cells. Both murine and human IL-5 augment IL-4-induced IgE synthesis and human IL-5 enhances IL-4-induced FcεRII expression on normal B cells (19,23). The enhancing effects of IL-5 were most pronounced at suboptimal IL-4 concentrations. The IgE production induced by combinations of IL-4 and IL-5 could be completely in-

Table 2   Biological activities of murine IL-4 and IL-5.

	IL-4	IL-5
T cell	TCGF* Thymocyte growth	Enhancement of IL-2- mediated killer cell induction
B cell	BCGFI* Ia induction* IgG1 enhancement* IgE enhancement* FcεRII induction*	BCGFII* IgA enhancement* IgM enhancement Enhancement of IL-4- induced IgE production*
Hemopoietic cells	MCGF Macrophage activation	Eosinophil-CSF*

*Activity confirmed in human.

hibited by IFN-γ. Use of antibodies or antagonists to IL-4 and IL-5 may be potentially useful to suppress allergic reactions. Although association between IL-5 and parasite infection in vivo is not established yet, IL-5 may play an important role in enhancing parasite killing by eosinophils.

Lymphokine network between hemopoietic cells and immunocompetent cells

Multipotential stem cells in the bone marrow generate multiple hemopoietic cell types including granulocytes, macrophages, mast cells, megakaryocytes, erythrocytes, eosinophils, T cells, and B cells. For a long time, functions of lymphocytes and hemopoietic cells have been studied independently by immunologists and hematologists, according to their own disciplines. However, as described above, helper T cells affect both hemopoiesis and the immune response through the production of lymphokines. IL-3 and GM-CSF stimulate hemopoietic stem cells whereas multifunctional lymphokines such as IL-4 and IL-5 stimulate both lymphocytes and hemopoietic cells. A general picture emerges indicating that there is a functional link in an immune response between lymphocytes and hemopoietic cells such as T cells, B cells, mast cells, macrophages, and eosinophils mediated by multiple and pleiotropic lymphokines produced by activated T cells (Fig 2). By studying the biological properties of molecularly cloned lymphokines, we can now begin to unravel the network organized between the 2 compartments responsible for inflammatory responses. All or a part of this network can be activated by antigen-specific or nonantigen-specific stimuli recognized by helper T cells through the production of a set of lymphokines. For clinical application of lymphokines, we have to consider this multifaceted cellular network.

Role of T cell lymphokines in hemopoiesis

Helper T cells produce 2 of the 4 major CSFs (IL-3 and GM-CSF) and Eo-CSF (IL-5). In addition, T cells produce other lymphokines and cytokines, such as IFN-γ, BSF-2 (IL-6), lymphotoxin, TGF-β, neuroleukin, IL-1, adult T cell leukemia-derived factor (ADF), and TNF-α, some of which were originally discovered in cells other than T cells. They all seem to affect proliferation, differentiation, and maturation of lymphocytes and hemopoietic cells. BSF-2 for example, which was previously thought to be a B cell-specific lymphokine, is identical to 26 KDa protein/IFN-γ2, hybridoma growth factor, and hepatocyte-stimulating factor (HSF) and is produced by macrophages, fibroblasts, and T cells. Neuroleukin, initially identified as a factor present in the salivary gland, stimulates the growth of neuronal cells and the production of immunoglobulin (23). In addition to these stimulatory factors, several factors such as TGF-β, PGE$_2$, and IFN-γ exert a negative effect on proliferation.

What then is the physiological role of T cell lymphokines in hemopoiesis? To avoid confusion, we have to distinguish steady state or "constitutive"

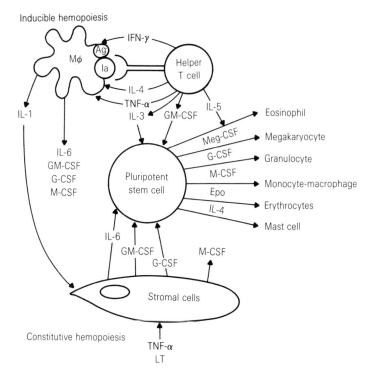

Inducible hemopoiesis

Fig 2 Possible role of lymphokines and cytokines in inducible and constitutive hemopoiesis.

hemopoiesis in the bone marrow microenvironment that occurs in the absence of an immunological stimulus, from "inducible" hemopoiesis, the hemopoietic activities associated with an inflammatory response in which T cells and macrophages play a major role (16) (Fig 2). Proliferation and maturation of hemopoietic cells occurs continuously in the bone marrow microenvironment under strict control mechanisms. It appears that T cell-derived lymphokines do not play a major role in the regulation of constitutive hemopoiesis. All hemopoietic progenitor cells are derived from self-renewing stem cells. In the bone marrow microenvironment, the interaction of stem cells with stroma cells may be important in the regulation of this constitutive hemopoiesis. Certain stroma cells produce M-CSF, G-CSF, GM-CSF (33), and BSF-2 (15). IL-1 strongly stimulates the production of GM-CSF, G-CSF, and BSF-2 by stroma cells. Interestingly, several stroma cells that support multipotential stem cells produce neither IL-3 nor GM-CSF (35), suggesting that this class of stroma cells produces a soluble factor(s) or cell surface molecule(s) which supports self-renewal and survival of stem cells.

The hemopoietic cascade triggered by T cell-derived lymphokines may play a major role in host defense reactions against the invasion of foreign substances.

In inducible hemopoiesis, T cells and macrophages may collaborate to produce a battery of lymphokines and cytokines that result in the rapid amplification and maturation of various hemopoietic cells at the site of inflammation (16). IL-3 and GM-CSF, produced by activated T cells, may stimulate early hemopoietic progenitor cells to amplify the cascade; IL-4 and IL-5 may coordinate the function of hemopoietic cells and lymphoid cells. IFN-γ produced by T cells may activate macrophages to produce G-CSF, M-CSF, and BSF-2. TNF-α and IL-1 produced by activated macrophage or T cells may stimulate endothelial cells, fibroblasts, and stroma cells. These reactions cease rapidly when antigen stimulation is abolished because lymphokine mRNA and protein disappear rapidly and hemopoietic cells die quickly after CSFs are depleted.

Role of lymphokines in IgE-mediated allergic response

Allergic reactions may be regulated at 2 levels: 1) the synthesis of IgE by B cells and 2) the interaction of IgE with the high affinity Fcϵ receptor (FcϵRI) on mast cells and basophils. Activation of this receptor initiates degranulation to release mediators contained in intracellular granules. The properties of IL-3, IL-4, and IL-5 suggest that these lymphokines play an important role in the regulatory circuit for IgE-mediated allergic responses (Fig 1). IL-4 is capable of stimulating both IgE synthesis and the target cells, ie, mast cells and basophils. In the mouse system, IL-4, in concert with IL-3, stimulates the growth of mast cells. Although human IL-3 stimulates basophils (30), the role of IL-3 and IL-4 in supporting mast cell growth remains to be established in the human system. Both mouse and human IL-4 stimulate IgE production, as well as the expression of a low affinity Fcϵ receptor (FcϵRII) on B cells. Since anti-CD23 (FcϵRII) antibody inhibited IgE production, expression of FcϵRII may be required for the induction of IgE by IL-4. The precise effects of CD23 or IgE-binding factors on IL-4-induced IgE production remain to be determined.

Two types of helper T cell clones recognized in the mouse system may play distinct roles in the regulation of the IgE response. IL-5, produced by T_H2 cells, enhances IL-4-induced IgE synthesis whereas IFN-γ, produced by T_H1 cells, is inhibitory (19,23). IFN-γ may also have an antagonistic effect on FcϵRII expression. Therefore, T_H1 cells may negatively regulate IgE synthesis through the production of IFN-γ. IgE synthesis in the human, like the mouse, is controlled by the balance of IL-4, IL-5, and IFN-γ. Production of these human lymphokines is affected by the mode of activation of T cells. Apart from its role in IgE and IgA synthesis, IL-5 stimulates proliferation and differentiation of eosinophils although the function of eosinophils in the regulatory network is unclear. It is likely that the inflammatory response which follows the invasion of foreign antigens or pathogens is controlled by the balance of positive and negative lymphokines produced by activated T cells.

Conclusions

The formation of antibodies by an animal after exposure to antigen involves multiple cellular interactions. At the beginning, an antigen processed by antigen-presenting cells is recognized by a T cell antigen receptor. At the end, B cells produce antibodies which can recognize the antigen that provoked their formation. In between the 2 antigen-specific events, T cells help B cells to make antibody by producing lymphokines. Unlike immunoglobulin or the T cell antigen receptor, lymphokines are not antigen specific. Therefore, helper T cells can be regarded as a "signal transduction machine," which receives antigen-specific signals and converts them into antigen-nonspecific mediators of the immune response. Understanding of lymphokines that stimulate B cells and hemopoietic cells may help to clarify the mechanisms underlying antigen-nonspecific inflammatory response.

If the functions of T cells and B cells are controlled by multiple lymphokines, how does the immune system maintain specificity for the original antigen in an immune response? It is possible that antigen-specific receptors on T and B cells play a key role in this process. For example, only T and B cells that receive a specific antigen signal may express functional receptor for a certain lymphokine and thereby become responsive to proliferation and/or differentiation signals.

Alternatively, antigen specificity can be mediated by cell-cell interaction. For example, B cells are capable of processing antigens via surface immunoglobulin and presenting them to T cells. The immune system, which is composed of both antigen-specific and -nonspecific receptors and mediators, provides an excellent model to study the basic principles in cell-to-cell communication and control of proliferation and differentiation of mammalian cells. It is to be hoped that basic molecular biology and cell biology research on lymphokines proves to be useful for the development of effective protocols for treatment of immunological and hematological disorders, such as autoimmune disease, allergy, and cancer.

Acknowledgment

We would like to thank our many colleagues in the Molecular Biology and Immunology Departments of DNAX and UNICET Immunology Laboratory.

References

1. Lee F, Yokota T, Otsuka, T, et al. Isolation and characterization of a mouse interleukin cDNA clone that expresses B-cell stimulatory factor 1 activities and T-cell- and mast-cell-stimulating activities. Proc Natl Acad Sci USA 1986;83:2061-5.
2. Noma Y, Sideras P, Naito T, et al. Molecular cloning of cDNA encoding the murine IgG1 induction factor by a novel strategy using SP6 promoter. Nature 1986;319:640-6.
3. Yokota T, Otsuka T, Mosmann T, et al. Isolation and characterization of a human

interleukin cDNA clone, homologous to mouse B-cell stimulatory factor 1, that expresses B-cell- and T-cell-stimulatory activities. Proc Natl Acad Sci USA 1986;83:5894–8.

4. Kinashi T, Harada N, Severinson E, et al. Cloning of complementary DNA encoding T-cell replacing factor and identity with B-cell growth factor II. Nature 1986; 324:70–3.

5. Azuma C, Tanabe T, Konishi, M, et al. Cloning of cDNA for human T-cell replacing factor (interleukin 5) and comparison with the murine homologue. Nucleic Acids Res 1986;14:9149–58.

6. Yokota T, Coffman RL, Hagiwara H, et al. Isolation and characterization of lymphokine cDNA clones encoding mouse and human IgA-enhancing factor and eosinophil colony-stimulating factor activities: Relationship to interleukin 5. Proc Natl Acad Sci USA 1987;84:7388–92.

7. Hirano T, Yasukawa K, Harada H, et al. Complementary DNA for a novel human interleukin (BSF-2) that induces B lymphocytes to produce immunoglobulin. Nature 1986;324:73–6.

8. Kishimoto T, Yoshizaki K, Kimoto M, et al. B cell growth and differentiation factors and mechanism of B cell activation. Immunol Rev 1984;78:97–118.

9. Gauldie J, Richards C, Harnish D, et al. Interferon $\beta2$/BSF-2 is identical to monocyte derived hepatocyte-stimulating factor and regulates the full acute phase protein response in liver cells. Proc Natl Acad Sci USA 1987;84:7251–5.

10. Okayama H, Berg P. A cDNA cloning vector that permits expression of cDNA inserts in mammalian cells. Mol Cell Biol 1983;3:280–9.

11. Takebe Y, Seiki M, Fujisawa J, et al. SRα promoter: an efficient and versatile mammalian cDNA expression system composed of the simian virus 40 early promoter and the R-U5 segment of human T-cell leukemia virus type 1 long terminal repeat. Mol Cell Biol 1988;8:466–72.

12. Miyajima A, Bond MW, Otsu K, et al. Secretion of mature mouse interleukin 2 by *Saccharomyces cerevisiae*: Use of a general secretion vector containing promoter and leader sequences of the mating pheromone α-factor. Gene 1985;37:155–61.

13. Miyajima A, Schreurs J, Otsu K, et al. Use of the silkworm, *Bombyx mori*, an insect baculovirus vector for high-level expression and secretion of biologically active mouse interleukin 3. Gene 1987;58:273–81.

14. Gray PW. Molecular characterization of human lymphotoxin. In: Webb DR, Goeddel DV, eds. Lymphokines, vol 13. Orlando, Florida: Academic Press; 1987:199–208.

15. Choy-Pik C, Moulds C, Coffman R, et al. Multiple biological activities are expressed by a mouse interleukin 6 cDNA clone isolated from bone marrow stromal cells. Proc Natl Acad Sci USA (in press).

16. Miyajima A, Miyatake S, Schreurs J, et al. Coordinate regulation of immune and inflammatory responses by T cell-derived lymphokines. FASEB J 1988;2:2462–73.

17. Ymer S, Tucker WQJ, Sanderson CJ, et al. Constitutive synthesis of interleukin-3 by leukemia cell line WEHI-3B is due to retroviral insertion near the gene. Nature 1985;317:255–8.

18. Miyatake S, Otsuka T, Yokota T, et al. Structure of the chromosomal gene for granulocyte-macrophage colony stimulating factor: Comparison of the mouse and human genes. EMBO J 1985;4:2561–8.

19. Yokota T, Arai N, de Vries J, et al. Molecular biology of interleukin 4 and interleukin 5 genes and biology of their products that stimulate B cells, T cells and hemopoietic cells. Immunol Rev 1988;102:137–87.

20. Otsuka T, Villaret D, Yokota T, et al. Structural analysis of the mouse chromosomal gene encoding interleukin 5 which expresses B cell, T cell and mast cell stimulating activities. Nucleic Acids Res 1987;15:333–44.

21. Arai N, Nomura D, Villaret D, et al. Nucleotide sequence of the gene encoding human interleukin 4 and its location on the human chromosome. J Immunol 1989;142:274–82.

22. Mosmann TR, Cherwinski H, Bond MW, et al. Two types of murine helper T cell clone. I. Definition according to profiles of lymphokine activities and secreted proteins. J Immunol 1985;126:2348–57.

23. Coffman RL, Seymour BWP, Lebman DA, et al. The role of helper T cell products in mouse B cell differentiation and isotype regulation. Immunol Rev 1988;102:5–28.

24. Hagiwara H, Yokota T, Luh J, et al. Reconstitution of inducible lymphokine production in BW5147-derived T cell hybridomas: Evidence that the AKR thymoma BW5147 is able to produce lymphokines. J Immunol 1987;138:2514–9.

25. Show G, Kamen R. A conserved AU sequence from the 3' untranslated region of GM-CSF mRNA mediates selective mRNA degradation. Cell 1986;46:659–67.

26. Ihle JN, Pepersack L, Rebar L. Regulation of T cell differentiation: in vitro induction of 20 alpha-hydroxysteroid dehydrogenase in splenic lymphocytes from athymic mice by a unique lymphokine. J Immunol 1981;126:2184–9.

27. Yokota T, Lee F, Rennick D, et al. Isolation and characterization of a mouse cDNA clone that expresses mast-cell growth-factor activity in monkey cells. Proc Natl Acad Sci USA 1984;81:1070–4.

28. Yang Y-C, Ciarletta AB, Temple PA, et al. Human IL-3 (Multi-CSF): Identification by expression cloning of a novel hematopoietic growth factor related to murine IL-3. Cell 1987;47:3–10.

29. Otsuka T, Miyajima A, Brown N, et al. Isolation and characterization of an expressible cDNA encoding human interleukin 3: Induction of IL-3 mRNA in human T cells. J Immunol 1988;140:2288–95.

30. Saito H, Hatake K, Dvorak AM, et al. Selective differentiation/proliferation of hematopoietic cells by recombinant human interleukins. Proc Natl Acad Sci USA 1988; 85:2288–92.

31. Donahue RE, Wang EA, Stone DK, et al. Stimulation of haemopoiesis in primates by continuous infusion of recombinant human GM-CSF. Nature 1985;321:872–5.

32. Groopman JE, Mitsuya RT, Deleo MJ, et al. Effect of recombinant human granulocyte-macrophage colony stimulating factors on myelopoiesis in the acquired immunodeficiency syndrome. N Engl J Med 1987;317:593–8.

33. Rennick D, Yang G, Gemmell L, Lee F. Control of hemopoiesis by a bone marrow stromal cell clone: LPS and interleukin 1 inducible production of colony stimulating factors. Blood 1986;69:682–91.

34. Coffman RL, Schrader B, Carty J, et al. A mouse T cell product that preferentially enhances IgA production. I. Biologic characterization. J Immunol 1987;139:3685–90.

35. McInnes A, Rennick DM. Interleukin 4 induces cultured monocytes/macrophages to form giant multinucleated cells. J Exp Med 1988;167:598–611.

36. Kodama H, Hagiwara H, Sudo H, et al. MC3T3/PA6 preadipocytes support in vitro proliferation of hemopoietic stem cells through a mechanism different from that of interleukin 3. J Cell Physiol 1986;129:20–6.

Biomolecular mechanisms of macrophage activation for tumor cell killing

Stephen W. Russell

University of Kansas Cancer Center, and Departments of Pathology/Oncology and Microbiology, University of Kansas Medical Center, Kansas City, Kansas, USA

The phenomenon of macrophage activation

Beginning with the observations of Metchnikoff (1), it has been apparent that phagocytic cells, including macrophages and other members of the mononuclear phagocyte lineage, are important in host defense against an assortment of pathogens. George Mackaness' recognition (2) that macrophages become much more efficient at eliminating microbial invaders when they become "activated" was a key step toward understanding conceptually how these cells provide protection.

The morphologic, functional, and biochemical changes that characterize activated macrophages have been the subject of intense investigation during the last 25 years, sometimes with surprising results. Cases in point are the discoveries of Alexander and Evans (3) and of John Hibbs Jr and his colleagues (4) that activated mouse macrophages could injure and kill tumor cells with which they were incubated. The many subsequent observations of Hibbs and his colleagues have provided an important foundation for current investigations into macrophage activation for tumor cell killing. They showed, for example, that contact between the activated effector and its target tumor cell is required for killing to occur (4,5); that cytolysis is mediated by extracellular (ie, nonphagocytic) rather than intracellular mechanisms (4); that the time needed either to damage or kill is relatively long (4,6) (measured in h rather than min as for complement- or T cell-mediated cytotoxicity); that once macrophages become activated in response to any stimulus, they have acquired the capacity to kill a variety of different tumor cells, without regard to immunologic (ie, antigenic) specificity (4, 5; similar to Mackaness' observation that activated macrophages have the capacity to kill a wide range of microbes, regardless of the immunologic stimulus that caused them to become activated [7]); and that activated macrophages can distinguish between malignant and nonmalignant cells, generally sparing those that are normal (8). This latter observation has been confirmed repeatedly in many different laboratories, but no more dramatically than by Meltzer and his colleagues (9), who recorded the phenomenon by time-lapse microcinematography in cultures that contained both normal and malignant cells.

The next major step was the demonstration by Piessens et al (10) of a secreted product of lymphocytes that activated macrophages, ie, a macrophage activating factor, or MAF. The existence of such a factor had been postulated earlier by Mackaness (11). Hibbs and coworkers (12,13) extended understanding of MAF's mechanism of effect by showing that elevation of macrophages to a cytolytic (ie, fully activated) state in vitro was due to the influence of at least 2 stimuli: one a lymphokine, and the other traces of endotoxin that often contaminated cell culture systems at that time. They demonstrated conclusively that when all vestiges of endotoxin were eliminated, macrophages exposed to MAF did not become cytolytic, as subsequently confirmed quantitatively by Pace and Russell (14). Recognition that, as part of the activation process, macrophages could be elevated to a noncytolytic but functionally altered state, either in vitro (12,13,15) or in vivo (16), led to the concept that activation for either microbial or tumor cell killing develops through a series of discrete steps. Figure 1 illustrates the current view of this process.

Stages of activation

The first identifiable stage in the activation sequence is one that is defined operationally as "responsive" or "inflammatory." Macrophages in this state have been elicited by any agent that provokes inflammation. They have distinct morphologic and biochemical differences when they are compared to unstimulated macrophages, such as increased size, vacuolation, and content of hydrolytic enzymes; however, the change that is most relevant to this brief review is that they respond more readily to activating stimuli than unstimulated macrophages do (17). The basis for this difference is not known, but it is likely due to exposure of macrophages at the site of inflammation to 1 or more of the many mediators that are present there; it is probably not an inherent difference in populations of cells at the site. For example, Lee et al (18) separated inflammatory macrophages on the basis of size differences and found that all subpopulations were equally responsive to activating stimuli. This would suggest that the entire population was changed, not just 1 group, such as smaller, newly immigrated mononuclear phagocytes (17). In Fig 1, the unstimulated and inflammatory populations have been combined for the sake of simplicity because either can be activated; it simply takes more of the stimulus if one begins with quiescent cells.

The name of the second stage, "primed," connotes that the macrophage has been prepared to mediate cytotoxicity, but will not do so unless something more is done to it. The "something" is application of a 2nd, "triggering" stimulus which can be provided by a variety of agents. Among these, endotoxin and bacterial lipopolysaccharide (specifically, the lipid A component of these molecules) are most often employed experimentally to provide this 2nd signal. The identity of the triggering stimulus in vivo is unknown; however, it would

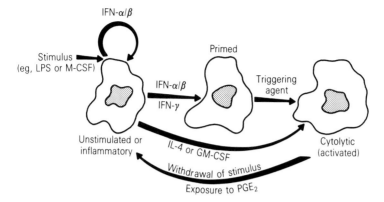

Fig 1 Stages of macrophage activation and mediators or conditions that regulate their appearance and disappearance. Under appropriate conditions, cytolytic macrophages that have lost their ability to kill can be reactivated (19). LPS, lipopolysaccharide; PGE_2, prostaglandin E_2.

most logically be a constituent of the plasma membrane or cell wall of the activated macrophage target. Were this true, only those macrophages that had a reason to become fully activated, ie, those that were in contact with their target, would develop a cytolytic capability. Such an arrangement would help guard against the indiscriminate activation of large numbers of macrophages, which could result in the injury of normal tissues.

The final cytolytic stage is maintained only when activating stimuli are continuously present. The noncytolytic cell to which an activated macrophage reverts after the removal of activators can be restimulated to kill again (19).

Activating stimuli

Interferon-γ

The stimulus for activation that has received the most attention is interferon-γ (IFN-γ), also known as either immune or type II interferon. It is produced by T lymphocytes in response to stimulation by either mitogen or antigen, and is likely to be the principal MAF. The type I interferons, α (IFN-α; also known as leukocyte interferon) and β (IFN-β; fibroblast interferon), are also activators of macrophages, but tend to be much less effective than IFN-γ when they are compared on the basis of antiviral units (20). Nevertheless, as will be seen, they may be important in regulating activation.

Schultz and Chirigos (21,22) were the first to recognize that there were similarities between the interferons and the activating factors that were found in the culture supernates of stimulated lymphocytes. Their observations set off intensive investigations in many different laboratories that were designed to verify or reject the hypothesis that MAF and interferon are the same. Results of purification and physicochemical characterization of MAF from lymphocytes (23–27), lymphocyte cell lines (28,29), and T cell hybridomas (30,31) strongly supported the hypothesis, especially when the studies included antibodies that were specific for the interferons and that would also neutralize the activation potential of lymphokine-containing supernates (21,27,29,32–34). The hypothesis was confirmed when several studies (34–37) showed that recombinant IFN-γ had all of the characteristics of native MAF. Functionally, it would "prime" macrophages for tumor cell killing, requiring an additional "triggering" stimulus in most instances to cause the expression of cytolytic activity. When the macrophages of certain strains of mice were used, or relatively high concentrations of the mediator were applied, IFN-γ had the capacity to activate fully, ie, to make macrophages cytolytic (37,38).

Interferon-α and -β

IFN-α and IFN-β can also affect macrophage activation for tumor cell killing. Appreciating that these type I interferons have such potential is important for 2 reasons. First, their capacity to activate must be remembered when any chemical or biological mediator is claimed to be an activator; such agents may simply be stimulating the macrophages to secrete IFN-α/β, which then activates the producer macrophages through an autocrine feedback mechanism. Bacterial lipopolysaccharide has its activating effect in this way (19,21). Second, the type I interferons can modulate the response of macrophages to IFN-γ. Pace and her colleagues first showed that preincubation of macrophages with IFN-β suppressed their subsequent responsiveness to IFN-γ (39), while simultaneous incubation of macrophages with IFN-β and -γ augmented their overall response (40). In these latter experiments, which utilized isobologram analysis, different concentrations of each of the 2 mediators were evaluated for their net effect on priming for tumor cell killing. The effect of combining the 2 interferons was, in most cases, greater than additive and in some instances synergistic. Yoshida et al (41) have recently reported similar kinds of agonistic and antagonistic effects of different concentration ratios of human IFN-γ and human IFN-α/β on mature human macrophages, using hydrogen peroxide-releasing capacity as their principal measure of effect.

Other activators

Throughout this intensive investigation of the interferons, sporadic reports appeared of activators that were apparently not members of the IFN family (28,29,42–48; Fig 1). Some of these studies have not been reproducible and others were not completely convincing because involvement of endogenous IFN-α/β had not been excluded. Recently, several reports have suggested that the biosynthetically produced growth regulators, interleukin 4 (IL-4; also known as BSF-1) (49) and granulocyte–macrophage colony-stimulating factor (GM-CSF) (49,50), have direct activating capabilities. Similar claims have been made (44,48) for another CSF, CSF-1 (M-CSF), although it is a known inducer of IFN-α/β (51,52). We have shown that recombinant murine IL-4 (rMuIL-4) remains an activator of macrophages, even when anti-IL-4 antibody is included in the system to minimize the possibility of autocrine activation by endogenously produced IFN-α/β (S. Caballero, B. Torres, S.W. Russell, unpublished observations). Similar experiments need to be performed with other non-IFN activators; however, to be absolutely certain that an autocrine effect of IFN-α/β is not involved, it will ultimately be necessary to examine macrophages that have been stimulated with non-IFN activators to ensure that there is not increased expression of the genes that code for IFN-α/β. If such experiments confirm that mediators such as IL-4 are directly activating macrophages, it will unequivocally show that there is more than a single pathway, at least in part, to the activated phenotype.

Transduction of activating signals

Receptors

Whether it is an interferon or a noninterferon activator, its effect is likely to begin through interaction with specific receptors on the surface of macrophages. The best studied of these is the receptor for IFN-γ, which appears to be of a single class (53,54) that is distributed ubiquitously among cell types. The binding protein in mouse macrophage plasma membranes is a glycoprotein of apparent relative molecular mass M_r 95 000 (55). It has an apparent homologue of M_r 90 000 in the cellular membranes of human beings (56,57). Smaller proteins (55, 57–59), some with binding activity (57,58), have also been described. However, these probably will prove to be degradation products of the larger binding protein rather than separate entities. Supportive of such conjecture is the fact that the smaller species can be eliminated when conditions are rigorously controlled to minimize proteolytic degradation during isolation of the receptor (55,57).

By most accounts, IFN-α and IFN-β share a single receptor which differs from the one for IFN-γ (reviewed in 60,61). The genetic information for these 2 receptors is located in human beings on chromosomes 21 (62) and 6 (63), respectively. Despite such evidence of distinctness, a number of reports have described competition between IFN-β and INF-γ for cellular binding (41,53,64–68). This led Thompson et al (67) to postulate that, while there are 2 receptors, both of which bind IFN-β, 1 of them also has the capacity to bind IFN-γ, while the other additionally binds IFN-α. A different model has recently been postulated by Yoshida et al (41), who described a novel, high-affinity receptor that was expressed on the surfaces of mature human macrophages which had been culture derived from monocytes. It bound all 3 species of interferon, but had a higher binding affinity for IFN-α and -β than for INF-γ. Depending on the ratio between the concentrations of IFN-γ and either IFN-α or -β, the effect on hydrogen peroxide-releasing capacity was either suppression, no effect, or augmentation of what could be expected with IFN-γ used alone.

One of the most intriguing questions currently before workers in the field of activation is whether or not a single binding protein for IFN-γ is sufficient to transduce the signal for priming and activation. Although no data currently bear directly on this question, there is evidence from Pestka's group (63) that more than the receptor is needed for IFN-γ to exert its inductive effect on the expression of major histocompatibility (MHC) antigens, either by hamster–human or mouse–human hybrid cells. Their conclusion was that chromosome 6, which bears the code for the receptor for human IFN-γ, was insufficient by itself to confer MHC inducibility on hybrid cells; a 2nd species-specific entity or "transducer" was needed, coded for by chromosome 21 (which also carries the genetic information for the receptor for HuIFN-α/β). The implications of these observations are great and will undoubtedly have an important influence on the directions of future research in this area.

Relatively little is known about the cellular receptor for IL-4, as summarized by Kishimoto and Hirano (69). The receptor exists on murine macrophages, as well as on B and T lymphocytes and mast cells. Cross-linking studies suggest that it consists of at least one chain of M_r 55–60.

Processing of signal for activation

After 1 of the interferons binds to its receptor, the complex is internalized (65,70–75). Evidence for this is both direct (ie, ultrastructural, showing association with coated pits) and indirect. Results of the latter kind have been derived either by elution of surface-bound ligand with acid or by degrading it with trypsin, with any residuum considered to be inside the cell. It is controversial whether or not binding of interferon per se is sufficient to signal cells, and 3 lines of evidence suggest that it may be insufficient. First, high-affinity nuclear binding sites have been demonstrated for interferon (74). No association with function has been made for these, however. Second, interacting cells with IFN-γ contained in liposomes, and thereby ostensibly bypassing the surface receptor, both activated the macrophages and abrogated the species specificity of the interferon (under these conditions, mouse IFN-γ efficiently activated human cells, and vice versa [76]). Third, and perhaps most compelling, is the discovery that mouse cells transfected with cDNA that had been engineered so that the human IFN-γ produced from it would lack the leader sequence required for its secretion, induced an interferon-dependent activity, namely, an antiviral state (77). Collectively, these observations raise the possibility that, at least for some functions stimulated by IFN, the receptor may act as nothing more than a carrier to facilitate internalization of the ligand.

It is difficult to conclude which 2nd messenger(s) is (are) related to signalling for activation, because most observations to date have been associative, rather than of a cause-and-effect nature. An exception may be those that relate calcium to the activation process. Gorecka-Tisera investigated RAW 264, a macrophage-like cell line that can be activated by lymphokine and lipopolysaccharide to kill tumor cells (78–80). She showed that a slow flux of Ca^{2+} from intracellular sources was needed to activate cells of this line for tumor cell killing. Hamilton et al (81) and Johnson and Torres (82), using mouse peritoneal and bone marrow culture-derived macrophages, respectively, showed that the calcium ionophore A23187 could mimic the priming activity of rMuIFN-γ. They differed only in that phorbol myristate acetate was required in one of the studies (81) in addition to Ca^{2+}. Since colony-stimulating factors may be able to influence the activation process (48–50), the difference between the results of the 2 groups could be attributable to the fact that 1 group (82) used macrophages that had recently been exposed to M-CSF (CSF-1).

Another subcellular biochemical change that results from exposing macrophages to activating stimuli is a selective one in the metabolism of RNA (83,84). While it is not certain that this alteration is causally related to activation, the likelihood is increasing that it is.

Protein kinase C (PK-C) was at first thought to be a participant in the biochemical pathway leading to macrophage activation by IFN-γ. The bases for this hypothesis were: 1) the finding that phorbol myristate acetate, a known activator of PK-C, was thought to be needed, along with Ca^{2+}, to mimic the priming effect of MuIFN-γ; and 2) the finding that activity of PK-C was increased in macrophages that had been stimulated with MuIFN-γ (81,85). Recent studies may cast doubt on this conclusion, however. Using 2 different inhibitors of PK-C, Radzioch and Varesio (86) showed that virtually complete inhibition of the enzymatic activity of PK-C had no inhibitory effect on the ability of MuIFN-γ to activate macrophages for tumor cell killing. By contrast, the effect of the inhibitors on activation induced by mouse IFN-β was dramatic: activation was inhibited in a strict dose-dependent manner. These results provide additional evidence that there may be at least 2 different biochemical pathways that lead to the phenotype of the activated cytolytic macrophage. Furthermore, they implicate PK-C as a required participant in the chain of events leading to activation for tumor cell killing which is initiated by IFN-β.

Other changes induced by activating stimuli

A great variety of changes occur in macrophages after they are exposed to activating stimuli. These include both cellular and subcellular alterations, as well as a wide range of functional modifications (reviewed in 87). Many of these are either unrelated to activation for tumor cell killing or are of unknown significance; the challenge is to sort out the ones that are relevant from the greater number that are not.

Modulation of expression of proteins

Cells exposed to either a priming agent, eg, an interferon, or a triggering agent, such as lipopolysaccharide, alter the expression of cellular and secreted proteins dramatically (19,88–95). In several instances, investigators have related such changes in the expression of proteins to the stages of macrophage activation for tumor cell killing (38,89,92,93,95). Changes in expression detected on 1- and 2-

dimensional gels have been both qualitative (ie, either complete loss of existing proteins or gain of new ones) and quantitative. The changes most closely associated with the activation process are in the expression of protein 47b (p47b) and the doublet protein(s) p71/73. Each of the 3 is absent before stimulation and is extensively expressed after. p47b appears to be a marker for the primed (ie,

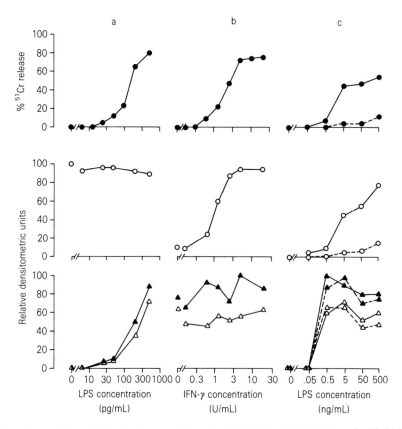

Fig 2 Comparison of levels of expression of p47b (○) and p71 (▲) and p73 (△) with cytolytic responses in bone marrow culture-derived macrophages. Macrophages were treated with varying concentrations of lipopolysaccharide (LPS, 0 to 400 pg/mL) in the presence of a constant amount (10 U/mL) of IFN-γ (column a); varying concentrations of IFN-γ (0–10 U/mL) in the presence of a constant concentration (400 pg/mL) of LPS (column b); or (column c) varying concentrations of LPS alone (0–500 ng/mL) either in the absence (——) or presence (- - -) of antiserum to IFN-α/β. The antiserum was used at a final concentration sufficient to neutralize 3000 U/mL IFN-α/β. Activation of macrophages for tumor cell killing (top row) measured as isotope release from ^{51}Cr-labeled P815 mastocytoma cells. Each point on the curves depicting levels of specific protein expression (middle and bottom rows) reflects the total optical density within the corresponding spot in fluorograms of 2-dimensional gels, and each point is given as percentage of maximal densitometric value for that protein during the series of treatments described here. Reproduced, with permission, from Mackay RJ, Russell SW (19).

interferon-stimulated) state, while p71/73 signals that a macrophage has been exposed to a triggering agent. The presence of both proteins is the phenotype of an activated cytolytic macrophage. These changes are found in mouse macrophages that have been activated either in vitro (19,95) or in vivo (93). Figure 2 illustrates the closeness of the linkage between the expression of these proteins and the development of cytolytic activity by bone marrow culture-derived mouse macrophages.

Thus far, it has not been possible to separate the expression of p47b and p71/73 from the development of the primed or activated state, in spite of many different approaches designed to do so. This has not been the case with another protein, p120. We have substantiated the report (92) that p120 is newly expressed by activated mouse peritoneal macrophages. Nevertheless, when bone marrow culture-derived macrophages are used instead of ones from the peritoneal cavity, noncytolytic stages, including those which have not been exposed to either priming or triggering stimuli, express the protein (95). Thus, the linkage between activation and the expression of p120 can be broken under certain conditions.

The importance of proteins that are faithful markers of activation stages is potentially great. First, their detection (eg, immunocytochemically using labeled monoclonal antibodies) would allow the process of activation to be followed in single cells, rather than in populations. Second, the activation status of macrophages in tumors (or in inflammatory lesions, such as immune granulomas) could be ascertained directly. Third, biological response modifiers could be evaluated in terms of how they affect the state of activation of macrophages within primary or metastatic neoplasms. And finally, an association of such closeness between protein expression and the development of cytolytic function suggests that the subject proteins could be causally related in some way to the regulation of macrophage activation.

Binding site for tumor cells

Another change that is particularly significant in the activation process is the acquisition of a binding site for neoplastic cells on primed and fully activated macrophages. The development of such a site probably explains how activated macrophages attach to and selectively kill malignant but not normal cells. The increased specific binding of tumor cells to activated macrophages was first observed by Piessens (96). His observation was subsequently confirmed and extended by Marino and his colleagues (97,98). These latter investigators showed that the site was sensitive to digestion by trypsin and that it was saturable with membranes from tumor cells. The precise nature of this component in or on the membranes of activated macrophages is not known, but clearly its characterization will be an important part of understanding the physiology of tumor cell killing by these cells. One possibility is a binding site that recognizes complex asparagine-linked oligosaccharides on the surfaces of neoplastic cells, as proposed by Mercurio (99).

Mechanism of killing tumor cells

The ultimate purpose of activation for tumor cell killing is, as the name implies, to confer on macrophages the ability to destroy malignant cells. Despite many attempts to elucidate the mechanism of killing, it has not been possible to single out a "silver bullet" that is solely responsible for mediating the effect. There have been many candidates, including transfer of lysosomes between the activated macrophage and its target (6,100); elaboration of a cytolytic proteinase (101); secretion of C3 with subsequent cleavage to cytolytic C3a (102); production of arginase (103); secretion of reactive oxygen intermediates, primarily hydrogen peroxide (104,105); interference with the oxidative metabolism of tumor cells (106,107); and elaboration of tumor necrosis factor (108,109). Each of these has some degree of merit; however, none will explain the killing of tumor cells by activated macrophages in all instances. Therefore, it is likely that more than a single mechanism is used by activated macrophages to dispatch malignant cells.

Conclusions

As can be discerned from this brief review, the biomolecular mechanisms of macrophage activation for tumor cell killing are just beginning to unfold. However, the pace at which new information is becoming available is quickening, primarily because of the wider availability of the techniques of molecular biology and immunology and the application of these techniques to the analysis of macrophage activation. Definitive answers to many open questions in the field should therefore soon be forthcoming.

Acknowledgments

This study was supported in part by research grants CA 31199 and CA 37187 from the National Cancer Institute, and the Wilkinson Endowment for the Advancement of Cancer Research.

References

1. Metchnikoff E. Immunity in infective diseases. Cambridge: Cambridge University Press; 1905.
2. Mackaness GB. The monocyte in cellular immunity. Semin Hematol 1970;7:172–84.
3. Alexander P, Evans R. Endotoxin and double stranded RNA render macrophages cytotoxic. Nature New Biol 1971;232:76–8.
4. Hibbs JB Jr, Lambert LH Jr, Remington JS. Possible role of macrophage-mediated non-specific cytotoxicity in tumour resistance. Nature New Biol

1972;235:48–50.

5. Hibbs JB Jr, Lambert LH Jr, Remington JS. In vitro nonimmunologic destruction of cells with abnormal growth characteristics by adjuvant activated macrophages. Proc Soc Exp Biol Med 1972;139:1049–52.

6. Hibbs JB Jr. Heterocytolysis by macrophages activated by bacillus Calmette-Guérin: lysosome exocytosis into tumor cells. Science 1974;184:468–71.

7. Mackaness GB. The immunological basis of acquired cellular resistance. J Exp Med 1964;120:105–20.

8. Hibbs JB Jr. Macrophage nonimmunologic recognition: target cell factors related to contact inhibition. Science 1973;180:868–70.

9. Meltzer MS, Tucker RW, Breuer AC. Interaction of BCG-activated macrophages with neoplastic and nonneoplastic cell lines in vitro: cinemicrographic analysis. Cell Immunol 1975;17:30–42.

10. Piessens WF, Churchill WH Jr, David JR. Macrophages activated in vitro with lymphocyte mediators kill neoplastic but not normal cells. J Immunol 1975;114:293–9.

11. Mackaness GB. The influence of immunologically committed lymphoid cells on macrophage activity in vivo. J Exp Med 1969;129:973–92.

12. Hibbs JB Jr, Taintor RR, Chapman HA Jr, Weinberg JB. Macrophage tumor killing: influence of the local environment. Science 1977;197:279–82.

13. Weinberg JB, Chapman HA Jr, Hibbs JB Jr. Characterization of the effects of endotoxin on macrophage tumor cell killing. J Immunol 1978;121:72–80.

14. Pace JL, Russell SW. Activation of mouse macrophages for tumor cell killing. I. Quantitative analysis of interactions between lymphokine and lipopolysaccharide. J Immunol 1981;126:1863–7.

15. Ruco LP, Meltzer MS. Macrophage activation for tumor cytotoxicity: development of macrophage cytotoxic activity requires completion of a sequence of short- lived intermediary reactions. J Immunol 1978;121:2035–42.

16. Russell SW, Doe WF, McIntosh AT. Functional characterization of a stable, noncytolytic stage of macrophage activation in tumors. J Exp Med 1977;146:1511–20.

17. Ruco LP, Meltzer MS. Macrophage activation for tumor cytotoxicity: increased lymphokine responsiveness of peritoneal macrophages during acute inflammation. J Immunol 1978;120:1054–62.

18. Lee K-C, Wong M, McIntyre D. Characterization of macrophage subpopulations responsive to activation by endotoxin and lymphokines. J Immunol 1981;126:2474–9.

19. MacKay RJ, Russell SW. Protein changes associated with stages of activation of mouse macrophages for tumor cell killing. J Immunol 1986;137:1392–8.

20. Pace JL, Russell SW, LeBlanc PA, Murasko DM. Comparative effects of various classes of mouse interferons on macrophage activation for tumor cell killing. J Immunol 1985;134:977–81.

21. Schultz RM, Chirigos MA. Selective neutralization by antiinterferon globulin of macrophage activation by L-cell interferon, *Brucella abortus* ether extract, *Salmonella typhimurium* lipopolysaccharide, and polyanions. Cell Immunol 1979;48:52–8.

22. Schultz RM, Chirigos MA. Similarities among factors that render macrophages tumoricidal in lymphokine and interferon preparations. Cancer Res 1978;38:1003–7.

23. Kelso A, Glasebrook AL, Kanagawa O, Brunner KT. Production of macrophage-activating factor by T lymphocyte clones and correlation with other lymphokine activities. J Immunol 1982;129:550–6.

24. Kleinschmidt WJ, Schultz RM. Similarities of murine gamma interferon and the lymphokine that renders macrophages cytotoxic. J Interferon Res 1982;2:291-9.
25. Roberts WK, Vasil A. Evidence for the identity of murine gamma interferon and macrophage activating factor. J Interferon Res 1982;2:519-32.
26. Le J, Prensky W, Yip YK, et al. Activation of human monocyte cytotoxicity by natural and recombinant immune interferon. J Immunol 1982;131:2821-6.
27. Männel DN, Falk W. Interferon-γ is required in activation of macrophages for tumor cytotoxicity. Cell Immunol 1983;79:396-402.
28. Meltzer MS, Benjamin WR, Farrar JJ. Macrophage activation for tumor cytotoxicity: induction of macrophage tumoricidal activity by lymphokines from EL-4, a continuous T cell line. J Immunol 1982;129:2802-7.
29. Meltzer MS, Gilbreath MJ, Crawford RM, et al. Macrophage activation factor from EL-4, a murine T-cell line: antigenic characterization by hamster monoclonal antibodies to murine interferon-γ. Cell Immunol 1987;107:340-7.
30. Pace JL, Russell SW, Schreiber RD, et al. Macrophage activation: priming activity from a T-cell hybridoma is attributable to interferon-γ. Proc Natl Acad Sci USA 1983;80:3782-6.
31. Schreiber RD, Pace JL, Russell SW, et al. Macrophage-activating factor produced by a T cell hybridoma: physiochemical and biosynthetic resemblance to γ-interferon. J Immunol 1983;131:826-32.
32. Le J, Vilcek J. Lymphokine-mediated activation of human monocytes: neutralization by monoclonal antibody to interferon-γ. Cell Immunol 1984;85:278-83.
33. Spitalny GL, Havel EA. Monoclonal antibody to murine gamma interferon inhibits lymphokine-induced antiviral and macrophage tumoricidal activities. J Exp Med 1984;159:1560-5.
34. Svedersky LP, Benton CV, Berger WH, et al. Biological and antigenic similarities of murine interferon-γ and macrophage-activating factor. J Exp Med 1984;159:812-27.
35. Pace JL, Russell SW, Torres BA, et al. Recombinant mouse γ interferon induces the priming step in macrophage activation for tumor cell killing. J Immunol 1983;130:2011-3.
36. Schultz RM, Kleinschmidt WJ. Functional identity between murine γ interferon and macrophage activating factor. Nature 1983;305:239-40.
37. Varesio L, Blasi E, Thurman GB, et al. Potent activation of mouse macrophages by recombinant interferon-γ. Cancer Res 1984;44:4465-9.
38. Pace JL, Varesio L, Russell SW, Blasi E. The strain of mouse and assay conditions influence whether MuIFN-γ primes or activates macrophages for tumor cell killing. J Leukocyte Biol 1985;37:475-9.
39. Pace JL, MacKay RJ, Hayes MP. Suppressive effect of interferon-β on development of tumoricidal activity in mouse macrophages. J Leukocyte Biol 1987;41:257-63.
40. Pace JL. Synergistic interactions between IFN-γ and IFN-β in priming murine macrophages for tumor cell killing. J Leukocyte Biol 1988;44:514-20.
41. Yoshida R, Murray HW, Nathan CF. Agonist and antagonist effects of interferon α and β on activation of human macrophages. Two classes of interferon γ receptors and blockade of the high-affinity sites by interferon α or β. J Exp Med 1988;167:1171-85.
42. Kniep EM, Domzig W, Lohmann-Matthes M-L, Kickhofen B. Partial purification and chemical characterization of macrophage cytotoxicity factor (MCF, MAF) and its separation from migration inhibitory factor (MIF). J Immunol 1981;127:417-

22.

43. Ratliff TL, Thomasson DL, McCool, RE, Catalona IJ. T-cell hybridoma production of macrophage activation factor (MAF). I. Separation of MAF from interferon gamma. J Reticuloendothel Soc 1982;31:393–7.

44. Wing EJ, Waheed A, Shadduck RK, et al. Effect of colony stimulating factor on murine macrophages. Induction of antitumor activity. J Clin Invest 1982;69:270–6.

45. Kleinerman ES, Zicht R, Sarin PS, et al. Constitutive production and release of a lymphokine with macrophage-activating factor activity distinct from γ-interferon by a human T-cell leukemia virus-positive cell line. Cancer Res 1984;44:4470–5.

46. Nacy CA, Oster CN, James SL, Meltzer MS. Activation of macrophages to kill rickettsiae and *Leishmania*: dissociation of intracellular microbicidal activities and extracellular destruction of neoplastic and helminth targets. Contemp Top Immunobiol 1984;13:147–70.

47. Lee JC, Rebar L, Young P, et al. Identification and characterization of a human T cell line-derived lymphokine with MAF-like activity distinct from interferon-γ. J Immunol 1986;136:1322–8.

48. Ralph P, Nakoinz I. Stimulation of macrophage tumoricidal activity by the growth and differentiation factor CSF-1. Cell Immunol 1987;105:270–9.

49. Crawford RM, Finbloom DS, Ohara J, et al. B cell stimulatory factor-1 (interleukin 4) activates macrophages for increased tumoricidal activity and expression of Ia antigens. J Immunol 1987;139:135–41.

50. Grabstein KH, Urda DL, Tushinski RJ, et al. Induction of macrophage tumoricidal activity by granulocyte-macrophage colony-stimulating factor. Science 1986;232:506–8.

51. Moore RN, Pitruzzello FJ, Robinson RM, Rouse BT. Interferon produced endogenously in response to CSF-1 augments the functional differentiation of progeny macrophages. J Leukocyte Biol 1985;37:659–64.

52. Warren MK, Ralph P. Macrophage growth factor CSF-1 stimulates human monocyte production of interferon, tumor necrosis factor, and colony stimulation activity. J Immunol 1986;137:2281–5.

53. Celada A, Gray PW, Rinderknecht E, Schreiber RD. Evidence for a gamma-interferon receptor that regulates macrophage tumoricidal activity. J Exp Med 1984;160:55–74.

54. Hayes MP, Russell SW, Trotta PP, Basu M. Enrichment and initial characterization of the solubilized receptor for mouse gamma interferon. Biochem Biophys Res Commun 1988;150:1096–105.

55. Basu M, Pace JL, Pinson DM, et al. Purification and partial characterization of a receptor protein for mouse gamma interferon. Proc Natl Acad Sci USA 1988;85:6282–6.

56. Sheehan KCF, Calderon J, Schreiber RD. Generation and characterization of monoclonal antibodies specific for the human interferon gamma receptor. J Immunol 1988;140:4231–7.

57. Calderon J, Sheehan KCF, Chance C, et al. Purification and characterization of the human interferon-γ receptor from placenta. Proc Natl Acad Sci USA 1988;85:4837–41.

58. Aguet M, Merlin G.Purification of human γ interferon receptors by sequential affinity chromatography on immobilized monoclonal antireceptor antibodies and human γ interferon. J Exp Med 1987;165:988–9.

59. Novick D, Orchansky P, Revel M, Rubinstein M. The human interferon-γ receptor. Purification, characterization, and preparation of antibodies. J Biol Chem

1987;262:8483-7.

60. Pestka S, Langer JA. Interferons and their actions. Annu Rev Biochem 1987;56:727-77.

61. Russell SW, Pace JL. The effects of interferons on macrophages and their precursors. Vet Immunol Immunopathol 1987;15:129-65.

62. Raziuddin A, Sarkar FH, Dutkowski R, et al. Receptors for human α and β-interferon but not for γ interferon are specified by human chromosome 21. Proc Natl Acad Sci USA 1984;81:5504-8.

63. Jung V, Rashidbaigi A, Jones C, et al. Human chromosomes 6 and 21 are required for sensitivity to human interferon γ. Proc Natl Acad Sci USA 1987;84:4151-5.

64. Anderson P, Yip YK, Vilcek J. Specific binding of ^{125}I-human interferon-γ to high affinity receptors on human fibroblasts. J Biol Chem 1982;257:11301-4.

65. Hannigan GE, Gewert DR, Williams BRG. Characterization and regulation of α-interferon receptor expression in interferon-sensitive and -resistant human lymphoblastoid cells. J Biol Chem 1984;259:9456-60.

66. Wahl LM, Katona IM, Wilder RL, et al. Isolation of human mononuclear cell subsets by counterflow centrifugal elutriation (CCE). I. Characterization of B-lymphocyte-, T-lymphocyte-, and monocyte-enriched fractions by flow cytometric analysis. Cell Immunol 1984;85:373-83.

67. Thompson MR, Zhang Z, Fournier A, Tan YH. Characterization of human β-interferon-binding sites on human cells. J Biol Chem 1985;260:563-7.

68. Zhang Z, Fournier A, Tan YH. The isolation of human β-interferon receptor by wheat germ lectin affinity and immunosorbent column chromatographies. J Biol Chem 1986;261:8017-21.

69. Kishimoto T, Hirano T. Molecular regulation of B lymphocyte response. Annu Rev Immunol 1988;6:485-512.

70. Aguet M, Blanchard B. High affinity binding of ^{125}I-labeled mouse interferon to a specific cell surface receptor. II. Analysis of binding properties. Virology 1981;115:249-61.

71. Branca AA, Faltynek CR, D'Alessandro SB, Baglioni C. Interaction of interferon with cellular receptors. Internalization and degradation of cell-bound interferon. J Biol Chem 1982;257:13291-6.

72. Zoon KC, Arnheiter H, Zur Nedden D, et al. Human interferon alpha enters cells by receptor-mediated endocytosis. Virology 1983;130:195-203.

73. Sarkar FH, Gupta SL. Interferon receptor interaction. Internalization of interferon α_2 and modulation of its receptor on human cells. Eur J Biochem 1984;140:461-7.

74. Kushnaryov VM, MacDonald HS, Sedmak JJ, Grossberg SE. Murine interferon-β receptor-mediated endocytosis and nuclear membrane binding. Proc Natl Acad Sci USA 1985;82:3281-5.

75. Celada A, Schreiber RD. Internalization and degradation of receptor-bound interferon-γ by murine macrophages. Demonstration of receptor recycling. J Immunol 1987;139:147-53.

76. Fidler IJ, Fogler WE, Kleinerman ES, Saiki I. Abrogation of species specificity for activation of tumoricidal properties in macrophages by recombinant mouse or human interferon-γ encapsulated in liposomes. J Immunol 1985;135:4289-96.

77. Sanceau J, Sondermeyer P, Beranger F, et al. Intracellular human γ-interferon triggers an antiviral state in transformed murine L cells. Proc Natl Acad Sci USA 1987;84:2906-10.

78. Gorecka-Tisera AM, McCulloch MA. Extracellular calcium is not an absolute re-

quirement for tumoricidal activation of RAW-264 macrophage-like cell line. J Leuk Biol 1986;40:203–14.

79. Gorecka-Tisera AM, Snowdowne KW, Borle AB. Implications of a rise in cytosolic free calcium in the activation of RAW-264 macrophages for tumor cell killing. Cell Immunol 1986;100:411–21.

80. Gorecka-Tisera AM, McCulloch MA, Borle AB. The effect of calmodulin antagonists on the activation of RAW-264 macrophage-like cells for tumor cell killing. Immunopharmacology 1986;12:59–67.

81. Hamilton TA, Becton DL, Somers SD, et al. Interferon-γ modulates protein kinase C activity in murine peritoneal macrophages. J Biol Chem 1985;260:1378–81.

82. Johnson HM, Torres BA. Mechanism of calcium ionophore A23187-induced priming of bone marrow-derived macrophages for tumor cell killing: relationship to priming by interferon. Proc Natl Acad Sci USA 1985;82:5959–62.

83. Varesio L. Imbalanced accumulation of ribosomal RNA in macrophages activated in vivo and in vitro to a cytolytic stage. J Immunol 1985;134:1262–7.

84. Radzioch D, Clayton M, Varesio L. Interferon-α, -β, and -γ augment the levels of rRNA precursors in peritoneal macrophages but not in macrophage cell lines and fibroblasts. J Immunol 1987;139:805–12.

85. Celada A, Schreiber RD. Role of protein kinase C and intracellular calcium mobilization in the induction of macrophage tumoricidal activity by interferon-γ. J Immunol. 1986;137:2373–9.

86. Radzioch D, Varesio L. Protein kinase C inhibitors block the activation of macrophages by IFN-β but not by IFN-γ. J Immunol 1988;140:1259–63.

87. Adams DO, Hamilton TA. The cell biology of macrophage activation. Annu Rev Immunol 1984;2:283–318.

88. Weil J, Epstein CJ, Epstein LB, et al. A unique set of polypeptides is induced by γ interferon in addition to those induced in common with α and β interferons. Nature 1983;301:437–9.

89. Grand-Perret T, Petit J-F, Lemaire G. Modifications induced by activation to tumor cytotoxicity in the protein secretory activity of macrophages. J Leukocyte Biol 1986;40:1–19.

90. Largen MT, Tannenbaum CS. LPS regulation of specific protein synthesis in murine peritoneal macrophages. J Immunol 1986;136:988–93.

91. Johnston PA, Jansen MM, Somers SS, et al. Maleyl-BSA and fucoidan induce expression of a set of early proteins in murine mononuclear phagocytes. J Immunol 1987;138:1551–8.

92. Johnston PA, Somers SD, Hamilton TA. Expression of a 120,000 dalton protein during tumoricidal activation in murine peritoneal macrophages. J Immunol 1987;138:2739–44.

93. MacKay RJ, Russell SW. Protein phenotypes of mouse macrophages activated in vivo for tumor cell killing. J Leukocyte Biol 1987;42:213–21.

94. Tannenbaum CS, Nurmi-McKernan L, Largen MT. Differential protein synthesis by murine peritoneal macrophages elicited by various stimuli. J Leukocyte Biol 1987;41:527–38.

95. MacKay RJ, Pace JL, Jarpe MA, Russell SW. Macrophage-associated proteins. Characterization of stimuli and conditions needed for expression of proteins 476, 71/73, and 120. J Immunol 1989;142:1639–45.

96. Piessens WF. Increased binding of tumor cells by macrophages activated in vitro with lymphocyte mediators. Cell Immunol 1978;35:303–17.

97. Marino PA, Adams DO. Interaction of bacillus Calmette Guérin-activated

macrophages and neoplastic cells in vitro. I. Conditions of binding and its selectivity. Cell Immunol 1980;54:11–25.

98. Marino PA, Whisnant CC, Adams DO. Binding of bacillus Calmette-Guérin-activated macrophages to tumor targets. Selective inhibition by membrane preparations from homologous and heterologous neoplastic cells. J Exp Med 1981;154:77–87.

99. Mercurio AM. Disruption of oligosaccharide processing in murine tumor cells inhibits their susceptibility to lysis by activated mouse macrophages. Proc Natl Acad Sci USA 1986;83:2609–13.

100. Bucana C, Hoyer LC, Hobbs B, et al. Morphological evidence for the translocation of lysosomal organelles from cytotoxic macrophages into the cytoplasm of tumor target cells. Cancer Res 1976;36:4444–58.

101. Adams DO, Kao K-J, Farb R, Pizzo SV. Effector mechanisms of cytolytically activated macrophages. II. Secretion of a cytolytic factor by activated macrophages and its relationship to secreted neutral proteases. J Immunol 1980;124:293–300.

102. Ferluga J, Schorlemmer HU, Baptista LC, Allison AC. Production of the complement cleavage product, C3a, by activated macrophages and its tumorolytic effects. Clin Exp Immunol 1978;31:512–7.

103. Currie GA. Activated macrophages kill tumour cells by releasing arginase. Nature 1978;273:758–9.

104. Nathan CF, Brukner LH, Silverstein SC, Cohn ZA. Extracellular cytolysis by activated macrophages and granulocytes. I. Pharmacologic triggering of effector cells and the release of hydrogen peroxide. J Exp Med 1979;149:84–99.

105. Nathan CF, Silverstein SC, Brukner LH, Cohn ZA. Extracellular cytolysis by activated macrophages and granulocytes. II. Hydrogen peroxide as a mediator of cytotoxicity. J Exp Med 1979;149:100–13.

106. Granger DL, Lehninger AL, Hibbs JB Jr. Aberrant oxygen metabolism in neoplastic cells injured by cytotoxic macrophages. Adv Exp Med Biol 1985;184:51–63.

107. Hibbs JB Jr, Vavrin Z, Taintor RR. L-arginine is required for expression of the activated macrophage effector mechanism causing selective metabolic inhibition in target cells. J Immunol 1987;138:550–65.

108. Old LJ. Tumor necrosis factor (TNF). Science 1985;230:630–2.

109. Urban JL, Shepard HM, Rothstein JL, et al. Tumor necrosis factor: a potent effector molecule for tumor cell killing by activated macrophages. Proc Natl Acad Sci USA 1986;83:5233–7.

Successful therapy of melanoma with a regimen of low-dose cyclophosphamide and interleukin 2

Malcolm S. Mitchell, Raymond A. Kempf, William Harel, Hungyi Shau, William D. Boswell, Susan Lind, Grace Dean, Jane Moore, Edward C. Bradley

Departments of Medicine, Microbiology, and Radiology, University of Southern California School of Medicine and Comprehensive Cancer Center, Los Angeles, and the Cetus Corporation, Emeryville, California, USA

Introduction

Malignant melanoma is a tumor whose incidence is increasing steadily, probably because of its association with intense, intermittent sun exposure among individuals with indoor occupations. Nearly 27 000 new cases will occur in 1988 in the USA (1). Melanoma is therefore not a rare tumor and, with better awareness of its early signs, the primary lesion is becoming more commonly recognized by internists, dentists, and ophthalmologists, as well as by the patients themselves. While surgery of primary melanoma can be curative in early stages, the treatment of advanced disease is extremely disappointing. Neither chemotherapy nor radiation therapy is particularly helpful, although there have been intermittent reports of successful intensive chemotherapy regimens.

The report by Rosenberg and colleagues in 1985 (2) of the usefulness of adoptive immunotherapy with lymphokine-activated killer (LAK) cells given together with interleukin 2 (IL-2) in the treatment of melanoma was met with appropriate enthusiasm. IL-2 was reported by Rosenberg and colleagues to elicit LAK cells from the leukocytes of patients with melanoma when the 2 were incubated for 4 days in vitro. These LAK cells upon reinfusion into the patient, together with varying doses of additional iv IL-2, were effective in causing 5 of 10 patients with melanoma to have significant regressions of their disease (2). The strategy of ex vivo activation was necessitated by that group's findings that IL-2 given by itself was incapable of activating LAK cells sufficiently to cause clinical responses (3). Most recently, however, the same group has reported preliminary success with high doses of IL-2 alone in vivo (4,5), although with a response rate of only 13% versus the 22% noted with LAK cell reinfusion.

While the regression of a highly resistant tumor such as melanoma was highly gratifying, the toxicity of the regimens that have been described has been substantial, even with modifications (6). In particular, elderly patients have been at a

61

significant risk of developing interstitial edema in the lungs, as part of a diffuse capillary leak syndrome, and 4 deaths have been attributable to the regimen (5). The cost and complexity of ex vivo activation of LAK cells are considerable, which militates against broad adoption of the technique, even in modern general hospitals. Finally, in vitro incubation of leukocytes with IL-2 for several days requires extensive tissue culture facilities, and carries a risk of hepatitis.

We have investigated whether IL-2 given directly to patients with melanoma could affect the disease. Because IL-2 is known to stimulate all subsets of T cells rather than simply the T helper and T cytolytic cells that one might want to activate preferentially, we designed a strategy that might decrease T suppressor cells before IL-2 was administered. This might permit the proliferation and maturation of the other subclasses unimpeded by suppressor influences. A dose of 350 mg/m^2 of cyclophosphamide was chosen for this purpose because of the work of others (7,8) as well as our own pilot investigations (9), which showed that this drug at doses of 300–500 mg/m^2 selectively depleted suppressor T cells in man. We further designed a schedule of administration of IL-2 that might be given to outpatients in a day-hospital setting that permitted close observation for 8 h or more, and which incorporated a week's respite from therapy after each of 3 2-week cycles of treatment.

Patients

Thirty-eight patients with disseminated malignant melanoma have been studied, unselected except by preestablished entry criteria. These included the presence of measurable lesions on physical examination or on X-rays or CT scans of the chest or abdomen, the absence of central nervous system involvement, a Karnofsky performance status of at least 70%, and either resistance to "standard" chemotherapy or a refusal of the patient to undergo such chemotherapy after a discussion with the referring physician. The ages of the patients ranged from 25 to 75, with 8 over the age of 50. No one was excluded because of age, except for those under 18 years old. Pregnancy and lactation were also criteria for ineligibility, as were psychological or social impediments to compliance. The diagnosis was always confirmed by our pathologists after review of the original slides. A written consent form was signed by each patient, after a full explanation of the study was given by the physician. All patients to be reported here were treated with at least 1 full cycle of cyclophosphamide plus IL-2, although the critical evaluation of a response to the treatment was performed after 3 complete cycles (1 full course).

Twenty-four patients were male and 14 were female. Sites of disease included subcutaneous and intradermal skin nodules (21 patients), pulmonary metastases (16 patients), lymph nodes (14 patients), liver metastases (10 patients), bone lesions (6 patients), pelvic mass (4 patients), adrenal metastases (4 patients), chest wall mass (1 patient), splenic metastasis (1 patient), and a renal metastasis (1 patient). The majority (26 patients) had not been treated with any chemotherapy. Twenty-two of the 38 had received some form of immunotherapy, including 15 who were treated with a lysate of melanoma cells and the immunological adjuvant DETOX (detoxified endotoxin and mycobacterial cell wall skeletons) (10) in a study to be reported separately (11). Four of the patients had no therapy other than surgery. No therapy of any kind was permitted within the 3 weeks prior to the start of the cyclophosphamide plus IL-2 regimen, during which time the patient had recovered from any side effects of previous treatment, and the disease was either stable or progressing.

Regimen

All treatment was administered in a day-hospital outpatient setting, where prolonged observation was possible without admitting the patient to a ward. Cyclophosphamide was given as an intravenous bolus of 350 mg/m^2 3 days before the start of the IL-2 treatment, on a Friday morning. Beginning 3 days later, on a Monday morning, IL-2 was given as a 15-min iv infusion. IL-2 was then repeated at the same level on the 2nd through 5th, and 8th through 12th days, with doses omitted on Saturday and Sunday. The dose of IL-2 during the 1st 2-week "cycle" was 3.6×10^6 U/m^2 per day. Each patient was observed for 8 h on the 1st day. By the 5th day, the patient was permitted to go home within 1–2 h if he or she had no serious toxicity, such as hypotension or uncontrollable fever. We found that pretreatment with paracetamol 650 mg, repeated every 4 h as needed, with indomethacin 25 mg if needed, was helpful in limiting the severity of the fever, although it did not entirely prevent it. Pethidine 25–50 mg iv given once or twice as required was helpful in controlling the shaking chills that preceded the fever. Indomethacin 25 mg was also given every 4 h if needed for severe arthritis or fever, unless gastrointestinal toxicity became intolerable. Medicines specifically excluded were corticosteroids and type 2 antihistamines.

The 2-week cycle of cyclophosphamide plus IL-2 was repeated at least twice more to complete a 3-cycle course of therapy. The dose most often used through all 3 cycles was 3.6×10^6 U/m^2. The attending physician could, at his discretion, increase the dose to 5.4×10^6 U/m for the 2nd and 7.2×10^6 U/m^2 for the 3rd, if the patient had tolerated earlier treatments without severe toxicity as explicitly defined by World Health Organization criteria, modified by Cetus. However, after the first 20 patients, we rarely increased the dose above the starting level. If patients had at least a minor response (see definitions of response in next section) after 3 2-week cycles, they were eligible for continuation of the treatment. Stable disease or progression after a full course of 3 cycles mandated a discontinuation of therapy. After a complete remission, 2 or 3 more cycles of treatment were given, after which treatment was stopped and the unmaintained response was followed. If patients had sustained a partial remission after 3 cycles, they were treated with at least 3 more cycles or until either a complete remission or progression occurred. Maintenance therapy, of 1 cycle of treatment every 6 weeks, was given to those who had a stable partial remission after more intensive treatment. In one instance, a patient with a partial response of lymph nodes, but a minor response of subcutaneous lesions, was kept on this maintenance regimen, and in fact has continued on maintenance beyond 18 months.

Except for the earliest patients, most were given at least a 2-week interval after the first 3 cycles, to provide a respite from the stresses of continual treatment. The oldest patients in the study and those treated for many months were often permitted a 4-week interval after each full course of 3 cycles.

Criteria of response

Standard criteria were used to judge the response to treatment. Thus, a complete remission was defined as the complete disappearance of all measured lesions for at least 4 weeks, and the failure of new lesions to appear during that time. A partial remission was defined as a 50% decrease in the sum of products of the greatest perpendicular dimensions of all measured lesions, lasting for at least 4 weeks, and without the appearance of new lesions. A minor response was at least a 25% but less than a 50% diminution in the sum of the products of the perpendicular diameters of all measured lesions, or a 50% decrease in that sum that lasted less than 4 weeks. A mixed response was greater than 50% shrinkage at one or more sites, eg, the skin or lymph nodes, but with no change or progression at another, eg, pelvic mass. Stable disease was no change, or a diminution of less than 25%, in the sum of the products of diameters of measured lesions. Progression was greater than 25% increase in the sum of the products of diameters of all measured lesions. "No response" to therapy, as used here, comprised both stable and progressive disease.

Immunologic studies

We monitored the immunologic effects of our regimen in several different ways. Natural killer (NK) cells and LAK cells were measured twice before, and on the last day of each 2-week cycle. Off-study immunologic measurements were also made 72 h after completion of the final 2-week cycle. Standard assays for these cells were used (12–14), except that the cells we have termed LAK cells were tested against *cultured* melanoma cells resistant to NK cells, rather than against *fresh* tumor cells, as described in the original paper by Grimm et al (12). With this proviso, we will refer to the cells as LAK cells. Besides melanoma, other NK-resistant tumor cells, such as Raji and Daudi B cell lymphomas and Bachle squamous lung carcinoma cells, as well as allogeneic lymphoblasts, were also tested in randomly chosen patients. The tumor cells, but not the lymphoblasts, were found to be lysed by the cytolytic mononuclear cells, supporting their close similarity, if not identity, with bona fide LAK cells. Various ratios of effector to target cell were tested, ranging from 200:1 to 25:1 for LAK cell assays and from 40:1 to 2.5:1 for NK assays. We calculated the number of "lytic units" of each type of killer cell by best-fit regression analysis, comparing linear, logarithmic, exponential, and power curves, with a computer program ("Curvefit") created by Mr Jeffrey S. Mitchell (Epstein, Mitchell, and Blackford, Computer Consultants, New Haven, Connecticut). The logarithmic and power curves proved most useful in this regard. The results were expressed in "lytic units" per 10 million effector cells, where 1 lytic unit is the number of cells that can kill 30% of the target cells in 4 h. Fisher's 2-tailed exact test was used to evaluate the statistical significance of differences between groups.

Serial measurements of concanavalin A-inducible suppressor T cells were made in 17 patients (15) immediately before cyclophosphamide and then 3 and 6 day later (ie, 3 days before IL-2 and then before the 1st and 4th doses).

Results

Therapeutic efficacy

Nine of the 38 patients (23.7%) sustained a partial or complete remission, and 1 (2.6%) has had a long-term, maintained minor remission that has lasted more than 18 months (Table 1). There were 2 complete remissions, 1 in a patient with extensive subcutaneous metastases, and 1 in a patient with 3 lung nodules and an enlarged hilar lymph node. There were also 7 partial remissions. One of the latter included disappearance of all lesions in the liver and skin, and of 2 of 3 lung nodules, with only a residual 1-cm pulmonary nodule. A 10th patient, a 50-year-old man, had a 50% decrease in size of a large inguinal lymph node, with a lesser degree of decrease of a large number of intradermal and subcutaneous nodules. His disease, which had been inexorably progressive despite several previous types of treatment, has been entirely stable for more than 18 months on maintenance cyclophosphamide plus IL-2 treatment. This long-term response has been highly significant clinically, even though technically a "minor response."

Minor responses were found in a total of 5 patients (13.1%), including this patient, and mixed responses were noted in another 4 patients (10.5%).

In general, softening or flattening of skin nodules was frequently discernible after the first 2-week cycle, but optimal responses usually required 6 cycles or more.

Table 2 shows the results of treatment by sites of disease. Of most interest to us

Table 1 Results of treatment (n = 38).

Response	n (%)		
Complete remission	2 (5.3)	} 23.7%	} 26.3%
Partial remission	7 (18.4)		
Long-term minor response	1 (2.6)		
Minor response	4 (10.5)		
Mixed response	4 (10.5)		
Progression	20 (52.6)		
Total	38 (100)		

Table 2 Results of treatment by site (n = 38).

Site of disease	No. of patients	Complete remission	Partial remission	Duration (mo)
Liver	10	2	2	CR: 20;7+ PR: 13;10
Lung	16	1	3	CR: 8 PR: 20;3;2
Subcutaneous	21	2	6	CR: 20;1.5 PR: 16;3;2;2; 1;1
Lymph node	14	1	3	CR: 8 PR: 15;18+;2
Bone	6	0	0	
Pelvic, renal	5	0	0	
Adrenal	4	0	0	

CR, complete remission; PR, partial remission. Durations of response are given from the date a CR was achieved, or the date therapy was begun for a PR, as per convention.

were the responses of the 4 of 10 patients with metastases to the liver, a site which, in melanoma, is rarely responsive to systemic treatment. There was a complete remission of 8 large liver metastases in a 42-year-old woman and in approximately 12 liver metastases, including 1 of 5 × 4 cm in a 45-year-old man. Both of those patients also showed disappearance of all of their 3–5 small skin nodules. The man had new disease in his bones, which led to discontinuation of his treatment, but has not had reappearance of liver lesions in over 9 months. The woman also had 2 of 3 lung nodules disappear. Although overall she had only a partial remission by strict criteria, with a residual 1-cm lung nodule, we elected to discontinue her treatment after 1 year (15 cycles). She remained in unmaintained remission for 8 months, relapsing with brain metastases. There was no recurrence in previously responsive sites outside the central nervous system. Her total dose of IL-2 was 540 × 10^6 U/m^2, the highest cumulative amount administered in our study. Two other patients had more than 50% shrinkage of liver lesions, which persisted for at least 6 months. Their responses lasted nearly a year, before they too died of brain metastases.

Seven of 21 patients with subcutaneous nodules responded, with 2 complete and 5 partial remissions. Two responders had long-term remissions lasting more than 18 months, on continual maintenance in one instance, and even upon discontinuation of treatment in another. A 3rd patient was nearing a complete remission but had pernicious anorexia and depression, which forced his removal from the study despite his continuing response. There were also minor responses in 6 patients.

Metastases to the lung were also responsive in 4 of 16 patients, 1 of whom had a complete remission in that site. He received 2 further cycles of treatment, and then was observed without treatment, as per protocol. He relapsed with brain metastases after 8 months and died shortly thereafter, but his lung nodules never returned. Among the partial responders was the oldest patient on study, a 75-year-old man, who tolerated 6 cycles of treatment.

Lymph node metastases responded in 4 of 14 instances, with 1 complete and 3 partial responses, and 4 other minor responses. The complete regression was that of a large hilar node in the patient noted above who had a complete remission of lung metastases. Three of the 4 responses persisted for 8 to more than 18 months, and the 4th response was limited by relapse in the brain, which forced temporary discontinuation of treatment.

Unresponsive sites comprised bone, adrenal, renal, and pelvic metastases, where none of 13 patients had a response. In fact, 3 patients developed or had exacerbations of bone pain that forced discontinuation of therapy that had beneficially affected other sites.

The median duration of complete or partial remissions is 9 months, with a mean of > 10.1 months. Four patients have had more than 12 months of remission on continued treatment.

Toxicity

The regimen we have described was generally well tolerated, although it was accompanied by moderate degrees of toxicity (Table 3). Severe side effects were

Table 3   Toxicity.

Toxic effect	No. of patients experiencing effect	No. with grade III toxicity (% of entire group)
Fatigue	40	6 (15)
Fever	39	4 (10)
Nausea, vomiting	38	5 (12)
Chills, rigors	34	3 (7)
Hypotension	28	4 (10)
Diarrhea	27	2 (5)
Allergies, rash	26	1 (2)
Fluid retention	25	2 (5)
Dry cough, dyspnea	25	1 (2)
Arthralgias, arthritis	24	2 (5)
Myalgia	23	2 (5)
Catarrhal symptoms	15	0 (0)
Anemia	12	1 (2)

Data shown on 41 patients entered into the study, including 3 not evaluable for a clinical response. WHO criteria used except for hypotension, which was modified as described in the text, and fluid retention (weight gain), which was a category specifically added for IL-2 protocols by Cetus.

found in 10–15% of 4 categories: fatigue, fever, nausea/vomiting, and chills/rigors, and in 0–9% in the remaining 9 categories. Only 2 patients required admission to hospital as a result of the toxicity; both were overnight stays either for repletion of fluids or for fatigue. Hypotension to some degree was found in two-thirds of the patients, but was usually mild to moderate. Severe hypotension (grade III) was found in only 4 patients (10% of the entire group). Episodes of severe hypotension occurred on 1 occasion during the treatments of 3 patients, all of whom then continued on study at reduced levels of IL-2. An episode of hypotension also occurred early in the treatment of patient #1, who subsequently tolerated a total of 15 cycles, all at $3.6 \times 10^6 \, U/m^2$. The elderly patients had the most difficulty with the regimen, requiring more encouragement to continue than did the others. Only 1 patient left the study because of a lack of tolerance, but diminution of dose and an increase in the interval between courses of 3 cycles were necessary for 2 of the oldest patients.

Shaking chills, fever to a maximum of 103°F (39.4°C), nausea and/or vomiting, and fatigue were nearly universally experienced. Fluid retention, arthralgia/arthritis, myalgia, diarrhea, dry hacking cough, and rash were also common. Diuresis often ensued spontaneously over the weekend following 5 days of treatment and, in any event, the fluid retention was always responsive to furosemide. The joint symptoms were severe in only 1 patient, and abated within a few days of cessation of a cycle of treatment. Indomethacin or ibuprofen was helpful in mitigating this symptom, but did not entirely counteract it. One patient with a previous history of rheumatoid arthritis developed an erythematous rash and a true arthritis with her 1st course of treatment, but on subsequent treatments only arthralgia without overt swelling or rash was noted. A dry hacking cough, responding to cough suppressants, and respiratory symptoms were also found in two-thirds of the group, which suggested an IL-2-induced bronchitis. Eosinophilia (>10% of total leukocytes) was noted in 20 patients, and 23 patients complained of myalgia. Many of these symptoms were those that might have been expected from a lymphokine active in inflammatory processes.

A mild to moderate decrease in hemoglobin was also found in 12 patients, but no significant changes in leukocytes or platelets were noted. The cyclophosphamide caused minor to moderate nausea lasting 1–3 days, in one-half of the patients, and frequently caused a flare-up in arthralgia. No toxic effects on hair, bone marrow, or bladder were found.

Immunologic studies

An increase in LAK cell activity was significantly correlated with a clinical response (p = 0.014) (Table 4A). All 9 patients with a partial or complete remission had a LAK activity that was increased to a level of 10 lytic units per 10^7 cells or higher. Conversely, none of the 14 patients who failed to develop an increase in LAK activity had a clinical remission. LAK activity was also increased in 15 nonresponding patients, indicating that the induction of LAK cells was necessary but not sufficient for remission. However, a failure to show an increase in LAK cells portended a failure to respond clinically.

Table 4 Immunologic correlates of clinical response.

A. Induction of LAK cell activity versus response

	Response*	No response	Total
LAK increased[†]	9	15	24
LAK not increased	0	14	14

B. Induction of NK cell activity versus response

NK increased >1000[‡]	7	18	25
NK increased <1000[‡]	2	11	13

*Comprises complete and partial remissions.
[†]>10 lytic units maximal increase during treatment.
[‡]Maximal increase in lytic units during treatment.
A, p=0.014; B, p=0.46 (Fisher's exact test).

In contrast, as indicated in Table 4B, NK cell activity was consistently stimulated in all patients and showed no significant correlation with clinical response (p = 0.46). An increase in NK activity to some degree above baseline occurred not only in the 9 responders, but also in all 29 nonresponders. Even considering those patients who had a large increase of more than 1000 lytic units per 10^7 cells, there was no significant correlation. Thus, although 7 of 9 responders had an increase of more than 1000 lytic units per 10^7 cells, 18 of the 29 nonresponders also showed such an increase.

There were no significant preexisting levels of LAK cells measurable in the circulation. After cyclophosphamide and IL-2, those patients who had an increase usually had an incremental increase in the levels of LAK cells with successive cycles, but there was a rapid fall-off within 3 days after the end of a 2-week cycle. This characteristic requirement for the continued presence of IL-2 lent further credence to their being LAK cells rather than another type of cytolytic lymphocyte, such as a cytotoxic T cell. However, 2 patients have been shown to have an elevation of cytotoxic T cells too. One was the woman who sustained a complete remission of her liver metastases and the other was the man with a long-term minor response. The former had a level of LAK cells at the highest level in the study, nearly 5000 lytic units, after her 15th and final cycle of treatment. Cold target competition assays performed during the last cycle of her treatment, and after the 17th month of treatment of the male patient, revealed the presence of cytolytic lymphocytes that were specifically inhibitable by melanoma cells. These cells, which are CD3 positive and can be blocked by antibodies to CD3, coexisted with LAK cells with a much broader reactivity against tumor cells.

Concanavalin A-inducible suppressor T cells were not consistently reduced by cyclophosphamide in the 17 patients studied. In 8 of the patients, there was a reduction of suppressor T cells 3 days after the cyclophosphamide, but on day 6,

3 days after IL-2 was begun, the suppressor cell activity had returned to its pretreatment level. These results contrasted with previous findings in patients who were given cyclophosphamide alone, where the decrease persisted at least until day 6 after cyclophosphamide (9), and usually until day 28 (10). Unfortunately, we did not have the opportunity to study patients given IL-2 alone, to determine what levels of suppressor activity would have been elicited by IL-2 had cyclophosphamide not been given.

Lack of influence of indomethacin or fever on clinical response

As shown in Table 5, there was no apparent influence either of high fever (temperature elevation to $> 101\,°F$) or the administration of the prostaglandin antagonist indomethacin on the clinical response to the regimen. It was conceivable that each of those influences might have acted independently to mediate the effects of the regimen. In particular, antagonism of prostaglandin synthetase might have affected suppressor macrophage function and thus augmented the immunologic stimulatory effects of IL-2. However, we could not find statistical evidence here that those patients who received indomethacin for high fevers or arthralgias fared differently from those who did not.

Discussion

This investigation has shown that a regimen of low-dose cyclophosphamide and low-dose IL-2 was effective in the treatment of advanced melanoma, including not only subcutaneous and lymph node metastases but also more ominous sites of involvement, such as the liver and the lung. The treatment was given in an outpatient setting and was generally tolerable, even by elderly patients, although there were undeniably significant side effects and toxicity, particularly cumulative fatigue and arthralgias. However, most patients were able to go home within 1 h after the IL-2 infusion was given. LAK cells were elicited in the circulation of these patients by the in vivo therapy.

The response of melanoma to chemotherapy is at most 20% in large series, and

Table 5 Indomethacin or fever $> 101°F$ vs response.

Response	Indomethacin	Fever
CR	2/2	2/2
PR	5/6	6/6
Minor	4/5	5/5
None	11/17	15/17

Indomethacin: CR + PR vs minor + none; $p=0.28$, Fisher's exact test; $p=0.28$, trend analysis. Fever: CR + PR vs minor + none; $p>0.20$, Fisher's exact test.

Table 6   Final results for all patients studied, including those of 1 additional patient, as described in Addendum.

Response	n (%)
Complete remission	2 (5.1)
Partial remission	8 (20.5)
Long-term "minor" response	1 (2.6)
Minor response	4 (10.3)
Mixed response	4 (10.3)
No response	20 (51.2)
Total	39 (100)

there is no discernible increase in the patients' survival. The regimen we have reported of low-dose cyclophosphamide and low-dose IL-2 appears to have a response rate of approximately 25%, which is at least equivalent to that found in the expanded trials of IL-2 and LAK cells at the NCI (5) and at university centers (19%) (D. Parkinson, personal communication). Our rate of remission in melanoma exceeds published rates with high-dose IL-2 given without LAK cells (13%) (4). The duration of response to cyclophosphamide plus IL-2 was also encouraging, with a median of 9 months. In particular, the long-term responses of 5 patients, 4 of them treated for at least a year, are particularly gratifying. It is worth emphasizing that patients could be treated repeatedly with cyclophosphamide plus IL-2, to attempt to improve the degree of response or to maintain stability of the disease at less than 50% of its original volume.

Various sites of disease appear to be differentially sensitive to the effects of IL-2, with subcutaneous, lymph node, and pulmonary metastases most responsive in several series (2,6). The striking response of large liver lesions in 4 patients was unique in our experience with systemically administered therapy. Two patients with liver involvement responded with complete resolution of substantial-sized lesions, while durable partial remissions were achieved in 2 others. In contrast, bone disease and adrenal lesions may prove to be most resistant to this form of treatment, judging not only from the lack of responses in these sites, but also from 3 patients in whom persistent bone pain caused us to stop treatment that had caused regression of disease at other sites, in order to administer pain-reducing radiation therapy. Even within the same patient, we have found 1 site to be resistant to treatment while another was responding. In fact, our 1st patient on study had 1 lung nodule persisting relatively unchanged months after 2 other lung nodules, skin, and liver lesions had all disappeared. It was also not uncommon to find several subcutaneous lesions regressing while others were unchanged. The reasons for this sort of divergent response are not at all obvious, but the phenomenon has also been observed by others with IL-2-containing regimens (6).

The major cause of death in our most successfully treated patients—those who had a complete or partial remission for more than 6 months—was progression in the brain or spinal cord, with a large single metastatic lesion in the brain being the most common presentation. Regardless of its systemic effectiveness, cyclophosphamide plus IL-2 cannot prevent or effectively treat lesions of the central nervous system. We are now attempting to devise a means of prophylaxis for the central nervous system in patients with a complete or stable partial remission, but the problem is not easily solved. High-dose chemotherapy, with autologous bone marrow replacement, is a measure with potential efficacy, but has not yet been tested prophylactically in melanoma.

An improvement in survival cannot be claimed for the entire group, but it is clear that the survival of all but 2 of the patients with a complete or partial remission was prolonged. In addition, the patient with a long-term, maintained minor response has certainly exceeded expectations for his survival. It was possible to treat 1 patient intensively for a year, and to maintain responses with 1 2-week cycle every 6 weeks for 10–18+ months in 4 other patients.

Among our 10 significant responders were 4 who had received our regimen of active specific immunotherapy (11) previously, but the other 6 had never received that therapy. Nevertheless, it will be interesting to combine these 2 potentially complementary types of treatment, particularly since cytolytic T cells are generated by active immunotherapy, and are amplified by IL-2, as we demonstrated in 2 of our patients.

Since LAK cells were elicited solely by in vivo administration of cyclophosphamide and IL-2, there seems little need, at least in melanoma, for ex vivo incubation of peripheral blood leukocytes with IL-2. Whether this will be true for other diseases, such as renal cell carcinoma and breast cancer, which appear to be sensitive to IL-2 and LAK cells, remains to be determined. In any event, a relatively low dose of IL-2 has allowed us to treat even elderly patients without medical difficulties of significant proportions. However, we should emphasize the necessity for strong psychological supportive care from nurses, physicians, and relatives to encourage all patients to complete the prescribed courses of treatment.

It remains to be proved that cyclophosphamide as we have administered it, in single low doses 3 days before each 2-week cycle, accounted for our therapeutic success with intravenously administered IL-2 in the absence of adoptive immunotherapy. Whether our hypothesis for the mechanism by which cyclophosphamide exerted its influence, via the inhibition of suppressor T cells, is correct also requires further study. Our assay for (concanavalin A-induced) suppressor T cells showed no significant change in their activity at 3 and 6 days after cyclophosphamide. Whether IL-2 alone would have stimulated even higher levels of suppressor cell activity in the absence of cyclophosphamide is uncertain.

LAK cells are easily measured, and may serve as convenient criteria for an immunologic effect of IL-2, but one should not ascribe the in vivo rejection of human tumors uniquely to their activity. Cytolytic and helper T cells, macrophages, and perhaps B lymphocytes may all play important roles. IL-2, which can directly or indirectly influence all of those cells, may cause beneficial responses through effects on several types of cell at once. Nevertheless, LAK cell activation correlated well with a clinical response to therapy, and appeared to be the most important parameter to monitor as a prognostic indicator. Nearly 38% (9/24) of the patients who had a rise in LAK cell activity of at least 10 lytic units per 10^7 mononuclear cells had a remission. More importantly for prognosis, none of the 14 patients who failed to have a rise in LAK cells in response to IL-2 achieved a useful clinical remission.

Ultimately, IL-2 will undoubtedly be used as an important part of a combination regimen involving not only other cytokines, but other types of biomodulators and probably chemotherapy as well. There is little doubt that several regimens involving IL-2, including the one we have described, are very useful now in the treatment of melanoma, heretofore a highly resistant form of cancer.

Addendum

Just after this manuscript was completed, final data became available on the last patient in the study. That patient, a 57-year-old woman who had received no systemic therapy previously, had a 60% regression of disease in her right adrenal gland, the 1st patient to respond at that site. In addition, there was a 70% shrinkage of a pulmonary nodule and complete disappearance of breast and ear lobe masses, with only a presternal nodule remaining at 24% of its previous size, all as measured by the products of perpendicular diameters. Unfortunately, the patient had transient amaurosis nearly from the outset, and despite receiving 1.8 $\times 10^6$ U/m^2 of IL-2 during cycles 2 and 3, she had worsening of the attacks. The toxicity forced us to abandon therapy after only 2 months. Repeat measurements at all sites performed 4 weeks after completion of treatment confirmed that a partial remission had in fact occurred.

Thus, the final figures in our study are as shown in Table 6.

Acknowledgments

This study was supported by a contract from the Cetus Corporation, USPHS grant R01 CA-36233, a grant from the Concern Foundation, and gifts from the Morey and Claudia Mirkin Foundation, Mr Alan Gleitsman, and the Lenihan Trust.

References

1. Silverberg E, Lubera J. Cancer statistics, 1988. CA 1988;38:5–22.
2. Rosenberg SA, Lotze MT, Muul LM, et al. Observations on the systemic administration of autologous lymphokine-activated killer cells and recombinant interleukin-2 to patients with metastatic cancer. N Engl J Med 1985;313:1485–92.
3. Lotze MT, Matory YL, Ettinghausen SE, et al. In vivo administration of purified human interleukin 2: II. Half life, immunological effects, and expansion of

peripheral lymphoid cells in vivo with recombinant interleukin 2. J Immunol 1985;135:1865–75.

4. Lotze MT, Chang AE, Seipp CA, et al. High-dose recombinant interleukin 2 in the treatment of patients with disseminated cancer. JAMA 1986;256:3117–24.

5. Rosenberg SA, Lotze MT, Muul LM, et al. A progress report on the treatment of 157 patients with advanced cancer using lymphokine-activated killer cells and interleukin-2 or high-dose interleukin-2 alone. N Engl J Med 1987;316:889–97.

6. West WH, Tauer KW, Yannelli JR, et al. Constant-infusion recombinant interleukin-2 in adoptive immunotherapy of advanced cancer. N Engl J Med 1987;316:898–905.

7. Berd D, Maguire HC Jr, Mastrangelo MJ. Impairment of concanavalin A-inducible suppressor activity following administration of cyclophosphamide to patients with advanced cancer. Cancer Res 1984;44:1275–80.

8. Berd D, Maguire HC Jr, Mastrangelo MJ. Potentiation of human cell-mediated and humoral immunity by low-dose cyclophosphamide. Cancer Res 1984;44:5430–43.

9. Hengst JCD, Mitchell MS. Unpublished.

10. Ribi E, Cantrell JL, Takayama K, et al. Lipid A and immunotherapy. Rev Infect Dis 1984;6:567–72.

11. Mitchell MS, Kan-Mitchell J, Kempf RA, et al. Active specific immunotherapy for melanoma: Phase I trial of allogeneic lysates and a novel adjuvant. Cancer Res 1988;48: 5883–93.

12. Grimm E, Mazumder A, Zhang HZ, et al. Lymphokine-activated killer cell phenomenon. Lysis of natural killer-resistant fresh solid tumor cells by interleukin 2-activated autologous human peripheral blood lymphocytes. J Exp Med 1982; 155:1823–41.

13. Timonen T, Reynolds CW, Ortaldo J, Herberman RB. Isolation of human and rat natural killer cells. J Immunol Methods 1982;51:269–77.

14. Pross HF, Baines MG, Rubin P, et al. Spontaneous human lymphocyte-mediated cytotoxicity against tumor target cells. IX. The quantitation of natural killer cell activity. J Clin Immunol 1981;1:51–63.

15. Shou L, Schwartz SA, Good RA. Suppressor cell activity after concanavalin A treatment of lymphocytes from normal donors. J Exp Med 1976;143:1100–10.

Immunomodulation by tumor necrosis factor

K. Hori,* M.J. Ehrke, E. Mihich

Grace Cancer Drug Center, Roswell Park Memorial Institute, New York State Department of Health, Buffalo, New York, USA

Introduction

Tumor necrosis factor (TNF) was initially discovered in the serum of BCG-primed, endotoxin-treated mice, as a protein which induced hemorrhagic necrosis of subcutaneously transplanted tumors (1) and selective cytostatic or cytotoxic effects in tumor cells in culture (2). This protein was shown to be produced mainly by cells of the monocyte-macrophage type and to have a variety of biological effects (3). Molecular studies of TNF from various mammalian sources indicated that the amino acid sequence of this protein is highly conserved (4). Despite the relative species preference detected in some TNF functions (5–7), this is not a general feature for all the biological activities of the molecule. Indeed, there is also immunological cross-reactivity among TNF from different species and recombinant human TNF (rHu-TNF) binds to the same receptor on certain cells as recombinant murine TNF (rMu-TNF). The development of these recombinant TNF molecules has led to the identification of their multiple actions (8). The overall evidence available is consistent with the possibility that TNF has regulatory functions in the response of host defenses to neoplasia, both immunological and phlogistic in nature (9,10). Recently, immunomodulating and regulatory functions of TNF have been identified in this laboratory (8,11–14). The activation of monocyte-macrophages and the modes of macrophage-mediated target cell killing induced by TNF are the main focus of this discussion. The interactions of TNF with T lymphocyte activation and function are also considered.

Activation of macrophages and killer function

The requirement for two signals in the in vitro activation of macrophages has

---

*Present address: Asahi Chemical Industry Co. Ltd., Life Science Laboratory, Fuji, Shizuoka, Japan.

recently been reviewed (15). The role of TNF as an effector for target cell killing has been reported by several investigators (9,16–20). This role was confirmed in our laboratory (11). In addition, by using a TNF-insensitive target cell, like P815 mastocytoma cells, it was shown that this mediator also activates macrophages to kill cells by a cell-dependent mechanism independent of the direct cytotoxic action of TNF (8,11). Thus, an autocrine as well as an effector function for TNF has been put in evidence in connection with the activation and cytotoxic activity of macrophages.

The lipopolysaccharide (LPS)-independent TNF-induced activation of resident peritoneal exudate cells (PECs) to become macrophage killers for P815 cells was found to be dependent on the presence of a concanavalin-A (Con A)-induced lymphokine preparation (LK) or interferon-γ (IFN-γ), with a dose-dependent response for each signal (8,13). There was no species preference in this effect. When, instead of using whole PEC populations, plastic-adherent cells were used, TNF plus IFN-γ was able to promote killer cell induction equal to that obtainable with whole PEC populations, but TNF plus LK (the latter at antiviral titers comparable to those of corresponding concentrations of IFN-γ) had only a minor effect (13). When adherent PECs were exposed to TNF plus LK in the presence of nonadherent PECs, the activation of killer cells was described by a dependence on the number of nonadherent cells added (8). Based on these results it was concluded that a helper factor is provided by whole PEC populations, which has no antiviral activity but can be replaced by IFN-γ, which is required for maximal activation of adherent PECs to become killer macrophages. The killer cells develop within the adherent population but require the participation of helper factor-secreting nonadherent cells for full activation.

Macrophages are also stimulated by TNF to produce interleukin 1 (IL-1) and vice versa (14). As IL-1 plus IFN-γ was able to activate killer macrophages to lyse TNF-insensitive P815 cells, the question was raised whether IL-1 mediated the analogous effect that had been observed with TNF. It was found, however, that monoclonal antibodies specific for IL-1 could inhibit the activation of macrophages induced by IL-1 plus IFN-γ, but not that induced by TNF plus IFN-γ; in contrast, antibody directed against TNF could inhibit activation induced by either combination. It was therefore concluded that IL-1 is not a proximal signal for the activation of killer macrophages but, in fact, acts through the induction of TNF secretion by macrophages triggering the autocrine function of this molecule (14).

As it had been found (8,11) that TNF could provide a signal for the activation of macrophages to kill TNF-insensitive P815 cells, it was necessary to obtain direct evidence for a TNF-independent target cell killing by the activated macrophages. An experiment was carried out to this end. Macrophages were placed in the outer well of a double chamber, separated from an inner well by a millipore filter partition. The macrophages were activated by exposure to TNF (10^4 U/mL) plus IFN-γ (2 U/mL) for 18 h. The ^{51}Cr-labeled target P815 cells were then added into the outer or inner well and cell kill was measured by standard ^{51}Cr-release assay 18 h later. As shown by the results summarized in the Table, only when target cells were added into the outer wells did lysis occur. The

Table Direct cell-cell contact between TNF/IFN-γ-activated macrophages and target cells for tumor cell lysis.

Treatment of Mø in outer wells	Addition of target		% Specific ^{51}Cr release
	^{51}Cr-P815	Cold P815	
None	Outer well	—	0.0 ± 1.5
TNF* alone	Outer well	—	2.2 ± 1.7
IFN-γ† alone	Outer well	—	6.3 ± 1.7
TNF + IFN-γ	Outer well	—	56.2 ± 4.2
TNF + IFN-γ	Inner well	—	3.7 ± 2.6
TNF + IFN-γ	Inner well	Outer well	5.7 ± 1.0
TNF + IFN-γ	Outer well	Inner well	52.0 ± 1.9

*TNF 10^4 U/mL; †IFN-γ 2 U/mL.

possibility that a lytic soluble factor may be released as a result of cell to cell contact was excluded by the fact that the addition of unlabeled P815 cells into the outer well did not lead to lysis of labeled target cells added into the inner well. It was thus confirmed that TNF may cause lysis of target cells through a direct action or through the activation of killer macrophages capable of lysing killer cells by a mechanism independent of TNF or other possible soluble lytic factors.

Interactions with T lymphocyte activation and function

The interactions of TNF with T lymphocyte activation and function are indicated by several consistent pieces of evidence. The in vitro generation of C57Bl/6 allospecific splenic cells cytotoxic for P815 target cells was augmented by the addition of TNF to the primary cultures (21). A bell-shaped curve described the TNF concentration dependence of the effect, with 100 units of rHu-TNF per 2 mL culture being the optimal concentration inducing maximum stimulation.

Experiments in tumor-bearing mice showed that with certain target tumors, such as Meth A sarcoma, TNF is ineffective in nude mice while being fully active in the corresponding normal mice. TNF was also ineffective in normal mice which had received immunosuppressive doses of total body irradiation (400 R) prior to tumor implantation (22). These results are consistent with the idea that in vivo T cells have a role in the antitumor effects of TNF.

Recently a strictly species-specific induction by TNF of thymocyte proliferation in response to phytohemagglutinin (PHA) was observed comparing rMu-TNF with rHu-TNF. In these experiments (12), thymocytes from C3H/HeJ mice could be stimulated to respond to PHA only after exposure to rMu-TNF. It was further shown that this stimulation can be abolished by the addition of anti-TNF antibody but not by anti-IL-1 antibody, thus verifying the independence of the T cell stimulation from the induction of IL-1 production by TNF.

Conclusions

As indicated by a number of studies in different laboratories, TNF has a multitude of effects inclusive of functional modifications of normal cells such as increased secretion of acute phase proteins and decreased drug metabolism in liver or increases in antigens or receptors on the surface of islet pancreatic cells or fibroblasts (4). On tumor cells in vitro it may cause growth stimulation or inhibition, depending on concentration, and can induce differentiation. Among cells of host defense systems, augmentation of functions of T cells, natural killer (NK) cells, lymphokine-activated (LAK) cells, and macrophages have all been observed (4,21). As briefly discussed above, TNF appears to have an autocrine function on macrophages as it induces activation of killer macrophages while also being secreted by activated macrophages and can directly kill certain target tumor cells. The mechanism of macrophage activation by TNF is complex and seems to require interaction with other cytokines providing second signals, which can also be provided by IFN-γ. Interactions of TNF with T cells do occur and may have a significant role in the in vivo antitumor effects of the molecule inasmuch as TNF has no effect against certain sensitive tumors in nude mice or in mice given immunosuppressive doses of X-irradiation. The interactions of TNF with other cytokines such as IFN-γ or IL-1 are of interest not only for their functional role in the regulation of the immune system, but also for their therapeutic potential.

Acknowledgments

The research from this laboratory summarized in this report was carried out with partial support from US Public Health Service Grants CA24538 and CA13038 awarded by the National Cancer Institute, Department of Health and Human Services, and from Asahi Chemical Industry Co. Ltd.

References

1. Carswell EA, Old LJ, Kassel RL, et al. An endotoxin-induced serum factor that causes necrosis of tumors. Proc Natl Acad Sci USA 1975;72:3666–70.
2. Takai Y, Wong GG, Clark SC, et al. B cell stimulatory factor-2 is involved in the differentiation of cytotoxic T lymphocytes. J Immunol 1988;140:508–12.
3. Old LJ. Tumor necrosis factor (TNF). Science 1985;230:630–2.
4. Le J, Vilcek J. Biology of disease. Tumor necrosis factor and interleukin 1: Cytokines with multiple overlapping biological activities. Lab Invest 1987;56:234–8.
5. Fransen L, Ruysschaert MR, Van Der Heyden J, Fiers W. Recombinant tumor necrosis factor: Specificity for a variety of human and murine transformed cell lines. Cell Immunol 1986;100:260–7.
6. Kramer SM, Aggarwal BB, Eessalu TE, et al. Characterization of the in vivo and in vitro species preference of human and murine tumor necrosis factor-α. Cancer Res 1988;48:920–5.
7. Smith RA, Kirstein M, Fiers W, Baglioni C. Species specificity of human and murine

tumor necrosis factor. J Biol Chem 1986;261:14871-4.

8. Hori K, Ehrke M, Mace K, et al. Effect of tumor necrosis factor on the induction of macrophage tumoricidal activity. Cancer Res 1987;47:2793-8.

9. Philip R, Epstein LB. Tumor necrosis factor as immunomodulator and mediator of monocyte cytotoxicity induced by itself, γ-interferon and interleukin-1. Nature 1986;323:86-9.

10. Klebanoff SJ, Vadas MA, Harlan JM, et al. Stimulation of neutrophils by tumor necrosis factor. J Immunol 1986;136:4220-5.

11. Mace K, Ehrke M, Hori K, et al. The role of TNF in macrophage activation and tumoricidal activity. Cancer Res 1988;48:5427-32.

12. Ehrke MJ, Ho RLX, Hori K. Species-specific TNF-induction of thymocyte proliferation. Cancer Immunol Immunother 1988;27:103-8.

13. Hori K, Ehrke MJ, Mace K, Mihich E. Effect of tumor necrosis factor on tumoricidal activation of macrophages: Synergism between tumor necrosis factor and interferon-γ. Cancer Res 1987;47:5868-74.

14. Hori K, Ehrke MJ, Mihich E. Role of tumor necrosis factor and interleukin-1 in interferon-γ promoted activation of tumoricidal macrophages. Cancer Res (in press).

15. Adams DO, Hamilton TA. The cell biology of macrophage activation. Annu Rev Immunol 1984;2:283-318.

16. Austgulen R, Espevik T, Hammerstrom J, Nissen-Meyer J. Role of monocyte cytotoxic factor in cytolysis of actinomycin D-treated WEHI 164 cells mediated by freshly isolated human adherent mononuclear blood cells. Cancer Res 1986; 46:4566-70.

17. Nissen-Meyer J, Austgulen R, Espevik T. Comparison of recombinant tumor necrosis factor and the monocyte-derived cytotoxic factor involved in monocyte-mediated cytotoxicity. Cancer Res 1987;47:2251-8.

18. Urban JL, Shepard HM, Rothstein JL, et al. Tumor necrosis factor: A potent effector molecule for tumor cell killing by activated macrophages. Proc Natl Acad Sci USA 1986;83:5233-7.

19. Ziegler-Heitbrock HWL, Moller A, Linke RP, et al. Tumor necrosis factor as effector molecule in monocyte mediated cytotoxicity. Cancer Res 1986;46:5947-52.

20. Feinman R, Henriksen-DeStefano D, Tsujimoto M, Vilcek J. Tumor necrosis factor is an important mediator of tumor cell killing by human monocytes. J Immunol 1987;138:635-40.

21. Ehrke M, Mace K, Maccubbin D, Mihich E. Regulatory role of human recombinant tumor necrosis factor on murine, control and adriamycin-modified, host defense functions. In: Eckhardt S, ed. Abstracts of lectures, symposia and free communications, XIV International Cancer Congress, Budapest, Hungary, vol. 3, Basel: S. Karger; 1986:916.

22. Otsuka Y, Bernacki R. Unpublished.

Nocardia rubra cell wall skeleton
and its clinical application

Immunologic and biochemical properties of bacterial fractions and related compounds with special reference to BCG cell wall skeleton and *Nocardia rubra* cell wall skeleton

Ichiro Azuma

Institute of Immunological Science, Hokkaido University, Sapporo, Japan

Introduction

A variety of biological response modifiers (BRMs) have been used for host stimulation against cancer, infectious diseases, and other immunologic disorders in both clinical and experimental situations (Table). Among these, bacterial cells and cell fractions, including both living and killed mycobacterial cells, the cells of *Corynebacterium parvum* (*Propionibacterium acnes*), and the lipopolysaccharide of gram-negative bacteria and its active principle, lipid A, are the immunoadjuvants most often used. In particular, the living cells of *Mycobacterium bovis* BCG were used extensively in the immunotherapy of human cancer and in experimental studies during the 1960s and 1970s, when various serious complications associated with treatment with live BCG were reported. Since 1971, we have have reported that the active immunoadjuvant component of bacterial cells such as mycobacteria, *Nocardia*, corynebacteria, propionibacteria, and *Listeria* is the cell wall skeleton (CWS), and we have examined in detail the immunologic properties of these fractions.

In this paper, the immunologic properties of bacterial CWS and synthetic adjuvants such as *N*-acetylmuramyl-L-alanyl-D-isoglutamine (MDP), trehalose dimycolate (TDM), and lipid A will be reviewed with special reference to cancer immunotherapy.

Bacterial fractions

More than 30 years ago, heat-killed mycobacterial cells suspended in mineral oil (Freund's complete adjvant) were recognized to be the most potent immunoadjuvants for the induction of cell-mediated immunity and humoral antibody formation (1). In 1971, we showed that the CWS fraction was the active immunoad-

Table BRMs for nonspecific immunotherapy of cancer and infectious diseases.

Bacterial and fungal cells and fractions	Synthetic compounds	Cytokines and others
A. BCG cells *Corynebacterium parvum* *(P. acnes)* *Streptococcus pyogenes* (OK432) B. BCG-CWS N-CWS Trehalose dimycolate (TDM) Mycobacterial DNA Endotoxin (lipid A) C. Glucans Krestin, lentinan Shyzophyllan	A. MDP derivatives MDP-Lys(L18), L18-MDP MTP-PE Quinonyl-MDP Murabutide FK-565, FK-156 B. TDM analogues C. Lipid A analogues D. Bestatin, forphencinol deoxyspugallin E. Levamisole F. Poly IC G. Maleic anhydride divinyl ester (MVE-II) H. Tuftsin	A. Interferons (α, β, γ) Interleukins (1, 2, etc) Tumor necrosis factors (TNFs) Lymphotoxin Colony-stimulating fac- tors (CSFs) B. Thymic factors C. Lymphokine-activated killer cells (LAK) Tumor infiltrating lymphocytes (TIL)

juvant component of the cells of mycobacteria and related bacteria (2,3). The chemical structure of the CWS of *M. bovis* BCG and its biological activities, especially adjuvant and antitumor activities, were examined in detail (4,5). We have also reported the purification and chemical structures of the CWS fractions of *Nocardia rubra* (6–8), *P. acnes* (9–11), and *Listeria monocytogenes* (12,13), and their relative usefulness as immunoadjuvants.

BCG-CWS

The structure of BCG-CWS is a mycolic acid-arabinogalactan-mucopeptide complex, and the biochemical properties of each component have been extensively investigated (4,5). The adjuvant activity of BCG-CWS was examined in our laboratory (5). The immunoadjuvant activity of BCG-CWS varied both quantitatively and qualitatively according to the form in which it was administered. In experimental and human cancer studies, BCG-CWS was used as an immunotherapeutic agent in the form of an oil-in-water emulsion, using either mineral oil (Drakeol 6VR) or metabolizable oils such as squalene or squalane. The antitumor activity of BCG-CWS was shown using transplantable tumor systems in mice, rats, and guinea pigs, and in autochthonous tumors in mice. The prevention of carcinogenesis in mice, rats, and rabbits was also reported. In addition, it was shown that depressed T cell function in tumor-bearing mice could be increased to normal by administration of BCG-CWS.

Oil (Drakeol 6VR)-treated BCG-CWS has been used in the immunotherapy of human cancers such as lung cancer, leukemia, malignant melanoma, and other neoplastic diseases in Japan. Yamamura et al (14) studied BCG-CWS in the treatment of lung cancer patients. A total of 455 patients with primary lung cancer who were admitted to the 11 hospitals in our collaborative group between April 1974 and December 1976 were treated with BCG-CWS. All patients initially received conventional therapy, including surgery, irradiation, and/or chemotherapy. The control group comprised 380 patients treated with conventional therapy between April 1971 and March 1974 at the same hospitals.

Immunotherapy with BCG-CWS was introduced following and, in some cases, during initial conventional therapy. The 50% survival periods of all patients were 13.5 and 8.5 months, and median survival periods were 11 and 8 months in the immunotherapy and control groups, respectively. The difference was statistically significant (p < 0.0001). A marked prolongation of survival period was observed in patients with malignant pleurisy who received repeated intrapleural injection of BCG-CWS.

Yasumoto and his group (15) have assessed the clinical effect of BCG-CWS treatment in lung cancer patients by comparing the survival of the BCG-CWS group (155 cases) with that of a historical control group based on 4 years' results. A significant prolongation of survival time was observed in clinical stages II, III (M_0), and III (M_1). However, most stage III patients who were given the BCG-CWS treatment eventually died of cancer following a marked prolongation of survival time; an increase in complete cure rate was observed only in stages I and II. Patients having undergone surgical resection were sensitive to treatment with BCG-CWS at any stage. Histologically, all types of lung cancer, including squamous cell carcinoma, adenocarcinoma, and anaplastic carcinoma, were sensitive to treatment with BCG-CWS. It was also shown in trials that intrapleural administration of BCG-CWS to patients with malignant pleurisy was effective in controlling the pleural effusion and prolonging survival time.

A clinical trial of chemoimmunotherapy using BCG-CWS was conducted in 28 patients—20 adults (16 acute myeloblastic leukemia [AML] and 4 acute lymphoblastic leukemia [ALL]), and 8 children (3 AML and 5 ALL) in complete remission (16). Chemotherapy consisted of monthly intensification therapy for 2 months and bimonthly thereafter. Immunotherapy with 200 μg of oil-attached BCG-CWS mixed with 10^7 autochthonous leukemic cells was given intradermally at either the upper or lower extremities every week, except when the patients were on maintenance therapy. An increase in immunologic reactivity of the patients receiving BCG-CWS was noted. Their skin test response to PPD, Varidase, and *Candida* extract showed a notable increase. The in vitro lymphocyte blastogenic response to PPD, concanavalin A, and pokeweed mitogen also showed a significant increase. Although the duration of remission of adult patients with AML who received BCG-CWS therapy was not prolonged, the survival period was apparently prolonged compared to our historical control patients with AML.

Ochiai et al (17) examined the effectiveness of BCG-CWS in a randomized controlled clinical trial in patients with gastric cancer who underwent gastrectomy at a single institution between January 1976 and December 1978. A total of 140 patients were randomized into 3 groups: chemotherapy plus immunotherapy (BCG-CWS), chemotherapy alone, and a nontreatment control group. Survival time in 138 of these patients was looked at in January 1983. Statistically significant differences in the survival curve were observed between the control and chemotherapy plus immunotherapy groups (p < 0.01) and between the chemotherapy and chemotherapy plus immunotherapy groups (p < 0.05).

Nocardia rubra *CWS*

Previously, we reported that CWS fractions of *Nocardia* have potent adjuvant activity in the immune response. In particular, *N. rubra* CWS (N-CWS) has been shown to be most effective for the immunotherapy of cancer in experimental syngeneic transplantable and autochthonous tumor studies (6–8). N-CWS was composed of nocardomycolic acid, arabinogalactan, and mucopeptide (6), and details of the chemical structure of each component examined (18,19).

N-CWS has various advantages as an immunotherapeutic agent in comparison with BCG-CWS. The strain of *N. rubra* that was recently reclassified as *Rhodococcus lentifragmentus* AN-115 is nonpathogenic and easily cultivated in synthetic and semisynthetic media within a few days, and N-CWS was obtained by a similar method to that of BCG-CWS. The adjuvant and antitumor activities of N-CWS have been shown to be more potent than those of BCG-CWS in experimental studies. N-CWS was also shown to be less toxic than BCG-CWS.

The adjuvant activity of N-CWS was examined in detail (6,20–31). N-CWS acted as an adjuvant on the induction of delayed-type hypersensitivity, allogeneic cell-mediated cytotoxicity, helper T cell function, humoral immune response in vivo and in vitro, and macrophage activation. Mitogenic activity on mouse spleen cells was also demonstrated. N-CWS showed antitumor activity for the suppression and regression of transplantable tumors in syngeneic mice, rats, and guinea pigs, comparable to that of BCG-CWS (6–8,32–37). The preventive effect of N-CWS was demonstrated using experimental models of chemical carcinogenesis in mice, rats, and rabbits, and spontaneous carcinogenesis in mice (38–42). It was suggested that N-CWS was effective for the production of cytokines such as macrophage activating factor (MAF), colony-stimulating factor (CSF), interleukin 1 (IL-1), interferon-α/β, interferon-γ, and tumor necrosis factor (TNF) in mice and human systems (43–46).

The in vitro and in vivo effects of N-CWS on the induction of serum factors such as ceruloplasmin, hemopexin complement, and interferon have previously been described (47). The protective effect of N-CWS against experimental infection with Friend leukemia virus, herpes simplex virus, *Pseudomonas aeruginosa, Escherichia coli*, and *Klebsiella pneumoniae* in normal and immunosuppressed mice has also been reported (48).

After a toxicological study (49), the clinical effectiveness of N-CWS was evaluated by randomized, controlled trial in patients with lung cancer (50,51) gastric cancer (52,53), and nonlymphocytic leukemia (54,55). The clinical effectiveness of oil (squalene)-treated N-CWS in inoperable lung cancer patients and patients with malignant pleural effusion was examined in a randomized controlled trial by Yamamura et al (50), in 5 institutions, between October 1978 and June 1981. All patients without pleural effusions were treated by conventional therapies, such as chemotherapy and/or radiotherapy, and patients with performance status 0 to 3 were randomized into either the N-CWS or the control group. In the immunotherapy group, either 400 μg of N-CWS was injected once or twice into the bronchial tumor using a fiberoptic bronchoscope, or 200 μg was injected intradermally once a month. Of 309 patients, 118 patients in the N-CWS group and 108 patients in the control group were eligible for statistical analysis. There was no statistically significant difference in survival rate between the 2 groups, although by histologic type, a significant prolongation of survival period was observed in patients with small cell carcinoma ($p < 0.05$).

The effectiveness of N-CWS on lung cancer patients with malignant pleural effusion was observed. The efficacy of tube draining versus that of tube draining plus N-CWS as initial local treatment was investigated in 97 patients with malignant pleural fluid due to primary lung cancer. The response rate for patients receiving N-CWS was 85.7% compared with 60.6% for patients not receiving N-CWS ($p < 0.05$). The survival time of patients receiving N-CWS was also significantly longer than that of patients in the control group ($p < 0.05$). These results suggest that intrapleural and intracutaneous injections of N-CWS, combined with tube drainage and local chemotherapy, are effective with respect to management of malignant pleural fluid and prolongation of patient survival.

Yasumoto et al (51) performed a randomized, controlled clinical study in patients with operable lung cancer carried out from November 1977 to June 1981. Immunotherapy consisted of an intrapleural injection of N-CWS 300 μg followed by serial intradermal injection of N-CWS 200 μg. A total of 119 patients were entered into trial, of whom there were 64 evaluable patients in the control group and 52 in the N-CWS group. Treatment with N-CWS was shown to be effective in terms of prolonged duration of remission for all operable patients, and a significant improvement in survival rate was observed in the curative operation group ($p < 0.05$), but not in patients at stages I and II ($p < 0.10$). The rate of occurrence of distant metastasis in the control and the N-CWS-treated groups was 34.0% and 18.9%, respectively. The local recurrence rate was 14.9% in the control group, but there was none in the N-CWS group ($p < 0.05$).

Ochiai et al (52) have reported a clinial trial of N-CWS in the treatment of gastric cancer. From September 1979 through March 1981, a total of 302 patients with gastric cancer who underwent gastrectomy were studied. The patients were stratified according to gross stage of cancer and degree of operative curability. They were then assigned randomly to either a chemotherapy group or a chemotherapy plus immunotherapy group. Immunotherapy consisted of intradermal injection of 400 μg of N-CWS which was given weekly for the the 1st month and monthly thereafter. The patients were classified by histologic stage of cancer and extent of surgical intervention into curative or noncurative groups. Survival time was assessed at follow-up in December 1981. There was no statistical difference in survival rates between the groups for patients in the curative category, probably because of the short observation period. The intergroup difference in survival rates, however, was statistically significant for patients in the noncurative category ($p < 0.01$). These results indicate the adjuvant effect of N-CWS as an immunotherapeutic agent in patients undergoing gastrectomy for gastric cancer.

Koyama et al (53) performed a randomized, controlled study of postoperative adjuvant immunochemotherapy with N-CWS and tegafur for gastric carcinoma between September 1979 and March 1983. A total of 309 patients were entered into this trial, of whom there were 98 evaluable in the chemotherapy group and 115 in the immunochemotherapy group. In both groups, tegafur was given as chemotherapy at a daily dose of 400 to 800 mg beginning 24–29 days after gastrectomy. In the immunochemotherapy group, 400 μg of N-CWS was injected intradermally within the 2nd postoperative week. It was given weekly during the 1st month and monthly thereafter for as long as practicable. The patients were surveyed for survival time in March 1985. The postoperative survival rate was analyzed for all cases, and for patients with various histopathologic stages of carcinoma, for comparison between the 2 treatment groups. The overall survival rate for all patients was significantly higher in the immunochemotherapy group than in the chemotherapy group ($p < 0.05$). Fifty-three patients from the chemotherapy group and 61 patients from the immunochemotherapy group who had stage III and IV disease were included in the analysis. A highly statistically significant difference in 5-year survival rate was observed between the 2 groups in patients with stage III and IV disease (28.8% and 52.4%, respectively). Thus the 50% survival period of patients with stage III and IV cancer was 1800 days or more in the immunochemotherapy group, whereas it was only 722 days in the chemotherapy group.

The effect of N-CWS on the maintenance chemotherapy of patients with acute nonlymphocytic leukemia (ANLL) was evaluated by a randomized clinical trial by the Kyushu N-CWS Leukemia Study Group (54). After complete remission was induced and consolidated with repeated courses of induction chemotherapy using mainly DCMP (daunorubicin, cytarabine, vincristine, and prednisolone) regimens, 41 patients were randomly divided into 2 groups, ie, an immunochemotherapy (N-CWS) group and a chemotherapy-alone group. For the first 5 doses, N-CWS 200–300 μg was injected intradermally into both sides of the preaxial and inguinal areas in the N-CWS group every 2 weeks, and every 4 weeks thereafter. The median survival time for the 17 N-CWS-treated patients (12 AML, 2 acute monoblastic leukemia [AMOL], and 3 acute promyelocytic leukemia [APL]) was 811 days and that for the 18 control patients (14 AML, 1 AMOL, and 3 APL) was 416 days. This difference was statistically significant ($p < 0.05$). The median duration of remission for the N-CWS-treated group and the control group was 349 days and 202 days, respectively, but this difference was not statistically significant. The 2nd remission was more easily obtained the N-CWS group (7/13) compared to that in in the control group (2/14).

The effect of immunotherapy with N-CWS on duration of remission and survival of adults with AML was studied in a prospective, randomized, controlled study by Ohno et al (55). Following induction and consolidation of complete remission, 73 patients were randomized to receive either maintenance chemotherapy or maintenance chemotherapy plus immunotherapy with N-CWS and irradiated allogeneic AML cells. Thirty-four patients in the chemotherapy group and 32 in the chemoimmunotherapy group were evaluable. Six months after the closure of the study, the immunotherapy showed a borderline beneficial effect on duration of remission (p=0.080) and survival (p=0.098). When the data were analyzed 30 months after entry, there was a marginally significant difference in duration of remission (p=0.080) between the 2 groups, with the 50% survival period prolonged by 100 days. However, there was no significant difference in survival time (p=0.314), although the 50% survival was 168 days longer in the chemoimmunotherapy group. Nevertheless, there were 4 (18.2%) 5-year relapse-free surviors among 22 patients (11 in each group) who had been diagnosed more than 5 years before the time of the present analysis, all of whom belonged to the chemoimmunotherapy group (p=0.090). Thus, immunotherapy with N-CWS and irradiated allogeneic AML cells seems to be active in the treatment of adult AML when used for maintenance therapy in combination with chemotherapy.

Sakai's group has examined by randomized, controlled study the effecttiveness of N-CWS on head and neck cancer patients (this volume, p 242), and it was found that N-CWS-treated patients in stages III and IV showed a trend toward prolongation of survival period and lower recurrence rate in comparison with those of the control group. Case reports of the effective treatment of N-CWS have also been described in patients with malignant melanoma, by Maeyama et al (56), and laryngeal cancer, by Yanagida et al (57).

Yamakido et al (58) reported that intradermal administration of N-CWS caused the stimulation of NK cell activity and antibody-dependent cell-mediated cytotoxicity of peripheral lymphocytes, and elevation of interferon titer in sera of lung cancer patients. Moritani (59) has reported an increase in the cytotoxicity of lymphocytes in cancer tissue and regional lymph nodes in which N-CWS had been given by endoscopic injection.

It is well recognized that the incidence of complications of respiratory diseases such as chronic bronchitis and malignant neoplasms is high among retired workers from the Okunojima poison gas factory, indicating there are many abnormalities in their immunologic competence (60). Yamakido et al (61) treated retired poison gas factory workers (187 cases) with N-CWS during the influenza period from fall 1981 to spring 1982 and compared the clinical symptoms of N-CWS-treated subjects with those of an equal number of control patients. A study of the therapeutic and immunologic effects of N-CWS on influenza led to the following conclusions. The incidence of fever and cough among N-CWS-treated patients was significantly lower than among the control patients. In the N-CWS-treated group, the incidence of influenza among those with increased cell-mediated immunity was lower than among those with decreased cell-mediated immunity, and antibody titers against influenza virus among N-CWS-treated patients tended to be higher than among the control patients. Matsuzaka et al (62) have reported a case of herpes zoster virus that was treated effectively with N-CWS.

Nakamoto et al (63) have reported the effective treatment of severe spontaneous pneumothorax with N-CWS. Intrapleural instillation of N-CWS was tried in 53 patients with complex spontaneous pneumothorax, postoperative prolonged air leakage, and postoperative residual air space, during the period of July 1978 through June 1983. Thirty of these were spontaneous pneumothorax (without surgical treatment due to low pulmonary function, pneumoconiosis, old age, etc. The remaining 23 cases had postoperative air leakage and residual air space; 17 had lung cancer and 4 had giant bullae. Of the 53 patients, 36 required only 1 instillation and the remaining 17 required an additional instillation; this resulted in a success rate of 98% and there were no recurrences. No analgesics were needed during the instillation, and no pleural thickening occurred. No significant side effects were noted during the treatment, except for a temporary elevation in temperature and LDH level. From these clinical observations, it was concluded that N-CWS is a safe and effective treatment for pleural air leakage.

P. acnes *CWS*

The CWS of the *Propionibacterium* species, including *P. acnes, P. granulosum*, and *P. avidem*, have been purified and their biochemical and immunologic properties investigated in our laboratory (9–11). *P. acnes*-CWS was shown to consist mainly of isopentadecanoic acid as the major fatty acid, acidic polysaccharide containing glucose, mannose, galactose, galactosamine, and diaminomannuronic acid, and peptidoglycan. *P. acnes*-CWS was shown to suppress the growth of fibrosarcomas, EL-4 leukemia, and MH-134 hepatoma in syngeneic mice, and to cause a regression in established fibrosarcoma tumor (MC-104) in C57BL/6J mice, and a hepatoma (line 10) in strain 2 guinea pigs (9). Tanio et al (64) have reported that intralesional or iv administration of *P. acnes*-CWS prevented the pulmonary metastasis of Lewis lung carcinoma (3LL) in C57BL/6 mice, and prolonged the survival period of tumor-bearing hosts. It was also suggested that the adjuvant activity of *P. acnes*-CWS on macrophage activation was correlated to the antitumor activity of *P. acnes*-CWS.

L. monocytogenes *CWS*

The CWS of *L. monocytogenes* was purified and its biochemical and immunologic properties were examined in our laboratory (12). *L. monocytogenes*-CWS is composed of ribitol teichoic acid and peptidoglycan, and has been shown to have potent antitumor activity in transplantable tumors in syngeneic mice and guinea pigs. It should be noted that the peptidoglycan moiety prepared from *L. monocytogenes*-CWS was as active as CWS or whole cells in the regression of Meth-A in BALB/c mice. It was also shown that *L. monocytogenes*-CWS and its peptidoglycan moiety acted on macrophage activation as an adjuvant and on mouse B lymphocytes as a mitogen (13).

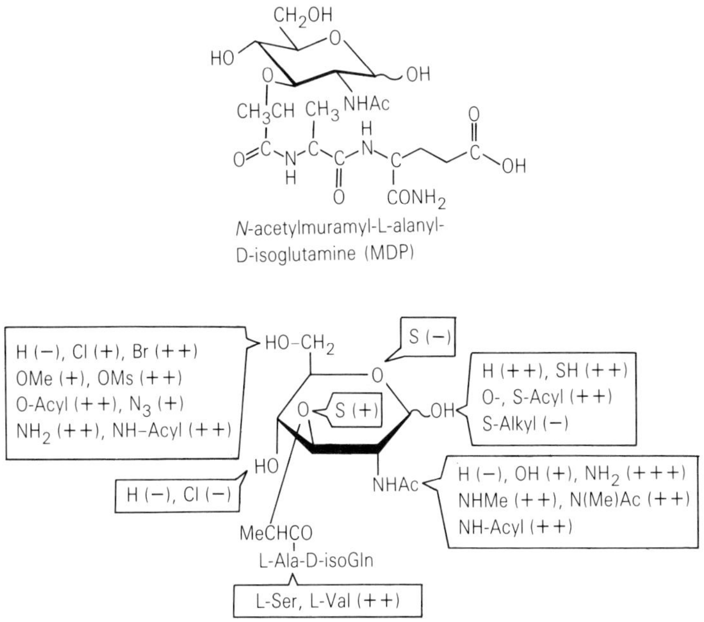

N-acetylmuramyl-L-alanyl-
D-isoglutamine (MDP)

Fig 1 MDPs: relationship between structure and adjuvant activity.

Synthetic *N*-acetylmuramyl dipeptides (MDP) and their acyl derivatives

Relationship between structure and adjuvant activity of MDP analogues and derivatives

In 1974, Ellouz et al (65) reported that the minimal adjuvant-active sub-unit of bacterial cell walls, including BCG-CWS, N-CWS, *P. acnes*-CWS, and *L. monocytogenes*-CWS, was *N*-acetylmuramyl-L-alanyl-D-isoglutamine (MurNAc-L-Ala-D-isoGln, MDP; Fig 1), and the biological activities of MDP were reported by several laboratories (66). A variety of MDP analogues and derivatives have been synthesized, and the relationship between their chemical structure and adjuvant activity has been examined (Fig 2). Although MDP and its analogues have potent adjuvant activities in vivo when they are administered as a water-in-oil emulsion together with antigen, MDP exhibits only limited adjuvant activity when administered as an aqueous solution in vivo, due to its rapid excretion into urine. We therefore synthesized several hydrophobic (acyl) derivatives of MDP analogues (67,68). From these acyl-MDP derivatives, 3 synthetic compounds were selected (Fig 2), a 6-quinonyl-MDP derivative for cancer immunotherapy and 2 kinds of stearoyl MDP derivatives as adjuvants for the nonspecific stimulation of host against bacterial and viral infections in cancer patients.

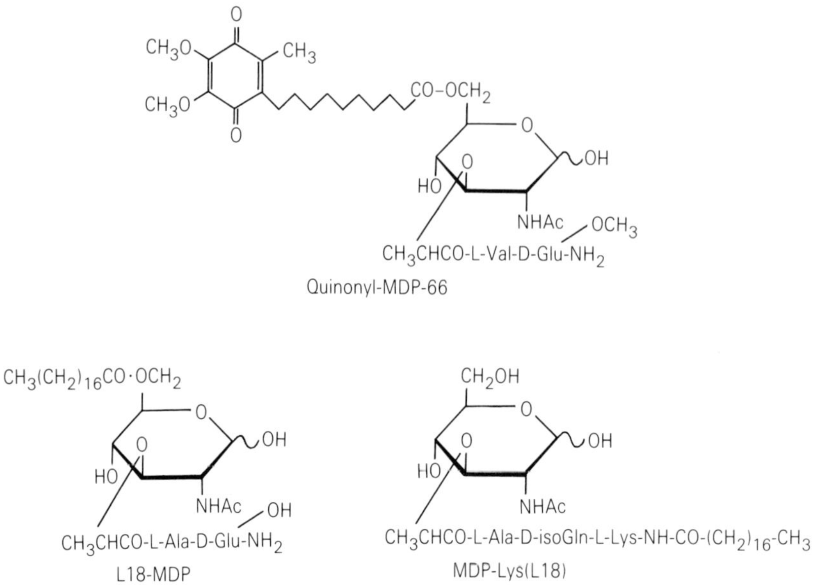

Quinonyl-MDP-66

L18-MDP

MDP-Lys(L18)

Fig 2 Acyl-MDP derivatives.

Antitumor activity of 6-O-quinonyl-MDP derivative

It has been clearly shown that ubiquinone and its related compounds, such as QS-10 [2,3-dimethoxy-5-methyl-6-(9′-carboxynonyl)-1, 4-benzoquinone], and Q acid-I[2,3-dimethoxy-5-methyl-6-(5′-carboxy-3′-methyl-2′-phenyl)-1,4-benzo-quinone], have various biological activities, such as effects on lysosomal membrane, on heart cAMP phosphodiesterase, restoration of a reduced succinate oxidase system, and immunoadjuvant activity. As a new lipophilic derivative of an MDP analogue, we synthesized a benzoquinonyl derivative of the *N*-acetylmuramyl-L-valyl-D-isoglutamine (MurNAc-L-Val-D-isoGln) methyl ester compound, which was named quinonyl-MDP-66 (68).

The adjuvant activity of quinonyl-MDP-66 and its parent compounds was examined in guinea pigs and mice. The quinonyl-MDP-66 was effective as an adjuvant for the induction of delayed type hypersensitivity, as well as for humoral antibody formation, allogeneic killer T cell induction, and macrophage activation. The antitumor activity of quinonyl-MDP-66 was examined by using syngeneic transplantable tumor systems, Meth-A-BALB/c mice and line 10-strain 2 guinea pigs. Quinonyl-MDP-66 was shown to be highly effective in the suppression of Meth-A growth in syngeneic (BALB/c) mice. The induction of systemic tumor immunity in mice in which tumor growth had been suppressed was demonstrated by the reinoculation of Meth-A cells (10^5). The results suggest that both lipophilic groups, the benzoquinonyl group and the methyl ester, play some roles in the manifestation of antitumor and adjuvant activities on the allogeneic cell-mediated cytotoxicity of MurNAc-L-Val-D-isoGln (69).

The antitumor activity of quinonyl-MDP-66 in the regression of line-10 hepatoma in strain-2 guinea pigs was examined (70). Tumor cells (10^6) were inoculated intradermally into strain-2 guinea pigs, and 10% squalene-treated quinonyl-MDP (400 or 100 μg) was injected intralesionally. Tumor growth at the inoculation site and metastasis of tumor into regional lymph nodes were examined. Repeated injections (4 times) of 10% squalene-treated quinonyl-MDP-66 completely suppressed tumor growth and prevented metastasis to regional lymph nodes. Even with only 2 injections of quinonyl-MDP-66, tumor growth was suppressed in 4 of 7 guinea pigs. More recently, we found that an oil-in-water emulsion containing quinonyl-MDP-66, 10% squalene, 5% detergent (HCO-60), and 5.5% mannitol in saline was the most effective and stable adjuvant form to manifest the antitumor activity (71).

It was found that quinonyl-MDP-66, as well as ubiquinone, could restore the reduced NAD oxidase and succinate oxidase activites of pentane- or acetone-treated beef heart mitochondrial preparations. Doxorubicin (Adriamycin) is an agent used widely in cancer treatment. However, a variety of serious complications of doxorubicin administration have been reported. Cardiotoxicity is the major factor limiting the prolonged use of doxorubicin. Several investigators have reported that doxorubicin-induced cardiotoxicity in cancer patients was prevented by the administration of ubiquinone-10(CoQ_{10}). We have reported the preventive effect of quinonyl-MDP-66 on doxorubicin-induced cardiotoxicity in rats (72).

Effects of acyl-MDP derivatives on host resistance against bacterial and viral infections

It is well recognized that the nonspecific host stimulation with immunostimulants is one of the most important factors for the treatment of immunosuppressed hosts such as cancer patients. Chedid et al (73) have reported that MDP and its derivatives stimulated host resistance against *Klebsiella pneumoniae* infection in mice. Several MDP derivatives and related compounds such as murabutide, stearoyl-MDP derivatives, MTP-PE (74), FK-565, FK-156 (75), and RP 40 639 (76) have been reported to have host-stimulating activities against bacterial infections in experimental models.

Matsumoto et al (77–79) have also examined 64 acyl-MDP derivatives as adjuvants for the stimulation of host resistance against nonspecific bacterial infection by using a sepsis type infection model with *E. coli* in mice; they selected 2 candidates, L18-MDP and MDP-Lys(L18) (Fig 2). The stimulatory effects of both stearoyl-MDP derivatives were examined in detail (80). Both were shown to be effective in the stimulation of host resistance against infection with *E. coli, Staphylococcus aureus, Pseudomonas aeruginosa*, and *Candida albicans*, but not effective for infections with *Salmonella typhimurium* and *L. monocytogenes*. It was also shown that both stearoyl-MDP derivatives stimulated immunosuppressed mice, rats, and guinea pigs. Both stearoyl-MDP derivatives had a synergistic effect in combination with antibiotics such as cephazolin, gentamicin, and amphotericin B.

On the mechanism of stimulation of the host with stearoyl-MDP derivatives, Osada et al (81) have shown that functions such as migration, phagocytosis, and production of superoxide of polymorphonuclear cells were stimulated by the administration of stearoyl-MDP derivatives. We have also demonstrated that both L18-MDP and MDP-Lys(L18) are effective for host stimulation against opportunistic infection with *Corynebacterium kutuscheri* infection in mice (82).

We have established models for host stimulation with immunoadjuvants against viral infection by using Sendai virus and herpes simplex type 1 virus in mice (83). Intranasal pretreatment with MDP, L18-MDP, and MDP-Lys(l18) dissolved in PBC augmented the nonspecific resistance to intranasal infection with Sendai virus in mice. Intranasal administration of MDP-Lys(L18) 10 μg 3 days and 1 day before intranasal challenge with Sendai virus resulted in 100% survival rates; however, administration of MDP-Lys(L18) 1 day after the infection showed effect in this experimental situation. It was also shown that intranasal administration of 10 μg and 1 μg of MDP-Lys(L18) was effective, but that 0.1 μg of MDP-Lys(L18) was not. Intranasal, intraperitoneal, and intravenous administration of MDP-Lys(L18) was effective but subcutaneous administration of MDP-Lys(L18) did not protect against Sendai virus infection in this model. The mechanism of action of MDP-Lys(L18) for protection against Sendai virus infection was investigated and discussed by Ishihara et al (84), and it was concluded that the growth of Sendai virus was suppressed by the treatment with MDP-Lys(L18) only at the early, nonspecific phase of infection, and that macrophages and interferon are the important elements activated by the MDP-LyS(L18) treatment. More recently, it has been shown that MDP-Lys(L18) was also effective on host resistance against herpes simplex virus (HSV) type 1 infection in cyclophosphamide-treated mice (Ishihara C. et al, unpublished data).

By using the same experimental model, we have shown the activity on host stimulation of other series of MDP derivatives such as the stearoyl derivatives of *N*-acetylglucosaminyl-*β*-(1→4)-*N*-acetylmuramyl tri- and tetrapeptide, compounds GM-50 and GM-53 (85), and multiprenylacetyl MDP derivatives, TDM-232 (86).

More recently, Tsubura et al (87) have examined the restorative effect of MDP-Lys(L18) in patients with leukopenia associated with anticancer chemotherapy and radiation therapy. MDP-Lys(L18) was most effective in augmenting the white blood cell population in patients receiving the drug subcutaneously every day in a 400-mg dose. MDP-Lys(L18) was considerably more effective in patients with a solid tumor than in those with hematologic malignancies. Considering both the efficacy and the side effect profile it was suggested that 200 μg/day on consecutive days was the optimal treatment regimen.

Trehalose mycolates

Trehalose-6,6'-dimycolate (TDM), a so-called cord factor, was originally discovered from a pathogenic mycobacterial lipid fraction by Bloch and his coworkers (88,89) as the mycobacterial toxic principle for mice when injected as an oil emulsion. Further investigation revealed that cord factor-like glycolipids were contained not only in pathogenic mycobacteria but also in the lipid fractions of related bacteria such as saprophytic mycobacteria, *Nocardia*, and corynebacteria. TDM was also shown to have a variety of biological activities such as a) toxic activity in mice, b) antitumor activity, c) stimulation of host resistance against infections by bacteria, fungi, viruses, and parasites, and d) synergistic potentiation of the antiinfectious and antitumor activities of other immunoadjuvants (90). Ribi et al (91) have reported that the adjuvant and antitumor activities of BCG-CWS, lipid A, or synthetic MDP derivatives were potently stimulated by the combination with TDM.

We have synthesized TDM and its analogues TD(L30), TD(B30), TD (BH32), TD(BH48), TD(BH28), TDNM, and TDN(BH32) (Fig 3) to examine in detail their adjuvant activity and the relationship between the chemical structure and their lethal and adjuvant activities. TDM and TDNM were 100% and 40% lethal, respectively, when injected intravenously into mice at a dose of 150 μg as a 9% oil-in-water emulsion, but the other analogues showed no lethal toxicity to mice at the same dose. The cytolytic activity of mouse peritoneal macrophages against tumor cell was potentiated by ip injection of TDM and its synthetic analogues. TDM and TD(BH32) also stimulated nonspecific host resistance against Sendai virus infection in BALB/c mice (92).

We have also synthesized 5 monoesters, TMM, GlcM, GlcNAcM, AraM, and GalM, by use of mycolic acid isolated from *Mycobacterium tuberculosis* strain Aoyama B. A single intravenous administration of 400 μg of TMM in a 9% oil-in-water emulsion killed 8 of 8 treated mice. The other analogues showed less lethal toxicity to mice at the same dose. Tumoricidal activity of mouse peritoneal macrophages was induced by intraperitoneal injection of TMM, GlcM, and GlcNAcM, respectively. In addition we have observed that 6-*O*-mycoloyl-1-deoxyl-*N*-acetylglucosamine was also as effective as TDM for mouse peritoneal macrophage activation, but was less toxic. Natural TDM is the 6,6′-dimycolate of trehalose(α,α). More recently, we have examined the immunoadjuvant efficacy of synthetic dimycolates of trehalose stereoisomers, such as trehalose(α,β), in collaboration with Kitajima's group at Toa Kasei Co., Ltd., (93). The results indicated that synthetic TDM(α,β) and TDM(β,β) were as effective as natural TDM(α,α) for the activation of mouse peritoneal macrophages, but were less toxic than natural TDM(α,α) (Azuma I. et al, unpublished).

Lipid A

It has been established that the lipopolysaccharide (LPS) of gram-negative bacteria has a variety of biological and immunomodulating activities, and that the active principle of LPS is the lipid A moiety. The chemical structure of lipid A has been extensively studied and that of lipid A of *E. coli* LPS described (94). The chemical synthesis of lipid A analogues and related compounds was reported by Shiba's group (95,96). The chemically synthesized compound 506 (Fig 4) possesses most of the biological activity of *E. coli* lipid A and LPS, in-

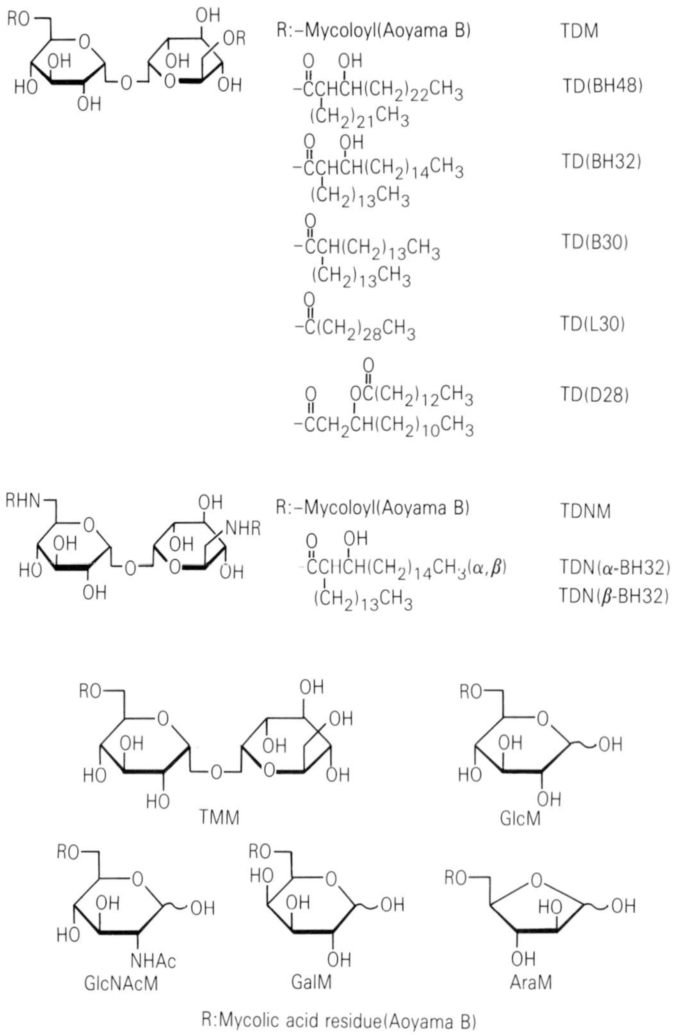

Fig 3   Synthetic TDM analogues.

cluding immunomodulating and toxic activity (97,98).

Hasegawa and his coworkers attempted to synthesize lipid A-related compounds, which are adjuvant active but less toxic, for application to immunomodulation in humans. Three acylated monosaccharide derivatives, GLA-27, GLA-59, and GLA-60, were selected as adjuvants (99,100). GLA-60 (Fig 4) was shown to have very potent adjuvant activity (101) for the induction of delayed type hypersensitivity in guinea pigs, activation of mouse peritoneal macrophages, induction of serum TNF in mice after priming with *P. acnes* or recombinant murine interferon-γ, and prevention of cancer metastasis in mouse

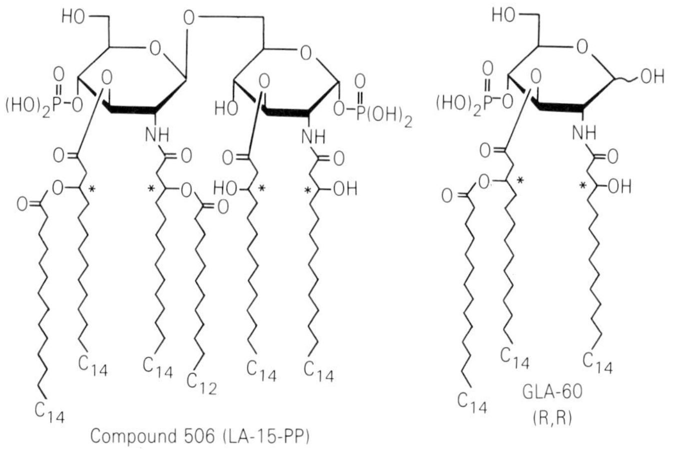

Fig 4 Synthetic lipid A (*E. coli*) and a related compound.

experimental models (102). GLA-60 was also demonstrated to have a very low adverse reaction rate (101). These results suggest that lipid A derivatives or related compounds having low toxicity will be useful immunoadjuvants for host stimulation in cancer patients.

Conclusions

Bacterial cells and their fractions have been shown to be the most important source of immunoadjuvants. In particular, mycobacterial cells, CWS, MDP, TDM, and lipid A have been widely used for experimental studies and clinical use in cancer patients. The chemical synthesis of analogues and derivatives of MDP, TDM, and lipid A has been extensively carried out and promising synthetic compounds have been developed. Most recent results clearly indicate that immunoadjuvants are a very useful tool for the treatment of patients with cancer and infectious diseases.

Acknowledgments

This work was supported in part by the following grants-in-aid. For Cancer Research: from the Japanese Ministry of Education, Science and Culture, and the Japanese Ministry of Health and Welfare for Comprehensive 10-Year Strategy for Cancer Control. For Scientific Recearch and for Developmental Scientific Research (No. 62870023) from the Japanese Ministry of Education, Science and Culture. For Scientific Research from the Japanese Ministry of Education, Science and Culture. This work was also supported by the Osaka

Foundation for Promotion of Clinical Immunology, the Yamanouchi Foundation for Research on Metabolic Disorders, and by a grant-in-aid for special project research from Hokkaido University, Sapporo, Japan.

References

1. Freund J. The mode of action of immunological adjuvants. Adv Tubercl Res 1956;1:130-48.
2. Azuma I, Kishimoto S, Yamamura Y, Petit J-F. Adjuvanticity of mycobacterial cell wall. Jpn J Microbiol 1971;15:193-7.
3. Azuma I, Kanetsuna F, Taniyama T, et al. Adjuvant activity of mycobacterial fractions. I. Purification and in vivo adjuvant activity of cell wall skeletons of *Mycobacterium bovis* BCG, *Nocardia asteroides* 131 and *Corynebacterium diphtheriae* PW8. Biken J 1975;18:1-13.
4. Azuma I, Ribi EE, Meyer TJ, Zbar B. Biological active components from mycobacterial cell walls. I. Isolation and composition of cell wall skeleton and componet P_3. J Natl Cancer Inst 1974;52:95-101.
5. Azuma I, Yamamura Y. Immunotherapy of cancer with BCG ccll-wall skeleton and related materials. Gann Monogr Cancer Res 1979;24:122-41.
6. Azuma I, Taniyama T, Yamawaki M, et al. Adjuvant and antitumor activities of *Nocardia* cell-wall skeletons. Jpn J Cancer Res (Gann) 1976;67:733-6.
7. Azuma I, Yamawaki M, Yasumoto K, Yamamura Y. Antitumor activity of *Nocardia* cell-wall skeleton preparations in transplantable tumors in syngeneic mice and patients with malignant pleurisy. Cancer Immunol Immunother 1978;4:95-100.
8. Yamawaki M, Azuma I, Saiki I, et al. Antitumor activity of squalene-treated cell-wall skeleton of *Nocardia rubra* in mice. Jpn J Cancer Res (Gann) 1978;69:619-26.
9. Azuma I, Yamawaki M, Yoshimoto T, et al. Antitumor activity of cell-wall skeleton of *Propionibacterium acnes* C7 in mice and guinea pigs. Jpn J Cancer Res (Gann) 1979;70:737-48.
10. Kamisango K, Fujii H, Yanagihara Y, et al. Structures of peptidoglycans of *Propionibacterium*. Microbiol Immunol 1983;27:635-40.
11. Nagaoka M, Kamisango K, Fujii H, et al. Structure of acidic polysaccharide from cell wall of *Propionibacterium acnes* strain C7. J Biochem 1985;97:1669-78.
12. Kamisango K, Fujii H, Okumura H, et al. Structural and immunochemical studies of teichoic acid of *Listeria monocytogenes*. J Biochem 1983;93:1401-9.
13. Saiki I, Kamisango K, Tanio Y, et al. Adjuvant activity of purified peptidoglycan of *Listeria monocytogenes* in mice and guinea pigs. Infect Immun 1982;38:58-66.
14. Yamamura Y, Sakatani M, Ogura T, Azuma I. Adjuvant immunotherapy of lung cancer with BCG cell-wall skeleton (BCG-CWS). Cancer 1979;43:1314-9.
15. Yasumoto K, Manabe H, Yanagawa E, et al. Nonspecific adjuvant immunotherapy of lung cancer with cell wall skeleton of *Mycobacterium bovis* Bacillus Calmette-Guérin. Cancer Res 1979;39:3262-7.
16. Ohno R, Ueda R, Imai K, et al. A clinical trial of cell-wall skeleton of BCG in chemoimmunotherapy of acute leukemia. Jpn J Cancer Res (Gann) 1978;69:179-86.
17. Ochiai T, Sato H, Hayashi R, et al. Postoperative adjuvant immunotherapy of gastric cancer with BCG-cell wall skeleton. Cancer Immunol Immunother 1983;14:167-71.

18. Fujioka M, Koda S, Morimoto Y. Novel glycosidic linkage between arabinogalactan and peptidoglycan in the cell wall skeleton of *Nocardia rubra* AN-115. J Gen Microbiol 1985;131:1323–9.

19. Koda S, Fujioka M, Shigi M, et al. Structural analysis of mycolic acids from the cell wall skeleton of *Rhodococcus lentifragmentus* AN-115. J Gen Microbiol 1986;132:1547–51.

20. Inamura N, Fujitsu T, Nakahara K, et al. Potentiation of tumoricidal properties of murine macrophages by *Nocardia rubra* cell wall skeleton (N-CWS). J Antibiotics 1984;37:244–52.

21. Ito M, Iizuka H, Masuno T, et al. Killing of tumor cells in vitro by macrophages from mice given injections of squalene-treated cell wall skeleton of *Nocardia rubra*. Cancer Res 1981;41:2925–30.

22. Ito M, Suzuki H, Nakano N, et al. Superoxide anion and hydrogen peroxide release by macrophages from mice treated with *Nocardia rubra* cell-wall skeleton: Inhibition of macrophage cytotoxicity by a protease inhibitor but not by superoxide dismutase and catalase. Jpn J Cancer Res (Gann) 1983;74:128–36.

23. Kawase I, Uemiya M, Yoshimoto T, et al. Effect of *Nocardia rubra* cell wall skeleton on T-cell-mediated cytotoxicity in mice bearing syngeneic sarcoma. Cancer Res 1981;41:660–6.

24. Masuno T, Ito M, Ogura T, et al. Activation of peritoneal macrophages by oil-attached cell-wall skeleton of BCG and *Nocardia rubra*. Jpn J Cancer Res Gann 1979;70:223–7.

25. Masuno T, Hayashi S, Ito M, et al. Mechanism(s) of in vitro macrophage activation with *Nocardia rubra* cell wall skeleton: The effects on macrophage-activating factor production by lymphocytes. Cancer Immunol Immunother 1986;22:132–8.

26. Ogura T, Namba M, Hirao F, et al. Association of macrophage activation with antitumor effect on rat syngeneic fibrosarcoma by *Nocardia rubra* cell wall skeleton. Cancer Res 1979;39:4706–12.

27. Sone S, Fidler IJ. In situ activation of tumoricidal properties in rat alveolar macrophages and rejection of experimental lung metastases by intravenous injection of *Nocardia rubra* cell wall skeleton. Cancer Immunol Immunother 1984;12:203–9.

28. Sone S, Pollack LA, Fidler IF. Direct activation of tumoricidal properties in rat alveolar macrophages by *Nocardia rubra* cell wall skeleton. Cancer Immunol Immunother 1980;9:227–32.

29. Sugimura K, Uemiya M, Azuma I, et al. Macrophage dependency of T-lymphocyte mitogenesis by *Nocardia rubra* cell-wall skeleton. Microbiol Immunol 1977; 21:525–30.

30. Yanagawa E, Yasumoto K, Manabe H, et al. Cytotoxic activity of peripheral blood monocytes against bronchogenic carcinoma cells in patients with lung cancer. Jpn J Cancer Res (Gann) 1979;70:533–9.

31. Yanagawa E, Yasumoto K, Ohta M, et al. Comparative study on antitumor effect of cell-wall skeleton of *Mycobacterium bovis* BCG and *Nocardia rubra*, with reference to T-cell dependency and independency. Jpn J Cancer Res (Gann) 1979;70:141–6.

32. Ogura T, Namba M, Yamamura Y, Azuma I. Immunotherapeutic effect of BCG and *Nocardia rubra* cell-wall skeletons on syngeneic tumors in rats. In: Terry WD, Yamamura Y, eds. Immunobiology and immunotherapy of cancer. New York: Elsevier North-Holland Publishers; 1979:259–309.

33. Tokuzen R, Okabe M, Nakahara W, et al. Effect of *Nocardia* and *Mycobacterium*

cell-wall skeletons on autochthonous tumor grafts. Jpn J Cancer Res (Gann) 1975;66:433–5.

34. Yamamura Y, Azuma I, Yamawaki M, et al. Immunotherapy of cancer with the cell-wall skeleton of *Nocardia rubra*. In: Terry WD, Yamamura Y, eds. Immunobiology and immunotherapy of cancer. New York: Elsevier North-Holland Publishers; 1979:279–94.

35. Haraguchi S, Kurakata S, Matsuo T, Yoshida T. Strain differences in the antitumor activity of an immunopotentiator, *Nocardia rubra* cell-wall skeleton, in B10 congenic and recombinant mice. Jpn J Cancer Res (Gann) 1985;76:400–13.

36. Kagawa K, Yamashita T, Tsubura E, Yamamura Y. Inhibition of pulmonary metastasis by *Nocardia rubra* cell wall skeleton, with special reference to macrophage activation. Cancer Res 1984;44:665–70.

37. Hirao F, Sakatani M, Nishikawa H, et al. Effect of *Nocardia rubra* cell-wall skeleton on the induction of lung cancer and amyloidosis by 3-methyl-cholanthrene in rabbits. Jpn J Cancer Res (Gann) 1980;71:398–401.

38. Inoue T, Yoshimoto T, Ogura T, et al. Effect of *Nocardia rubra* cell-wall skeleton treatment on tumor formation in two-stage chemical carcinogenesis of mouse skin. Cancer Immunol Immunother 1981;11:207–10.

39. Namba M, Yoshimoto T, Ogura T, et al. Effect of *Nocardia rubra* cell-wall skeleton on the induction of lung cancer in ACI/N rats. Jpn J Cancer Res (Gann) 1979;70:55–62.

40. Nagasawa H, Yanai R, Azuma I. Suppression by *Nocardia rubra* cell wall skeleton of mammary DNA synthesis, plasma prolactin level, and spontaenous mammary tumorigenesis in mice. Cancer Res 1978;38:2160–2.

41. Nagasawa H, Yanai R, Azuma I. Inhibitory effect of *Nocardia rubra* cell-wall skeleton on carcinogen-induced mammary tumorigenesis in rats. Eur J Cancer 1980;389–93.

42. Hayashi S, Masuno T, Hosoe S, et al. Augmented production of colony-stimulating factor in C3H/H3eN mice immunized with *Nocardia rubra* cell wall skeleton. Infect Immun 1986;52:128–33.

43. Izumi S, Hirai O, Hayashi K, et al. Induction of a tumor necrosis factor-like activity by *Nocardia rubra* cell wall skeleton. Cancer Res 1987;47:1785–92.

44. Izumo S, Ueda H, Okuhara M, et al. Effect of *Nocardia rubra* cell wall skeleton on murine interferon production *in vitro*. Cancer Res 1986;46:1960–5.

45. Inamura N, Nakahara K, Kuroda Y, et al. Effect of *Nocardia rubra* cell wall skeleton on interleukin 1 production from mouse peritoneal macrophages. Int J Immunopharmacol 1988;10:547–54.

46. Mine Y, Watanabe Y, Tawara S, et al. Effect of *Nocardia rubra* cell wall skeleton on human and cellular factors related to immune response in mice and guinea pigs. Arzneimittelforschung 1986;36:1774–8.

47. Mine Y, Yokota Y, Kikuchi H. Inhibitory effect of *Nocardia rubra* cell wall skeleton on splenomegaly induced by Friend leukemia virus in mice. Arzneimittelforschung 1985;35:1563–4.

48. Mine Y, Yokota Y, Nonoyama S, Kikuchi H. Protective effect of *Nocardia rubra* cell wall skeleton on experimental infection in normal and immunosuppressed mice. Arzneimittelforschung 1986;36:1489–92.

49. Fukuhara K, Iwanami K, Fujii T, et al. Toxicological studies of N-CWS. Kiso to Rinsho 1983;17:129–45. (In Japanese)

50. Yamamura Y, Ogura T, Sakatani M, et al. Randomized controlled study of adjuvant immunotherapy with *Nocardia rubra* cell wall skeleton for inoperable lung

cancer. Cancer Res 1983;43:5575-9.

51. Yasumoto K, Yaita H, Ohta M, et al. Randomly controlled study of chemotherapy versus chemoimmunotherapy in postoperative lung cancer patients. Cancer Res 1985;45:1413-7.

52. Ochiai T, Sato H, Sato H, et al. Randomly controlled study of chemotherapy versus chemoimmunotherapy in postoperative gastric cancer patients. Cancer Res 1983;43:3001-7.

53. Koyama S, Ozaki A, Iwasaki Y, et al. Randomized controlled study of postoperative adjuvant immunotherapy with *Nocardia rubra* cell wall skeleton (N-CWS) and tegafur for gastric carcinoma. Cancer Immunol Immunother 1986;22:148-54.

54. Kyushu N-CWS Leukemia Study Group. Adjuvant activity of *Nocardia* cell-wall skeleton on maintenance chemotherapy of acute non-lymphatic leukemia. Acta Haematol Jpn 1983;46:1093-8. (In Japanese)

55. Ohno R, Nakamura H, Kodera Y, et al. Randomized controlled study of chemoimmunotherapy of acute myelogeneous leukemia (AML) in adults with *Nocardia rubra* cell-wall skeleton and irradiated allogeneic AML cells. Cancer 1986;57:1483-8.

56. Maeyama T, Ohyama M, Katsuda K, et al. Combined treatment with cryosurgery and immunotherapy for malignant melanoma originating in the nose and paranasal sinus. Jibi Rinshou 1980;73:173-84. (In Japanese)

57. Yanagida J, Ishika S, Matsuzaka S, et al. A case of laryngeal cancer completely regressed with N-CWS. Rinshou Men-eki 1984;16:882-9. (In Japanese)

58. Yamakido M, Ishioka S, Onari K, et al. Changes in natural killer cell, antibody-dependent cell-mediated cytotoxicity and interferon activities with administration of *Nocardia rubra* cell wall skeleton to subjects with high risk of lung cancer. Jpn J Cancer Res (Gann) 1983;74:896-901.

59. Moritani Y. Distribution of lymphocyte subpopulation and natural killer activity in gastric cancer tissue, normal stomach and various tissues of gastric cancer patients. Nippon Geka Gakkai Zasshi 1984;85:132-42. (In Japanese)

60. Nishimoto Y, Yamakido M, Shigenobu T, et al. Long term observation of poison gas worker with special reference to respiratory cancers. Sangyo Ika Daigaku Zasshi 1983;5(suppl):89-94.

61. Yamakido M, Matsuzaka S, Yanagida J, et al. Effect of N-CWS injection against influenza virus infection in the retired workers of the Okunojima poison gas factory. Hiroshima J Med Sci 1984;33:547-51.

62. Matsuzaka S, Ishioka S, Yanagida J, et al. A case of herpes zoster treated by N-CWS. Rinshou Men-eki 1984;16:426-32. (In Japanese)

63. Nakamoto K, Sawamura K, Mori T, et al. Chemical pleurodesis with *Nocardia rubra* cell wall skeleton (N-CWS) for management of pleural air leakage. Nippon Kyoubu Geka Gakkai Zassi 1984;32:2090-4. (In Japanese)

64. Tanio Y, Yamamura Y, Saiki I, et al. Antimetastatic effect of cell-wall skeleton of *Propionibacterium acnes* C7 on Lewis lung carcinoma in C57BL/6J mice. Jpn J Cancer Res (Gann) 1981;72:403-10.

65. Ellouz F, Adam A, Ciorubaru R, Lederer E. Minimal structural requirements for adjuvant activity of bacterial peptidoglycan subunits. Biochem Biophys Res Commun 1974;59:1317-25.

66. Adam A, Lederer E. Muramyl peptide immunomodulators, sleep factors, and vitamins. Med Res Rev 1984;4:111-52.

67. Kusumoto S, Okada S, Yamamoto K, et al. Synthesis of long chain fatty acid esters

of *N*-acetylmuramyl-L-alanyl-D-isoglutamine in relation to antitumor activity. Tetrahedron Lett 1978;49:4899–902.

68. Azuma I, Yamawaki M, Uemiya M, et al. Adjuvant and antitumor activities of quinonyl-*N*-acetylmuramyldipeptides. Jpn J Cancer Res (Gann) 1979;70:847–8.
69. Saiki I, Tanio Y, Yamawaki M, et al. Adjuvant activity of quinonyl-*N*-acetylmuramyl-dipeptides in mice and guinea pigs. Infect Immun 1981;31:114–21.
70. Tanio Y, Souma H, Tokushima Y, et al. Regression of line-10 hepatocarcinoma with synthetic quinonyl muramyl dipeptide in strain-2 guinea pigs. Jpn J Cancer Res (Gann) 1983;74:192–5.
71. Azuma I, Ogawa Y, Igari Y, et al. Antitumor activity of quinonyl-MDP-66 on line 10 hepatoma in strain 2 guinea pigs. In: Tohno S et al, eds. Immunochemotherapy of cancer. Hirosaki: Hirosaki University School of Medicine; 1986:4–14.
72. Shimamoto N, Tanabe M, Shino A, et al. Preventive effect of a quinonyl derivative of *N*-acetylmuramyl dipeptide, QMDP-66, against adriamycin-induced ECG abnormalities in rats. Int J Immunopharmacol 1983;5:245–51.
73. Chedid L, Parant M, Lefrancier P, et al. Enhancement of nonspecific immunity to *Klebsiella pneumoniae* infection by a synthetic immunoadjuvant (*N*-acetylmuramyl-L-alanyl-D-isoglutamine) and several analogs. Proc Natl Acad Sci USA 1977;74:2089–93.
74. Shumann G. Biological activities of a lipophilic muramyl peptide (MTP-PE). In: Azuma I, Jollès G, eds. Immunostimulants: Now and tomorrow. Tokyo/Berlin: Japan Scientific Societies Press/Springer; 1987:71–7.
75. Goto T, Aoki H. The immunomodulatory activities of acylpeptides. In: Azuma I, Jollès G, eds. Immunomodulators: Now and tomorrow. Tokyo/Berlin: Japan Scientific Societies Press/Springer; 1987:130–48.
76. Floc'h F, Poirier J, Fizames C, Woehrle R. Pemelautide (R.P. 40 639). From experimental results to clinical trials: An illustration. In: Azuma I, Jollès G, eds. Immunomodulators: Now and tomorrow. Tokyo/Berlin: Japan Scientific Societies Press/Springer; 1988:193–204.
77. Matsumoto K, Ogawa H, Kusama T, et al. Stimulation of nonspecific resistance to infection induced by 6-O-acyl muramyl dipeptide analogs in mice. Infect Immun 1981;32:748–58.
78. Matsumoto K, Ogawa H, Nagase O, et al. Stimulation of nonspecific host resistance to infection induced by muramyldipeptides. Microbiol Immunol 1981;25:1047–58.
79. Matsumoto K, Otani T, Une T, et al. Stimulation of nonspecific resistance to infection induced by muramyl dipeptide analogs substituted in the *γ*-carboxyl group and evaluation of *N*^{α}-muramyl dipeptide-*N*^{ε}-strearoyllysine. Infect Immun 1983;39:1029–40.
80. Matsumoto K, Osada Y, Une T, et al. Anti-infectious activity of the synthetic muramyl dipeptide analogue MDP-Lys(L18). In: Azuma I, Jollès G, eds. Immunomodulators: Now and tomorrow. Tokyo/Berlin: Japan Scientific Societies Press/Springer; 1987:79–97.
81. Osada Y, Tsuyoshi O, Sato M, et al. Polymorphonuclear leukocyte activation by a synthetic muramyl dipeptide analog. Infect Immun 1982;38:848–54.
82. Ishihara C, Yamamoto K, Hamada H, Azuma I. Effect of stearoyl-*N*-acetylmuramyl-L-alanyl-D-isoglutamine on host resistance to *Corynebacterium kutuscheri* infection in cortisone-treated mice. Vaccine 1984;2:261–4.
83. Ishihara C, Hamada H, Yamamoto K, et al. Effects of muramyl dipeptide and its stearoyl derivatives on resistance to Sendai virus infection in mice. Vaccine

1985;3:370–4.

84. Ishihara C, Mizukoshi N, Iida J, et al. Suppression of Sendai virus growth by treatment with N^α-*acetylmuramyl-L-alanyl-D-isoglutaminyl-N*$^\varepsilon$-stearoyl-L-lysine in mice. Vaccine 1987;5:295–301.

85. Iida J, Saiki I, Ishihara C, Azuma I. Prophylactic activity against Sendai virus infection and macrophage activation with lipophilic derivatives of *N*-acetylglucosaminylmuramyl tri- or tetra-peptides. Vaccine (in press).

86. Azuma I, Saiki I, Iida J, et al. Immunological activities of multiprenylacetyl derivatives of muramyldipeptides. Vaccine 1988;6:339–42.

87. Tsubura E, Nomura T, Niitani H, et al. Restorative activity of muroctasin on leukopenia associated with anticancer treatment. Arzneimittelforschung 1988;38:1070–4.

88. Bloch H. Studies on the virulence of tubercle bacilli. Isolation and biological properties of a constituent of virulent organisms. J Exp Med 1950;91:197–217.

89. Noll H, Bloch H, Asselineau J, Lederer E. The chemical structure of the cord factor of *Mycobacterium tuberculosis*. Biochim Biophys Acta 1956;20:299–399.

90. Lemaire G, Tenu J-P, Petit J-F, Lederer E. Natural and synthetic trehalose diesters as immunomodulators. Med Res Rev 1986;6:243–72.

91. Ribi E, Mclaughlin CA, Cantrell JL, et al. Immunotherapy for tumors with microbial constituents of their synthetic analogues. A review. In: M.D. Anderson Hospital & Tumor Institute, eds. Immunotherapy of human cancer. New York: Raven Press; 1978:131–54.

92. Numata F, Nishimura K, Ishida H, et al. Lethal and and adjuvant activities of cord factor (trehalose-6,6'-dimycolate) and synthetic analogs in mice. Chem Pharm Bull 1985;33:4544–55.

93. Numata F, Ishida H, Nishimura K, et al. Lethal toxicity and adjuvant activity of synthetic trehalose monomycolate and related compounds. J Carbohydr Chem 1986;5:127–38.

94. Imoto M, Yoshimura H, Kusumoto S, et al. Chemical synthesis of phosphorylated tetraacyl disaccharide corresponding to a biosynthetic precursor of lipid A. Tetrahedron Lett 1985;26: 907–8.

95. Imoto M, Yoshimura H, Kusumoto S, Shiba T. Total synthesis of lipid A, active principle of bacterial endotoxin. Proc Jpn Academy Ser B 1984;60:285–8.

96. Imoto M, Yoshimura H, Shimamoto T, et al. Total synthesis of *Escherichia coli* lipid A, the endotoxically active principle of cell-surface lipopolysaccharide. Bull Chem Soc Jpn 1987;60:2205–14.

97. Kotani S, Takada H, Tsujimoto M, et al. Synthetic lipid A with endotoxic and related biological activities comparable to those of a natural lipid A from an *Escherichia coli* Re murant. Infect Immun 1985;49:225–37.

98. Takahashi I, Kotani S, Takada H, et al. Requirement of a properly acylated β(1-6)-D-glucosamine disaccharide bisphosphate structure for efficient manifestation of full endotoxic and associated bioactivities of lipid A. Infect Immun 1987;55:57–68.

99. Kiso M, Tanaka S, Fujita M, et al. Synthesis of the optically active 4-O-phosphono-D-glucosamine derivatives related to the nonreducing sugar subunit of bacterial lipid A. Carbohydr Res 1987;162:127–40.

100. Kiso M, Tanaka S, Fujita M, et al. Synthesis of nonreducing-sugar subunit analogs of bacterial lipid A carrying an amide-bound (3R)-3-acyl-oxytetradecanoyl group. Carbohydr Res 1987;162:247–56.

101. Kumazawa Y, Nakatsuka M, Takimoto H, et al. Importance of fatty acid substituents of chemically synthesized lipid A-subunit analogs in the expression of im-

munopharmacological activity. Infect Immun 1988;56:149–55.

102. Saiki I, Maeda H, Sakurai T, et al. Induction of endogenous tumor necrosis factor in mice by murine recombinant interferon-γ combined with low toxic lipid A analogs. Cancer Immunol Immunother (in press).

Molecular and cellular multihit attack against tumor cells with immunostimulants

Takato O. Yoshida, Soichi Haraguchi, Tetsumichi Matsuo

Department of Microbiology and Immunology, Hamamatsu University School of Medicine, Hamamatsu, Japan

Introduction

Experimental immunotherapy of cancer in animals has been widely attempted using immunomodulators or immunostimulants and the modes of action have been elucidated in detail (1). Such an accumulation of experimental data has led to clinical applications in human cancer. Marked progress in research in immunology has been made, especially in immunogenetics. In research on complex immunological phenomena, mice with well-known immunogenetic constitutions have been useful. Congenic and recombinant mice are expected to be powerful tools for use in researching the modes of action of immunomodulators or immunostimulants.

It has been reported that host responses to immunomodulators or immunostimulants such as lipopolysaccharides (LPS) (2,3), BCG (4–6), levamisole (7), and muramyl dipeptide (MDP) (8) are genetically controlled. However, with the exception of some reports on the antitumor effect of BCG by Tokunaga et al (9), lentinan by Zákány et al (10), and BCG for childhood acute lymphocytic leukemia (ALL) by Tursz et al (11), there has been little research on the antitumor effect of immunopotentiators or immunostimulants using an immunogenetic approach.

We have been extensively involved in studies on the immunogenetic recognition of and resistance to non-virus-producing tumor cells induced by the Schmidt-Ruppin strain of Rous sarcoma virus (RSV) in syngeneic, H-2 congenic, and H-2 recombinant B10 mice (12–16). Using this system, we have undertaken a new evaluation and in vitro analysis of the antitumor activity of immunopotentiators or immunostimulants from an immunogenetic viewpoint (17–20).

In this paper we first summarize the antitumor activity of *Nocardia rubra* cell wall skeleton (N-CWS) and the host genetic influences on that activity existing within RSV-induced syngeneic tumor systems. We also suggest how the cellular immune response in vitro might be reflected in the in vivo antitumor activity, focusing on the difference in antitumor effect of N-CWS in responding B10 and nonresponding B10.A strains of mice (19). Second, we analyze tumor rejection mechanisms using N-CWS in nude mice and suggest that molecular and cellular multihit attacks against tumor cells are necessary for tumor immunotherapy.

Materials and methods

The advantages of using RSV-induced mouse syngeneic tumor systems for studies of the host immunogenetic influence on immunostimulant activity are the following:

1. Common tumor-specific surface antigens exist among RSV-induced tumor cell lines derived from rats and mice detected by the complement-dependent cytotoxicity method, but do not exist on other tumor cells and normal mouse cells, as shown in Table 1 (14).

2. Common tumor-specific surface antigens related to tumor rejection in vivo exist on RSV-induced tumor cells derived from B10 congenic and recombinant strains, and inbred strains of mice, but not on methylcholanthrene (MC)-induced tumor cells tested in BALB/c nu/nu mice, reconstituted with CSA9F-immune T lymphocytes, as shown in Table 2.

Mice

Eight- to 20-week-old male and female C57BL/10 (B10) (H-2^b), B10.BR (H-2^k), B10.D2 (H-2^d), B10.A (H-2^a), and B10.A(5R) (H-2^{i5}) inbred mice were maintained in our laboratory. Six- to 8-week-old male and female BALB/cCr inbred and BALB/cCr nu/nu mice were supplied by the Shizuoka Agricultural Cooperative Association for Laboratory Animals (Hamamatsu). The reciprocal F1 hybrid male and female mice, (B10.A × BALB/c)F1 hybrid mice, and (BALB/c × B10.A)F1 hybrid mice were bred in our laboratory.

Tumors and cultured cell lines

Subcutaneous tumors, S1018(B10) and B10SA2F from female B10 mice, S623(BR) from a female B10.BR mouse, S908(D2) from a male B10.D2 mouse, S826(BA) and B10ABr1F from female B10.A mice, S322(5R) from a female B10.A(5R) mouse, CSA9F from a female BALB/cCr mouse, and CSA1M from a male BALB/cCr mouse were all initially induced in newborn mice using the Schmidt-Ruppin strain of RSV (12). MC-induced intramuscular tumors, MCSA4M from a male BALB/cCr mouse, MCSA6M from a male B10.D2 mouse, MCSA1M from a male B10.A, and MCSAB10(5R) from a male B10.A(5R) mouse were initially induced in adult mice. These cell lines were established as monolayer cell cultures for each tumor. Meth A from a BALB/c mouse, an established cultured tumor cell line, was used. They were maintained in RPMI-1640 supplemented with 5–10% fetal calf serum, penicillin G (100 U/ mL), and streptomycin (100 µg/mL). These cells are usually non-RSV-producing, except in chickens where the virus is produced. They carried the RSV *src*

Table 1 Cytotoxic sensitivity of rat and mouse cells to antisera against RSV structural components and syngeneic antiserum against a rat fibroblast cell line transformed by an *env* gene deletion mutant of SR-RSV (NY8-3Y1). Reprinted, with permission, from Kuzumaki N, Minakawa H, Matsuo T, et al (14).

Cells	Cytotoxic titer* with antisera against		
	AMV gp85[env]	RSVPr76[gap]	NY8-3Y1
Rat ASV tumors			
SR–3Y1	—	—	320
NY8–3Y1	—	—	640
ts68–3Y1 (p)[†]	—	—	80
ts68–3Y1 (np)[‡]	—	—	—[§]
B77–3Y1	160	—	20
Other rat tumor			
Sp6	—	—	—
Normal rat cells			
3Y1	—	—	—
Mouse RSV tumors			
CSA1M	—	—	40
CSA9F	—	—	20
CBr2F	—	—	80
S908D2	—	—	40
B6SA1M	—	—	80
B6SA3F	—	—	80
C3SA1F	—	—	40
Other mouse tumors			
MCSA1F	—	—	—
MCSA4M	—	—	—
RL♂1	—	—	—
BW5147	—	—	—
Normal mouse cells			
BAL/c embryo cells	—	—	—
BALB/c splenocytes	—	—	—

*Reciprocal of serum dilution producing more than 0.20 of cytotoxic index. Mean value of 3 repeated experiments. [†]Cultivated at the permissive temperature. [‡]Cultivated at the nonpermissive temperature. [§]No positive reaction at 1:10 serum dilution.

gene product pp60 as detected by the SDS-PAGE method, and possessed tumor-specific surface antigen (TSSA) related to pp60[src]. They did not carry the RSV envelope gp85 as determined by a cytotoxicity test with complement using rabbit anti-gp85 antibody (14).

N-CWS

N-CWS was used as a lyophilized preparation formulated with N-CWS 2 mg,

Table 2 Growth (+) and regression (−) of various tumors in BALB/c nu/nu mice, reconstituted with CSA9F-immune lymphocytes.

Mouse	RSV-induced tumor*	MC-induced tumor*	Experiment				
			1	2	3	4	5
BALB/c	CSA9F		−	−	−	−	
	CSA1M		−				
		MCSA4M	+	+	+		
		Meth A	+			+	
B10	S1018B10			−	−		
B10BR	S623BR			−	−		
B10D2	S908D2			−	−		−
		MCSA6M					+
B10A	S826BA			−	−		−
		MCSA1M					+
B10A(5R)	S3225R			−	−	−	
		MCSAB10(5R)	+	+	+		

*All tumors grew in nontreated nude mice, and killed the hosts.
No. of injected tumor cells: 2×10^5 or 5×10^5.

squalene 4 mg, polysorbate 80 1 mg, and mannitol 28.2 mg (21). A placebo with the same formulation without N-CWS was used as a control (donated by Fujisawa Pharmaceutical Co., Osaka). Both preparations were reconstituted and suspended in saline in doses equivalent to those of N-CWS, for instance, placebo "100 μg" corresponded to N-CWS 100 μg.

Mixed inoculation of N-CWS with tumor cells

Live cultured tumor cells (2×10^5) mixed with N-CWS 100 μg or placebo in 0.1 mL were inoculated intradermally into the shaved right flank of mice in the syngeneic system. The resulting tumors were measured for growth at weekly or more frequent intervals.

Intratumoral administration of N-CWS for tumor treatment

Mice were pretreated using the following procedures. 1) N-CWS 100 μg in 0.1 mL was administered intradermally into the skin of the left flank of mice 3 weeks before tumor cell inoculation, and then subcutaneously in the left groin area 1 week before the inoculation. Placebo was given as a control in the same way. 2) N-CWS 100 μg was mixed with mitomycin C (MMC; Kyowa Hakko, Tokyo)-treated tumor cells (1×10^6) in 0.1 mL, and intradermally inoculated into the left flank of mice 3 weeks before inoculation with tumor cells. Three groups served as the controls; 1 was given a mixed inoculation of placebo and tumor cells, the 2nd was given an inoculation of N-CWS alone, and the 3rd was given an inoculation of placebo alone.

All the pretreated mice were inoculated intradermally with tumor cells (5×10^5 in 0.1 mL) into the shaved flank opposite to the pretreatment side (right side). About 1 week later, when the tumors had grown to a diameter of 3–5 mm, 0.05 mL (100 μg) of N-CWS or placebo in saline was injected into each tumor once a week for 5 to 6 weeks using a 27-gauge needle. Just before each intratumoral injection of N-CWS, the tumor mass was measured at its widest (2a) and narrowest (2b) diameters with a caliper. The tumor size was calculated as follows: tumor size (mm^3) = $4/3\pi ab^2$. Tumor growth or regression was followed weekly for 17 weeks (11–12 weeks after completion of N-CWS treatment).

Mitogenic assay

The spleens of 2 untreated mice were aseptically excised and teased apart on a glass slide in RPMI-1640 medium containing 5% FCS. Spleen cells were then separated from the crude mixture by a conventional density-gradient centrifugation. Using a U-type microplate (no. 163320, Nunc, Denmark), mouse spleen cells (2×10^6/well) were cultured with 10 μg of N-CWS in 0.2 mL of RPMI-1640 containing 10% FCS for 48 h at 37°C in 5% CO_2. Then ^{3}H-TdR was added at 0.5 μCi/well and the plate was incubated for another 18 h. The mitogenic activity of N-CWS was assayed from the ^{3}H-TdR uptake into spleen cells, measured by the same procedure as that for the above cytostatic assay, and expressed as follows: Δcpm = cpm in the N-CWS group – cpm in the placebo group.

Analysis of tumor rejection mechanisms in nude mice, mixed inoculation of N-CWS with tumor cells, and additional intratumoral administration of immune T cell subsets and factors

Live cultured CSA9F tumor cells (2 or 5×10^5) mixed with N-CWS 100 μg or placebo in 0.1 mL were intradermally inoculated into female BALB/cCr nu/nu mice, and 4 or 5 days after inoculation of the mixture, CSA9F-immune or -nonimmune T cell subsets (1×10^6), and recombinant human interleukin 2 (IL-2) and recombinant A/D interferon (A/D IFN) were inoculated into the tumors consisting of tumor cells and inflammatory cells.

Treatment of BALB/c nu/nu mice with antiasialo GM1

Rabbit anti-AGM1 and normal rabbit serum were intraperitoneally inoculated into BALB/c nu/nu mice to decrease natural killer (NK) cell and macrophage activity.

Results

Antitumor activity of N-CWS within RSV-induced syngeneic tumor systems of B10, B10.BR, B10.D2, B10.A, and B10.A(5R) mice

The antitumor activity of N-CWS against RSV-induced mouse tumors in 5 syngenic systems is shown in Table 3. The development and growth of the tumors in both males and females of B10 strain mice were completely suppressed in all test mice (100%); the tumors in B10.A(5R) mice were completely suppressed in 23 of the 25 mice tested (92%); and the tumors in B10.BR mice were completely suppressed in 7 of the 14 mice tested (50%). In each of these cured mice, the tumor inoculation site was slightly swollen in the 1st week, with tumor suppression being complete within 2 to 4 weeks following the mixed inoculation with N-CWS. In contrast, the tumors in B10.D2 mice and the tumors in B10.A mice were not suppressed at all (0%). In all experiments with mice given a mixture of tumor cells and placebo, all animals died with tumors within 3 to 6 weeks following inoculation.

These results by themselves indicate that there is a strain difference in the antitumor activity of N-CWS in mice, suggesting that the genetic makeup of the host and major histocompatibility complexes may play an important role.

Antitumor activity of N-CWS in B10.A F1 hybrid mice

A simple question arose from analyzing the results in Table 3, ie, was the suppression of tumor development and growth mainly related to different tumor sensitivities or to the genetic makeup of the host? In an attempt to answer this question, further studies were conducted using B10.A F1 hybrid strains reciprocally bred with a strain responding to N-CWS, BALB/c, as shown in Table 4. These data strongly suggest that the tumor cell suppression mechanisms induced in mice by N-CWS are related to the genetic makeup of the host.

Effect of intratumoral administration of N-CWS on syngeneic tumors in B10 and B10.A mice

The following experiments focused on the strain difference in tumor response to N-CWS previously observed between B10 and B10.A strains. In contrast to the previous experimental protocol, tumor cells were first inoculated, and, after reaching a certain size, N-CWS was injected into each tumor (see "Materials and methods").

The results for B10 mice bearing syngeneic S101B(B10) tumors are shown in Fig 1 and for B10.A mice bearing syngeneic S326(BA) tumors in Fig 2. In N-CWS-pretreated B10 mice (Fig 1A), a significant antitumor effect on S1018(B10) tumors was observed with intratumoral N-CWS in 4 of the 5 mice; tumor growth began dramatically to regress, beginning 3–4 weeks after the last dose of N-CWS, and attaining complete regression at 12 weeks. No tumor regression was seen in either the placebo-treated or the nontreated group. In the placebo-pretreated B10

Table 3 Antitumor activity of N-CWS within RSV-induced syngeneic tumor systems of B10, B10.BR, B10.D2, B10.A, and B10.A(5R) mice.* Reprinted, with permission, from Haraguchi S, Kurakata S, Matsuo T, Yoshida TO (19).

Mouse		Tumor	Experiment no.	Sex	Complete suppression[†]	
H-2 region (KAESD)					N-CWS	Placebo
B10	bbbbb	S1018(B10)	1	M	4/4	0/3
				F	4/4	0/3
			2	M	5/5	0/4
				F	5/5	0/4
			Total (%)‡		18/18 (100)	0/14 (0)
		B10SA2F	1	M	6/6	0/2
				F	7/7	0/2
			Total (%)		13/13 (100)	0/4 (0)
B10.BR	kkkkk	S623(BR)	1	M	ND	ND
				F	2/5	0/5
			2	M	3/5	0/2
				F	2/5	0/5
			Total (%)		7/14 (50)	0/12 (0)
B10.D2	ddddd	S908(D2) (B10)	1	M	0/4	0/4
				F	0/2	0/2
			2	M	0/4	0/2
				F	0/4	0/1
			Total (%)		0/14 (0)	0/9 (0)
B10.A	kkkdd	S826(BA)	1	M	ND	ND
				F	0/5	0/4
			2	M	0/5	0/4
				F	0/5	0/5
			3	M	0/7	0/6
				F	0/4	0/3
			4	M	0/5	0/3
				F	0/5	0/4
			Total (%)		0/36 (0)	0/29 (0)
		B10ABr1F	1	M	0/6	0/3
				F	0/6	0/4
			Total (%)		0/12 (0)	0/7 (0)
B10.A(5R)	bbkdd	S322(5R)	1	M	ND	ND
				F	3/3	0/3
			2	M	2/3	0/2
				F	3/3	0/2
			3	M	11/12	0/3
				F	4/4	0/2
			Total (%)		23/25 (92)	0/12 (0)

*A mixture of N-CWS 100 μg and tumor cells (2 × 10⁵) was inoculated intradermally into syngeneic mice. [†]No. of tumor-free mice/no. of mice inoculated. ‡%: Percent of mice in which tumor cell growth was completely suppressed. ND, not done.

Table 4 Antitumor activity of N-CWS in F1 hybrid mice.* Reprinted, with permission, from Haraguchi S, Kurakata S, Maatsuo T, Yoshida TO (19).

Tumor	Mice	Experiment no.	Sex	Complete suppression[†]	
				N-CWS	Placebo
S826(BA)	B10A	1	M	0/7	0/6
			F	0/4	0/3
		2	M	0/3	0/3
			F	0/3	0/3
		Total (%)[‡]		0/17(0)	0/15(0)
	(BA × C)F1[§]	1	M	7/7	0/4
			F	7/10	0/3
		2	M	3/3	ND
			F	5/5	ND
		Total (%)		22/25(88)	0/7(0)
	(C × BA)F1[§]	1	M	5/6	0/3
			F	5/7	0/3
		2	M	2/2	ND
			F	5/5	ND
		Total (%)		17/20(85)	0/6(0)
CSA9F	BALB/c	1	M	4/4	0/3
			F	5/5	0/3
		Total (%)		9/9(100)	0/6(0)
	(BA × C)F1	1	M	5/5	0/3
			F	2/2	ND
		2	M	ND	ND
			F	4/5	0/3
		Total (%)		11/12(92)	0/6(0)
	(C × BA)F1	1	M	4/5	0/2
			F	8/8	0/4
		Total (%)		12/13(92)	0/6(0)

*A mixture of N-CWS 100 μg and tumor cells (2 × 10^5) was inoculated intradermally into syngeneic mice and F1 reciprocal hybrid mice. [†]No. of tumor-free mice/no. of mice inoculated. [‡]%: Percent of mice in which tumor cell growth was completely suppressed. [§](BA × C)F1: (B10.A × BALB/d)F1/ (C × BA)F1: (BALB/c × B10.A)F1. ND, not done.

mice (Fig 1B), complete tumor regresssion was seen in 2 of 5 mice given intratumoral N-CWS, but it was not seen in either the placebo-treated or non-treated groups. In the B10 mice pretreated with MMC-treated S1018(B10) tumor cells and/or test agent (Fig 1C), subsequent intratumoral N-CWS completely regressed tumor growth in 2 of 5 mice in the N-CWS-pretreated group and in 3 of 4 mice in the N-CWS plus MMC-treated tumor cell-pretreated group. Com-

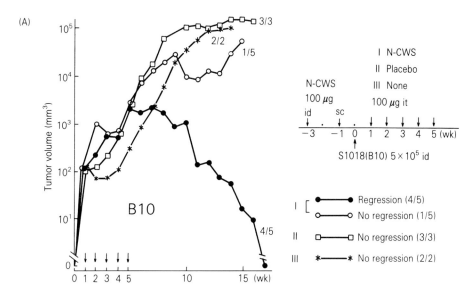

Fig 1 Effect of intratumoral injection of N-CWS on sygeneic tumors in B10 mice. (A) N-CWS-pretreated mice.

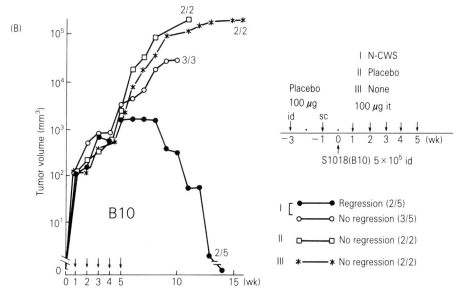

Fig 1 Effect of intratumoral injection of N-CWS on sygeneic tumors in B10 mice. (B) Placebo-pretreated mice.

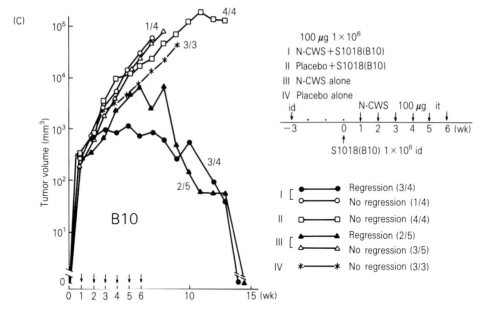

Fig 1 Effect of intratumoral injection of N-CWS on sygeneic tumors in B10 mice. (C) Mice pretreated with MMC-treated S1018 (B10) tumor cells and/or test agent.

plete tumor regression was not seen in the placebo-pretreated group, even after intratumoral administration of N-CWS.

A similar evaluation of the effect of N-CWS on tumor regression was made in the B10.A-S826(BA) tumor system. As shown in Fig 2A, 2B, and 2C, however, none of the mice showed complete tumor regression.

Thus, as in the experiments with simultaneous inoculation of N-CWS and live tumor cells, the antitumor activity of N-CWS was evident in B10 mice but not at all in B10.A mice, even with intratumoral administration.

Mitogenic activity of N-CWS on spleen cells of B10 congenic mice

Table 5 shows the results of the investigation of the mitogenic activity of N-CWS on spleen cells of B10, B10.BR, B10.D2, and B10.A mice. A significant strain difference in the splenocyte mitogenic activity of N-CWS was observed between B10 and B10.A mice. N-CWS showed moderate mitogenic activity on splenocytes of B10.BR and B10.D2 mice.

Antitumor activity of N-CWS combined with immune T cell subsets in BALB/c nu/nu mice

Table 6 summarizes the results of the analysis of tumor rejection mechanisms in BALB/c nu/nu mice. In BALB/c nu/nu mice, the mixed inoculations of N-CWS

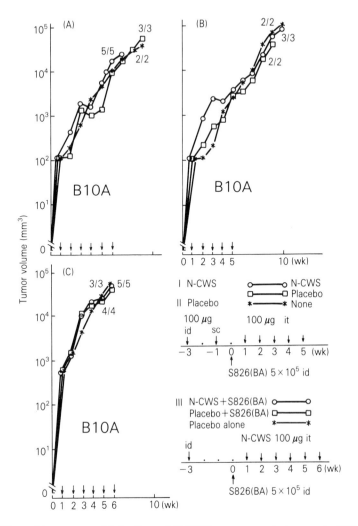

Fig 2 Effect of intratumoral injection of N-CWS on syngeneic tumors in B10.A mice.

with syngeneic CSA9F tumor cells did not suppress tumor growth at all (Fig 3). Therefore, additional intratumoral administration of T cells, recombinant human IL-2, and A/D IFN were administered to induce the suppression of tumor development and growth.

The additional intratumoral administration of immune Lyt2⁻ T cells (S.T Lyt2⁻) completely suppressed tumor growth in all test mice (100%) (Table 6, Fig 4). The additional intratumoral administration of immune Lyt1⁻ T cells (S.T Lyt1⁻) completely suppressed tumor growth in 3 of the 18 mice tested (17%). In contrast, each additional intratumoral administration of immune L3T4⁻ T cells (S.T L3T4⁻), normal Lyt1⁻, Lyt2⁻, and L3T4⁻ cells (N.T Lyt1⁻, N.T Lyt2⁻,

Table 5 Mitogenic activity of N-CWS on spleen cells of B10 congenic mice.* Reprinted, with permission, from Haraguchi S, Kurakata S, Matsuo T, Yoshida TO (19).

Experiment no.	Mice	Incorporation of ^{3}H-TdR (cpm)		Δcpm[†]
		Placebo	N-CWS	
1	B10	161 ± 11[‡]	1610 ± 128	1449
	B10.A	114 ± 15	339 ± 61	225
2	B10	106 ± 21	596 ± 11	490
	B10.A	232 ± 27	265 ± 76	33
3	B10	522 ± 24	2598 ± 787	2076
	B10.A	217 ± 18	792 ± 53	575
4	B10	143 ± 31	611 ± 61	468
	B10.BR	93 ± 15	267 ± 10	174
	B10.D2	106 ± 18	272 ± 6	166
	B10.A	64 ± 4	148 ± 6	84

*Mouse spleen cells (2 × 10^5) were cultured with N-CWS 10 μg for 6 h. Mitogenic activity of N-CWS in vitro was assessed in terms of ^{3}H-TdR (0.5 μCi/well) uptake into mouse spleen cells during the last 18 h of culture. [†]Δcpm = cpm in the N-CWS group − cpm in the placebo group. [‡]cpm ± SE.

Table 6 Antitumor activity of N-CWS combined with immune T cell subsets in BALB/c nu/nu mice.

Tumor cell	Immuno-stimulant	T cell subset	Experiment no.						Total
			1–3	4	5	6	7	8	
CSA9F	N-CWS		0/15*	0/3	0/1	0/2	0/21*		
2 × 10^5	Placebo		0/6	0/2			0/1	0/1	0/10
cells	N-CWS	S.T Lyt1$^-$		1/5	2/5	0/5	0/3		3/18
//	//	S.T Lyt2$^-$		5/5	5/5	4/4	3/3	5/5	22/22
//	//	S.T L3T4$^-$						0/5	0/5
//	//	N.T Lyt1$^-$				0/3	0/3		0/6
//	//	N.T Lyt2$^-$				0/3	0/3		0/6
//	//	N.T L3T4$^-$						0/2	0/2
//	Placebo	S.T Lyt1$^-$				0/2	0/2		0/4
//	//	S.T Lyt2$^-$				1/2	0/2		1/6
//	//	S.T L3T4$^-$						0/2	0/2
//	//	N.T Lyt2$^-$						0/2	0/2
//	//	N.T L3T4$^-$						0/2	0/2

*No. of complete suppressions/no. of tumors inoculated.

and N.T L3T4$^-$) did not suppress tumor growth at all (0%). The mixed inoculations of placebo with CSA9F cells, and each intratumoral administration of S.T Lyt1$^-$ and L3T4$^-$ cells, and N.T Lyt2$^-$ and L3T4$^-$ cells did not suppress tumor

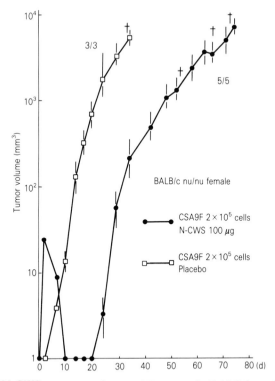

Fig 3   Effect of N-CWS on syngeneic CSA9F tumors in BALB/c nu/nu mice.

growth at all (0%), but S.T Lyt2⁻ cell group completely suppressed tumor growth in 1 of the 6 mice tested. Each additional intratumoral administration of IL-2 or A/D IFN showed a slight suppression of tumor development, but not of tumor growth (data not shown).

These data suggest that the tumor suppression mechanisms induced in mice by N-CWS are related to tumor-specific immune Lyt2⁻, L3T4⁺ cells.

Effect of NK cells and macrophages on the development of tumors in BALB/c nu/nu mice

Rabbit anti-AGM1 was intraperitoneally injected once before the mixed inoculations of N-CWS with CSA9F cells and 3 times after the inoculations into BALB/c nu/nu mice. Rabbit normal serum was used as the control in same protocol. Development of the tumors admixed with N-CWS was not inhibited in anti-AGM1-injected BALB/c nu/nu mice compared with normal rabbit serum-injected BALB/c nu/nu mice (Fig 5).

These data suggest that the activity of NK cells and macrophages decreases in

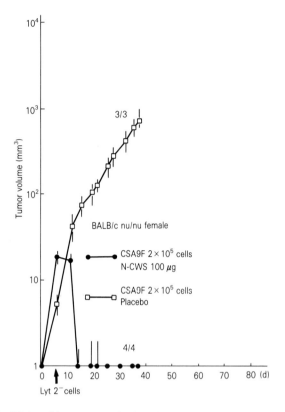

Fig 4 Effect of additional intratumoral administration of immune Lyt2 T cells into the admixed inoculation of N-CWS and CSA9F tumor cells in BALB/c nu/nu mice (experiment 6 in Table 6).

BALB/c nu/nu mice injected with anti-AGM1, and that tumor development is not suppressed by them.

Conclusions

An immunogenetic evaluation of the antitumor activity of the immunostimulant N-CWS was performed using non-virus-producing tumors induced by the Schmidt-Ruppin strain of RSV in B10 congenic and recombinant mice. Live tumor cells mixed with either N-CWS or a placebo control were inoculated intradermally into the right flank of syngeneic mice. With N-CWS, the development and growth of B10 mouse tumors in B10(H-2^b) mice were completely inhibited in all test mice. B10.A(5R) mouse tumor was completely suppressed in 23 of 25 B10.A(5R) (H-2^{i5}) mice, and B10.BR mouse tumor was completely suppressed in 7 of 14 B10.BR(H-2^k) mice. However, B10.D2 mouse tumor in B10.D2(H-2^d) mice and B10.A mouse tumorS in B10.A(H-2^a) mice were not sup-

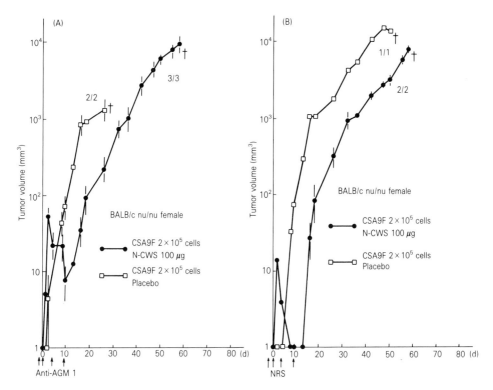

Fig 5 Effect of anti-AGM1 antibody on N-CWS-induced and -activated inflammatory cells in BALB/c nu/nu mice. Inhibition effects of tumor development by N-CWS-induced inflammatory cells, mainly NK cells and macrophages, were reduced by the administration of rabbit anti-AGM1 serum in BALB/c nu/nu mice (A), but were not reduced by the administration of rabbit normal serum (B).

pressed at all by N-CWS. N-CWS showed a marked antitumor effect in B10 mice, not only in mixed inoculation with the tumor cells but also with intratumoral administration. These effects were not seen in B10.A mice. Mitogenic activity of N-CWS on spleen cells was significantly different among B10 congenic mice; N-CWS induced greater blastogenesis of spleen cells from B10 mice than of those from B10.A mice, corresponding to the in vivo results showing strain differences. These results suggest that the immunogenetic background of the host may play an important role in cancer therapy with immunostimulants.

In addition, for analysis of tumor rejection mechanisms, the mixed inoculation of N-CWS with syngeneic RSV-induced tumor cells and additional intratumoral administration of immune T cell subsets and factors in BALB/c nu/nu mice were carried out. These data suggest that molecular and cellular multihit attack against tumor cells with immunostimulants is necessary for cancer therapy (Fig 6). This effect and/or model may be applied in the treatment of various kinds of tumor, especially tumor cells that are highly heterogenous.

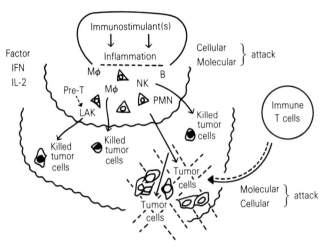

Fig 6 Molecular and cellular multihit attack against tumor cells.

Acknowledgments

We are most grateful to Professor Y. Yamamura and Professor I. Azuma for their encouragement of the N-CWS studies, and to Professor S. Fujimoto for supplying RSV-induced mouse tumor cell lines S1018(B10), S90B(D2), S623(BR), S826(BA), and S322(5R). This study was supported in part by a Grant-in-Aid for Cancer Research from the Ministry of Education, Science and Culture, Japan.

References

1. Terry WD, Yamamura Y, eds. Developments in immunology. Immunobiology and immunotherapy of cancer, vol 6. New York: Elsevier North-Holland; 1979.
2. McAdam KPWJ, Ryan JL. C57BL/10/CR mice: Nonresponders to activation by the lipid A moiety of bacterial lipopolysaccharide. J Immunol 1978;120:249–53.
3. Watson J, Kelly K, Largen M, Taylor BA. The genetic mapping of a defective LPS response gene in C3H/HeJ mice. J Immunol 1978;120:422–4.
4. Allen EM, Moore VL, Stevens JO. Strain variation in BCG-induced chronic pulmonary inflammation in mice. I. Basic model and possible genetic control by non-H-2 genes. J Immunol 1977;119:343–7.
5. Nakamura RM, Tokunaga T. Strain difference of delayed-type hypersensitivity to BCG and its genetic control in mice. Infect Immun 1978;22:657–64.
6. Goto Y, Nakamura RM, Takahashi H, Tokunaga T. Genetic control of resistance to *Mycobacterium intracellulare* infection in mice. Infect Immun 1984;46:135–40.
7. Renoux G, Renoux M, Gullaumin JM. Genetic and epigenetic control of levamisole-induced immunostimulation. Int J Immunopharm 1979;1:43–8.
8. Staruch MJ, Wood DD. Genetic influences on the adjuvanticity of muramyl dipeptide in vitro. J Immunol 1982;128:155–60.

9. Tokunaga T, Yamamoto S, Nakamura RM, et al. Mouse-strain difference in immunoprophylactic and immunotherapeutic effects of BCG on carcinogen-induced autochthonous tumors. Jpn J Med Sci Biol 1978;31:143–54.
10. Zákány J, Chihara G, Fachet J. Effect of lentinan on tumor growth in murine allogeneic and syngeneic hosts. Int J Cancer 1980;25:371–6.
11. Tursz T, Hors J, Lipinski M, Aamiel JL. HLA phenotypes in long-term survivors treated with BCG immunotherapy for childhood ALL. Br Med J 1978;1:1250–1.
12. Yoshida TO, Haraguchi S, Miyamoto H, Matsuo T. Recognition of RSV-induced tumor cells in syngeneic mice and semisyngeneic reciprocal hybrid mice. Gann Monogr 1979;23:201–12.
13. Kuzumaki N, Minakawa H, Miyazaki T, et al. Individually distinct tumor-specific cell surface antigen identified by monoclonal antibody on a Rous sarcoma virus-induced mouse tumor. J Natl Cancer Inst 1982;69:527–30.
14. Kuzumaki N, Minakawa H, Matsuo T, et al. Correlation between tumor-specific surface antigens and src gene expression in Rous sarcoma virus-induced rat tumors. Eur J Cancer Clin Oncol 1983;19:401–9.
15. Haraguchi S, Kurakata S, Fujii T, et al. Recognition of Rous sarcoma virus-induced tumor antigens by cytotoxic T lymphocytes (CTL): Studies on specificity of killing by CTL employing H-2 congenic and recombinant mouse tumor cells. Cell Immunol 1987;105:340–54.
16. Haraguchi S, Fujii T, Matsuo T, Yoshida TO. Mechanism of target cell lysis by cytotoxic T lymphocytes (CTL) employing RSV-induced H-2 congenic and recombinant mouse tumor cells: Demonstration of soluble mediators released from H-2-restricted CTL clones. Cell Immunol 1988;112:279–92.
17. Yoshida TO, Haraguchi S, Matsuo T, et al. Evaluation of antitumor activity of immunopotentiator, *N. rubra*-CWS within syngeneic tumor system of B10 congenic and recombinant mice. Cancer Immunol Parasite Immunol, INSERM 1980;97:105–14.
18. Yoshida TO, Haraguchi S, Matsuo T, et al. Antitumor activity of *N. rubra*-CWS within syngeneic tumor system of B10 congenic and recombinant mice. In: Yamamura Y, Kotani S, Azuma I, et al, eds. Immunomodulation by microbial products and related synthetic compounds. Tokyo: Excerpta Medica;1982:377–80.
19. Haraguchi S, Kurakata S, Matsuo T, Yoshida TO. Strain differences in the antitumor activity of an immunopotentiator, *Nocardia rubra* cell-wall skeleton, in B10 congenic and recombinant mice. Jpn J Cancer Res (Gann) 1985;76:400–13.
20. Yoshida TO, Haraguchi S, Matsuo T. Immunogenetic evaluation of antitumor activity of OK-432 within syngeneic tumor system of B10 congenic mice. In: Ishida N, ed. Mechanisms of antitumor effects of OK-432. Tokyo: Excerpta Medica;1986:228–39.
21. Yamawaki M, Azuma I, Saiki I, et al. Antitumor activity of squalene-treated cell-wall skeleton of *Nocardia rubra* in mice. Jpn J Cancer Res (Gann) 1978;69:619–26.

Chemical structure of *Nocardia rubra* cell wall skeleton

Shigetaka Koda, Mamoru Fujioka, Yukiyoshi Morimoto

Analytical Research Laboratories, Fujisawa Pharmaceutical Co., Ltd., Osaka, Japan

Introduction

Nocardia rubra cell wall skeleton (N-CWS) is the purified cell wall skeleton from *N. rubra* (1) strain no. AN-115, consisting of 3 major components. The mode of linkage between the components and the constituents of each component is presented in Fig 1. (Organisms labeled *N. rubra* should now properly be considered as members of the genus *Rhodococcus*, species *lentifragmentus*.)

Mycolic acids are long-chain α-branched β-hydroxy fatty acids, and those in N-CWS have from 38–50 carbon atoms with a saturated straight chain at the α-position (α-chain) and an unsaturated straight chain at the β-position (β-chain) containing 1 or 2 double bonds (2). Arabinogalactan is a polysaccharide composed of D-arabinose and D-galactose, together with small amounts of neutral sugars such as mannose, glucose, and rhamnose (3–5). N-CWS contains only rhamnose as a minor component. Peptidoglycan comprises a glycan moiety composed of disaccharide units, *N*-acetyl-D-glucosamyl-*N*-glycolyl-D-muramic acid, and a tetrapeptide moiety composed of D- and L-alanine, D-glutamic acid, and *meso*-diaminopimelic acid. In addition to these components, lipopeptide, which seems to be essential to N-CWS, has recently been identified (6).

Mycolic acids are bound to the arabinose residue of arabinogalactan by an ester linkage. The presence of a phosphodiester linkage has been demonstrated in various bacterial walls (4,5,7,8), and this is also the case in N-CWS. As well as the phosphodiester linkage, a glycosidic linkage between the *N*-acetyl-D-glucosamine residue of peptidoglycan and arabinogalactan is present in the wall of N-CWS (9). Structure and linkage details are discussed below.

Source and preparation

N. rubra (family Nocardiaceae, order Actinomycetales), found mainly in the soil, is a gram-negative and weakly acid-fast bacterium, easily cultured aerobical-

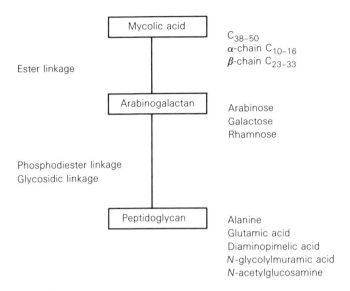

Fig 1 Constituents of N-CWS (major components in frames).

ly in synthetic media. Strain no. AN-115, found in the soil of Takarazuka City, Japan, was selected for the preparation of N-CWS.

The organisms are grown in neutral medium containing dextrose, polypeptone, yeast extract, and inorganic salts such as KH_2PO_4 and $MgSO_4$. After incubation is terminated, the cells are harvested by centrifugation, washed with water, and disrupted mechanically in a mill. The disrupted cells are then treated with deoxyribonuclease and ribonuclease in barbital (Veronal) buffer solution (pH 7.5) to remove nucleic acids. The enzyme-treated cell suspensions are centrifuged and the cell wall fraction is collected. This fraction is washed successively with acetone, a detergent solution (Triton X-100), and a mixture of ethanol and water to remove lipids and cell membranes. The residue is collected by centrifugation, washed with water, and deproteinated with protease in barbital/HCl buffer solution (pH 9.5). The sedimented cell walls are washed with water and a mixture of 1,2-dichloroethane and ethanol, and finally dried in vacuo. These are broken up in a mill, passed through a sieve (125 μm), and the resulting materials designated N-CWS. The chemical composition of N-CWS thus obtained is presented in Table 1 (9).

Structure of mycolic acids

Mycolic acids are lipids characteristic of the cell walls of the gram-positive bacteria *Corynebacterium*, *Mycobacterium*, *Nocardia*, and *Rhodococcus*, and can be obtained from ether extracts of alkali hydrolysates of the cell walls. Even

Table 1 Chemical composition of N-CWS.

Component		Content (%)
Lipid	Mycolic acid	27.6
Arabinogalactan	Arabinose	15.2
	Galactose	8.9
	Rhamnose	0.9
Peptidoglycan	Muramic acid	6.2
	Glutamic acid	5.8
	Alanine	8.5
	Diaminopimelic acid	7.2
	Glucosamine	4.8
	Other amino acids*	7.0
Total phosphorus		0.09
Residue on ignition		0.46
Loss on drying		7.2

*Threonine, serine, glycine, leucine, and phenylalanine.

among the same genera and strains there are structural differences resulting from varying chain lengths and from the nature of substituents particularly on the main chain (10–15). Mycolic acids from *Nocardia* are collectively known as nocardic acids and are characterized by carbon numbers ranging from C_{40} to C_{60}, and chain structures in which the α-chain is a saturated straight chain and the β-chain is an unsaturated straight chain containing 1 to 3 double bonds (15).

Structure elucidation of mycolic acids is routinely carried out by gas chromatography and mass spectrometry (GC/MS) after conversion of the acids to trimethylsilylated methyl mycolates (16). To characterize the mycolic acids isolated from N-CWS, we successfully applied field desorption mass spectrometry, a recently developed soft ionization technique which usually requires no derivatization (17).

Molecular species were shown to be distributed from C_{38} to C_{50}, and major components were C_{44}, C_{46}, and C_{48} mono- and dienoic β-hydroxy fatty acids. Pyrolysis GC/MS (18) of N-CWS methyl mycolates revealed that the α-branch is mainly a saturated straight C_{12} or C_{14} chain, and that the main chain (β-chain) has C_{29} or C_{31} carbons with 1 or 2 double bonds. Longer chain components tended to contain greater numbers of double bonds (14). These structures were similar to those of the mycolic acids of *N. rubra* previously reported by Yano et al (19) and Tomiyasu et al (20).

Proton nuclear magnetic resonance (NMR) spectroscopy of the N-CWS mycolic acids showed that the double bonds in the β-chain have *cis* conformations exclusively.

A method developed by Asselineau and Asselineau (21) and Tocanne and Asselineau (22) for determining the absolute configuration of mycolic acids was applied to the N-CWS mycolic acids, and it was shown that the absolute configurations of the α- and β-asymmetric carbon atoms are R. The chemical structure of the mycolic acid, with C_{46} and 2 double bonds, is shown in Fig 2 as an example of an N-CWS mycolic acid (2).

Structure of arabinogalactan

Arabinogalactan is a common polysaccharide of the cell walls of *Corynebacterium*, *Mycobacterium*, and *Nocardia*, and is regarded as the main antigenic polysaccharide (23). Mild alkaline hydrolysis under anaerobic conditions is generally used to liberate the arabinogalactan fraction from the cell wall (24,25).

The N-CWS arabinogalactan fraction was obtained by alkaline hydrolysis (NaOH 1M at 70°C for 72 h under anaerobic conditions) followed by dialysis, and was then purified by column chromatography on Dowex 50 W × 8 model and DEAE-cellulose. The relative molecular mass of the isolated main fraction of N-CWS arabinogalactan was found to be 50 000 by high-performance gel permeation chromatography on a G-2000 SW column (Toso Co., Ltd., Japan). This value was similar to that obtained from *Mycobacterium* reported by Misaki et al (23).

Rhamnose (Rha) was found to be one of the intrinsic constituents of the N-CWS arabinogalactan in which the molar ratio of Ara, Gal, and Rha was 2.5 : 1.0 : 0.1.

Misaki et al (23) studied the immunologic and chemical properties of arabinogalactans isolated from various *Mycobacterium* strains, finding that they were immunologically identical and chemically very similar, including their compositions. They proposed a general structure for those arabinogalactans that was based on the results of mass spectrometry and on using the techniques of permethylation and Smith degradation. Abou-zeid et al (26) also reported the structure of arabinogalactans isolated from a group of corynebacteria. Some minor differences in structure were observed, but the basic structures are likely to be common among *Mycobacterium*, *Corynebacterium*, and *Nocardia*.

The configuration of the D-galactose residues in the arabinogalactan still remains ambiguous (23,26–29). Misaki et al (23) have postulated that galactose

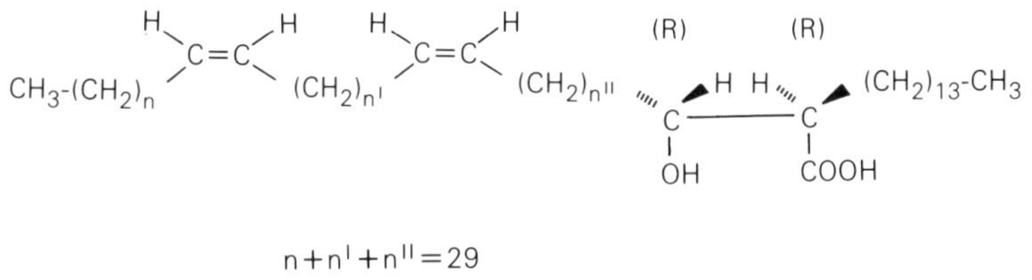

$$n+n^I+n^{II}=29$$

Fig 2 Structure of the $C_{46:2}$ mycolic acid of N-CWS. Reprinted, with permission, from Koda S, Fujioka M, Shigi M, et al (2).

residues exist in a galactopyranose form in the arabinogalactan of *Mycobacterium* strains. Vilkas et al (29) reported a galactofuranose residue in the arabinogalactan of *Mycobacterium tuberculosis* by identifying 6-O-D-galactofuranosyl-D-galactose using a partial acid hydrolysis of the walls and wax D fraction. Recently we have demonstrated by ^{1}H- and ^{13}C-NMR studies that the galactose residues of the N-CWS arabinogalactan are β-galactofuranoses and not β-galactopyranoses (30). In our study, the isolated and purified arabinogalactan was directly analyzed without introducing any derivatization techniques that could cause unfavorable structural changes. Therefore β-galactofuranose is the most plausible form in the N-CWS arabinogalactan. Our GC/MS study on galactose-oligomers isolated from a partial acid hydrolysate of the N-CWS arabinogalactan showed that at least the nonreducing terminal of the galactose residues takes a furanose configuration (31), agreeing with the NMR results.

Field desorption mass spectrometry on the partial hydrolysate revealed a galactose-pentadecamer and an arabinose-nonadecamer, which indicates the existence of monopolysaccharide partial structures in the N-CWS arabinogalactan. Permethylation and Smith degradation studies showed that -5(Araf)1-, -2(Araf)1-, (Araf)1-, -6(Galf)1-, -5(Galf)1-, and -3(Galf)1- are the straight-chain constituents, and -5(Araf)1-, -6(Galf)1-, and -6(Galf)1- are the branch-point residues. On the basis of these results, a ramified structure could be proposed for the N-CWS arabinogalactan (Fig 3).

Structure of peptidoglycan

Peptidoglycan, a highly cross-linked large molecule, is common to all bacterial cell walls. In the walls of *Mycobacterium*, *Corynebacterium*, and *Nocardia*, the

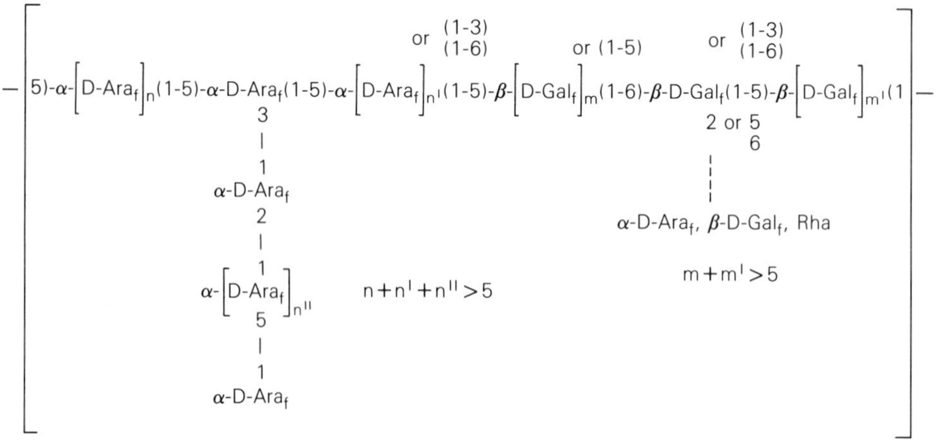

Fig 3 Structure of the N-CWS arabinogalactan.

peptidoglycan monomer consists of either *N*-acetylglucosamine (GlcNAc) linked 1–4 to *N*-acetylmuramic acid (MurNAc), or *N*-glycolylmuramic acid (MurNGl), to which a tetrapeptide chain—usually L-alanine-D-glutamic acid-*meso*-diaminopimelic acid-D-alanine (L-Ala-D-Glu-*meso*-Dap-D-Ala)—is attached (4,32–34). These monomer units are linked 1–4 at the disaccharide portion to form a linear polysaccharide backbone with the peptide side-chains. The linear polysaccharides are then cross-linked at the peptide portion, usually by a linkage between the COOH-terminal group of D-Ala and the ε-amino group of Dap. In some cases, other types of linkage between the 2 tetrapeptides such as Dap-Dap and Dap-Dap-Dap (in this case, the 2nd Dap is an intervening Dap residue) have been identified (35). Vacheron et al (34) demonstrated that the carboxyl groups of Glu and Dap that were not engaged in peptide bonds were amidated by mass spectrometry of permethylated and perdeuteriomethylated derivatives of purified tetrapeptide from the walls of *Nocardia* sp.

We studied the structure of the peptidoglycan of N-CWS mainly by mass spectrometry. Mild acid hydrolysis decomposed the arabinogalactan part, and the resulting material was washed with organic solvents and water repeatedly to obtain a purified peptidoglycan fraction of N-CWS.

Amino acid analysis of the isolated peptidoglycan showed that Mur, GlcN, Ala, Glu, Dap, and ammonia were in a molar ratio of 0.9 : 0.9 : 2.0 : 1.0 : 1.1 : 1.4. The glycan part was shown to be constituted by *N*-acetylglucosamyl-(1–4)-*N*-glycolylmuramic acid units when compared with the mass spectrum of the permethylated derivative of lysozyme-digested N-CWS and that of the permethylated disaccharide from *Mycobacterium smegmatis*, reported by Vacheron (34).

The tetrapeptide structure of the N-CWS was confirmed by GC/MS on trifluoroethyl *O*-trimethylsilyl polyamino alcohol derivatives (36) of the partial acid hydrolysate. The linkage between the glycan part and the tetrapeptide, as well as the cross-linkage between the peptide units, was also confirmed by the same experiment. Once the sequences of Ala-Glu, Glu-Dap, and Dap-Ala were respectively identified, it was shown that the tetrapeptide sequence is Ala-Glu-Dap-Ala. Besides those oligopeptides, the lactylalanine sequence was found in the hydrolysate. Lactic acid must be an acid degradation product of the MurNGl constituent of the glycan, which therefore establishes that the NH_2-terminal alanine residue of the tetrapeptide is linked to the carboxyl group of the MurNGl of the glycan part by an amide bond.

Sequences Ala-Dap, Ala-Dap-Ala, and Dap-Dap were also found in the hydrolysate, which suggests that 2 types of cross-linkages occur between the COOH-terminal group of Ala and the ε-amino group of Dap, and between the ε-amino group of Dap and either the ε- or α-carboxyl group (in this case, the COOH-terminal Ala is absent) of Dap.

To determine the absolute configuration of the amino acids, we isolated 2 peptide fragments, Ala-Glu and Dap-Ala, by high performance liquid chromatography (HPLC) from the partial acid hydrolysate of peptidoglycan, and then hydrolyzed them completely. The absolute configurations of the Ala and Glu residues were determined by comparing the retention times with those of the authentic Ala and Glu in HPLC, by using an eluent containing a copper-L-amino acid derivative complex (37). The absolute configuration of the Dap residue was found to be *meso* in the same way. The tetrapeptide sequence of the monomer was thus determined to be L-Ala-D-Glu-*meso*-Dap-D-Ala in the N-CWS peptidoglycan. The Glu and Dap carboxyl groups not involved in peptide bonds are supposed to be amidated on the basis of the amino acid composition. A tentative structure of the N-CWS peptidoglycan dimer is shown in Fig 4.

As a way of estimating the degree of cross-linkage, the number of Dap residues having free amino groups has been determined by the dansylation technique (38) on the N-CWS peptidoglycan solubilized by lysozyme. The portion of Dap residues with free amino groups was estimated to be 20% of the total Dap residues, and therefore the portion with cross-linkage is 80%. This means that 5 units of the peptidoglycan monomer are linked together through Dap-Ala and Dap-Dap linkages (39).

Linkage between mycolic acid and arabinogalactan

The presence of arabinose mycolate fractions from human tubercle bacillus Aoyama B by Azuma and Yamamura (40) suggested that an ester linkage would exist between mycolic acid and arabinogalactan. After Azuma et al (41) and Markovits and Vilkas (42) independently showed that mycolic acid was attached to the C-5 position of the terminal arabinose residues of the arabinogalactan in *Mycobacterium tuberculosis* Aoyama, the arabinose mycolates have been identified not only from the walls of the mycobacteria, but also from *Nocardia brasiliensis* (43). Thus the ester linkage is undoubtedly the usual linkage form between mycolic acids and arabinogalactan.

Mild acid hydrolysis would cause random cleavage of glycosidic linkages in arabinogalactan, and would yield a complex of mycolic acids and oligosaccharides degraded from the arabinogalactan. Chloroform extracts of the hydrolysate of the N-CWS, which contains a complex mixture of glycolipids, was purified by thin layer chromatography and analyzed. ^{1}H-NMR spectroscopy of the complex revealed the presence of a lipid moiety and sugars. Gas chromatographic analyses of lipids and sugars of a complete acid hydrolysate of the complex showed the presence of mycolic acids and arabinose. The infrared absorption spectrum of the complex had a characteristic ester band (1720 cm^{-1}) which indicates that the mycolic acids are linked to the arabinogalactan through an ester bond in N-CWS.

Linkage between arabinogalactan and peptidoglycan

Since Liu and Gotschlich (7) showed the presence of a phosphodiester linkage between arabinogalactan and peptidoglycan by the isolation of muramic acid 6-phosphate in the walls of *Mycobacterium butyricus*, many studies have been carried out to identify the phosphodiester linkage in other bacterial walls (4,7,27,44).

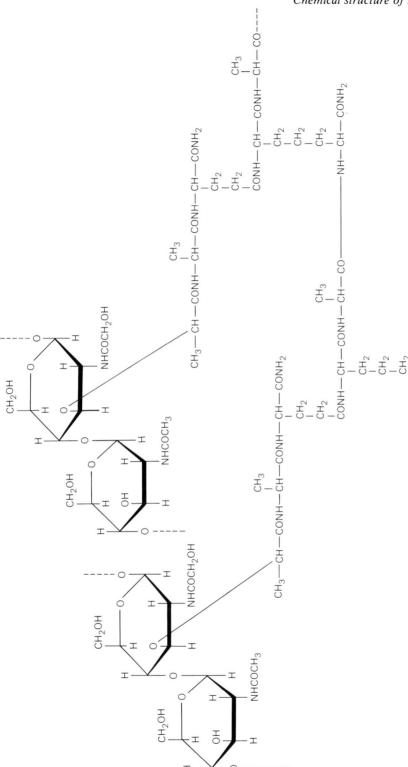

Fig 4   Structure of the N-CWS peptidoglycan dimer.

Finally, Amar and Vilkas (45) reported the isolation of an alkali-stable arabinose phosphate from the walls of *M. tuberculosis* H37Ra. These investigations resulted in the suggestion that arabinogalactan is linked to peptidoglycan through the phosphodiester bond between the arabinose residue and the muramic acid residue. Since muramic acid 6-phosphate has recently been isolated from N-CWS, and identified by ^{13}C-NMR study (46), the presence of a phosphodiester linkage between the arabinogalactan and the peptidoglycan in N-CWS could also be inferred.

Kanetsuna and Blas (27) reported that a glycosidic linkage might exist between the *N*-acetyl-D-glucosamine residue of the peptidoglycan and arabinogalactan in addition to the phophodiester linkage in the cell walls of *Mycobacterium*. However, there was insufficient evidence to prove this glycosidic linkage. We have recently found that alkaline treatment of N-CWS liberates not only the arabinogalactan fraction, but also large amounts of an additional polymer fraction composed of both arabinogalactan and peptidoglycan constituents (arabinogalactan-containing defective peptidoglycan). The isolated arabinogalactan still was contaminated by a very small amount of glucosamine, despite purification efforts. Since the phosphodiester linkage was readily broken by this alkaline treatment, these findings convinced us that other linkages besides the phosphodiester are present between the arabinogalactan and the peptidoglycan. Considering all the evidence obtained, we believe there might be a glycosidic linkage between the glucosamine residue of the peptidoglycan and the arabinogalactan.

Structural determination, which utilized GC/MS of a partial acid hydrolysate from the arabinogalactan-containing defective peptidoglycan from N-CWS, identified Gal-Rha-(1–3)-GlcNAc and Rha-(1–3)-GlcNAc as the oligosaccharides. As mentioned above, both Gal and Rha are constituents of the arabinogalactan, whereas GlcNAc is a constituent of the peptidoglycan. Thus, the presence of these 2 oligosaccharides strongly suggests a novel glycosidic linkage between the arabinogalactan and the peptidoglycan in N-CWS (9). A galactose-hexamer containing a Rha residue at the reducing terminal was identified in the partial acid hydrolysate by field desorption mass spectrometry (31). Therefore, it is deduced that the glycosidic linkage occurs at an end of the branched galactose oligomer of the arabinogalactan.

Other components (lipopeptide fraction)

Sohler et al (47) found large amounts of amino acids such as arginine, aspartic acid, glycine, lysine, serine, threonine, valine, phenylalanine, leucine, and isoleucine, which do not belong to the peptidoglycan in the walls of *N. rubra* strain 3639. Beaman (48) reported that there were amino acid complexes which could be extracted from the cell walls with an alkaline ethanol treatment, and concluded that these amino acids existed as peptides or proteins which were associated with lipids. Beaman et al (49) also have shown that the precise composition of the lipopeptide—the amino acids and lipids—varied with both culture age and the strain of *Nocardia*. The appearance of such lipopeptides was recently determined in various bacteria, including *N. rubra* (49,50), however, little is known about the biological function or structure of these lipoproteins, owing to the instrinsic complexities described above. The only exception is the lipoprotein from the gram-negative bacterium, *Escherichia coli* (51).

Significant amounts of nonpeptidoglycan amino acids have also been found in N-CWS, suggesting the presence of a lipopeptide fraction. We succeeded in isolating the lipopeptide fraction by 3% KOH/ethanol treatment of N-CWS, revealing a peptide moiety rich in phenylalanine, glycine, alanine, valine, leucine, isoleucine, serine, and threonine but lacking basic and acidic amino acids. The lipid moiety mainly consists of C_{18} to C_{24} fatty acids having double bonds.

The lipopeptide of N-CWS was ninhydrine negative, so the NH_2-terminal of the peptide must be blocked by the lipid moiety.

The now available partial structure is as follows: NH_2-terminal amino acid sequences were established to be mainly lipid-Gly-Phe by negative-ion fast-atom bombardment combined with tandem mass spectrometry (6). The Edman degradation of oligopeptide obtained from partial acid hydrolysis, followed by HPLC separation, revealed a characteristic sequence of -(Ala)$_5$-Gly-(Ala)$_6$-Gly-(Ala)$_5$-. Further investigations of the structure are now in progress.

References

1. Tsukamura M. Priority of *Rhodococcus lentifragmentus* (Kruse 1896; Tsukamura et al 1975) Tsukamura 1978 comb. nov. over *Rhodococcus rubra* (Kruse 1896) Goodfellow and Alderson 1980. Int J Syst Bacteriol 1985;35:124–5.
2. Koda S, Fujioka M, Shigi M, et al. Structural analysis of mycolic acids from the cell wall skeleton of *Rhodococcus lentifragmentus* AN-115. J Gen Microbiol 1986;132:1547–51.
3. Cummins CS. Chemical composition and antigenic structure of cell walls of *Corynebacterium*, *Mycobacterium*, *Nocardia*, *Actinomyces*, and *Arthrobacter*. J Gen Microbiol 1962;28:35–50.
4. Cunto G, Kanetsuna F, Imaeda T. Chemical analysis of the mucopeptide of *Mycobacterium smegmatis*. Biochim Biophys Acta 1969;192:358–60.
5. Kotani S, Yanagida I, Kato K, Matsuda T. Studies on peptides, glycopeptides and antigenic polysaccharide–glycopeptide complexes isolated from an L-11 enzyme lysate of the walls of *Mycobacterium tuberculosis* strain H37Rv. Biken J 1970;13:249–75.
6. Fujioka M, Sentoh F, Koda S, Morimoto Y. FAB MS/MS analysis of a complex mixture of lipo-oligopeptides from *Nocardia rubra* cell wall skeleton. Unpublished paper presented at the 36th American Society for Mass Spectroscopy conference on mass spectrometry and allied topics, San Francisco, 1988; Abstracts:p 223.
7. Liu T-Y, Gotschlich E. Muramic acid phosphate as a component of the mucopeptide of gram-positive bacteria. J Biol Chem 1967;242:471–6.
8. Kanetsuna F. Chemical analysis of mycobacterial cell walls. Biochim Biophys Acta 1968;158:130–43.
9. Fujioka M, Koda S, Morimoto Y. Novel glycosidic linkage between arabinogalactan and peptidoglycan in the cell wall skeleton of *Nocardia rubra* AN-115. J Gen

Microbiol 1985;131:1323–9.

10. Bordet C, Etémadi AH, Michel G, Lederer E. Structure des acides nocardiques de *Nocardia asteroides*. Bull Soc Chim Fr 1965;234–5. (In French)

11. Lederer E. The mycobacterial cell wall. Pure Appl Chem 1971;25:135–65.

12. Barksdale L, Kim KS. *Mycobacterium*. Bacteriol Rev 1977;41:217–372.

13. Minnikin DE, Goodfellow M. Lipid composition in the classification and identification of acid-fast bacteria. In: Goodfellow M, Board RG, eds. Microbiological classification and identification. London: Academic Press; 1980;189–256.

14. Yano I, Toriyama S. Gas chromatographic and mass spectroscopic analysis of mycolic acids (C_{60-80} very long-chain fatty acids) from mycobacteria and related acid-fast bacteria. Shitsuryobunseki 1979;27:69–82.

15. Michel G, Bordet C. Cell walls of nocardiae. In: Goodfellow M, Brownell GH, Serrano JA, eds. The biology of the nocardiae. New York: Academic Press; 1976;141–59.

16. Batt RD, Hodges R, Robertson JG. Gas chromatography and mass spectrometry of the trimethylsilyl ether methyl ester derivatives of long chain hydroxy acids from *Nocardia corallina*. Biochim Biophys Acta 1971;239:368–73.

17. Schulten H-R. Advances in field desorption mass spectrometry. In: Morris HR, ed. Soft ionization biological mass spectrometry. London: Heyden; 1981:6–38.

18. Etémadi AH. The use of pyrolysis gas chromatography and mass spectroscopy in the study of the structure of mycolic acids. J Gas Chromatogr 1967;5:447–56.

19. Yano I, Kageyama K, Ohno Y, et al. Separation and analysis of molecular species of mycolic acids in *Nocardia* and related taxa by gas chromatography mass spectrometry. Biomed Mass Spectrom 1978;5:14–24.

20. Tomiyasu I, Toriyama S, Yano I, Masui M. Changes in molecular species composition of nocardomycolic acid in *Nocardia rubra* by the growth temperature. Chem Phys Lipids 1981;28:41–54.

21. Asselineau C, Asselineau J. Stéréochemie de l'acide corynomycolique. Bull Soc Chim Fr 1966;1992–9. (In French)

22. Asselineau C, Tocanne G, Tocanne J-F. Stéréochemie des acides mycoliques. Bull Soc Chim Fr 1970;1456–9. (In French)

23. Misaki A, Seto N, Azuma I. Structure and immunological properties of D-arabino-D-galactans isolated from cell walls of *Mycobacterium* species. J Biochem 1974;76:15–27.

24. Misaki A, Yukawa S. Studies on cell walls of Mycobacteria. II. Constituents of polysaccharides from BCG cell walls. J Biochem 1966;59:511–20.

25. Azuma I, Kimura H, Niinaka T, et al. Chemical and immunological studies on mycobacterial polysaccharides. 1: Purification and properties of polysaccharides from human tubercle bacilli. J Bacteriol 1968;95:263–71.

26. Abou-zeid C, Voiland A, Michel G, Cocito C. Structure of the wall polysaccharide isolated from a group of corynebacteria. Eur J Biochem 1982;128:363–70.

27. Kanetsuna F, Blas GS. Chemical analysis of a mycolic acid-arabinogalactan-mucopeptide complex of mycobacterial cell wall. Biochim Biophys Acta 1970;208:434–43.

28. Vilkas E, Markovits J, Amar-Nacasch C, Lederer E. Sur la présence d'unités de D-galactofuranose dans l'arabinogalactane des parois et des cires D de souches humaines de *Mycobacterium tuberculosis*. C R Acad Sci Paris 1971; 273C:845–8. (In French)

29. Vilkas E, Amar C, Markovits J, et al. Occurrence of a galactofuranose disaccharide in immunoadjuvant fractions of *Mycobacterium tuberculosis* (cell walls and wax D).

Biochim Biophys Acta 1973;297:423–35.

30. Shigi M, Koda S, Morimoto Y. Structure of the arabinogalactan of *Nocardia rubra* cell wall skeleton. Unpublished paper presented at 23rd NMR Toronkai, Sendai; 1984:Abstracts pp 156–9.

31. Fujioka M, Koda S, Morimoto Y. Structural studies of *Nocardia rubra* cell wall skeleton (N-CWS). Structure of arabinogalactan and linkage with peptidoglycan. Unpublished paper presented at 8th Japanese Society for Medical Mass Spectrometry meeting, Yonago; 1983:Abstracts pp 227–30.

32. Kato K, Strominger JL, Kotani S. Structure of the cell wall of *Corynebacterium diphtheriae*. I. Mechanism of hydrolysis by the L-3 enzyme and the structure of the peptide. Biochemistry 1968;7:2762–73.

33. Azuma I, Ohuchida A, Taniyama T, et al. The mycolic acids of *Mycobacterium rhodochrous* and *Nocardia corallina*. Biken J 1974;17:1–9.

34. Vacheron M-J, Guinand M, Michel G, Ghuysen G-M. Structural investigations on cell walls of *Nocardia* sp. The wall lipid and peptidoglycan moieties of *Nocardia kirovani*. Eur J Biochem 1972;29:156–66.

35. Wietzerbin J, Das BC, Pitit J-F, et al. Occurrence of D-alanyl-(D)-*meso*-diaminopimelic acid and *meso*-diaminopimelyl-*meso*-diaminopimelic acid interpeptide linkages in the peptidoglycan of Mycobacteria. Biochemistry 1974;13:3471–6.

36. Carr SA, Herlihy WC, Biemann K. Advances in gas chromatographic mass spectrometric protein sequencing. 1—Optimization of the derivatization chemistry. Biomed Mass Spectrom 1981;8:51–61.

37. Lam S, Karmen A. Resolution of optical isomers of Dns-amino acids by high-performance liquid chromatography with L-histidine and its derivatives in the mobile phase. J Chromatogr 1982;239:451–62.

38. Hartley BS, Massey V. The active centre of chymotrypsin. I. Labelling with a fluorescent dye. Biochim Biophys Acta 1956;21:58–70.

39. Fujioka M, Kihara N, Koda S, Morimoto Y. Structural analysis of the peptide moiety of *Nocardia rubra* cell-wall skeleton (N-CWS) by mass spectrometry. Unpublished paper presented at the Pittsburgh Conference and Exposition on Analytical Chemistry and Applied Spectroscopy, Atlantic City, New Jersey; 1984: Abstracts p 840.

40. Azuma I, Yamamura Y. Studies on the firmly bound lipids of human tubercle bacillus. I: Isolation of arabinose mycolate. J Biochem 1962;52:200–6.

41. Azuma I, Yamamura Y, Misaki A. Isolation and characterization of arabinose mycolate from firmly bound lipids of mycobacteria. J Bacteriol 1969;98:331–3.

42. Markovits J, Vilkas E. Étude des cires D d'une souche humaine virulente de *Mycobacterium tuberculosis*. Biochim Biophys Acta 1969;192:49–54. (In French)

43. Lanéelle MA, Asselineau J. Caracterisation de glycolipides dans une souche de *Nocardia brasiliensis*. FEBS Lett 1970;7:64–8. (In French)

44. Kotani K, Wiegeshaus E, Smith DW. Demonstration of mycolic acid and phthiocerol dimycocerosate in "in vivo grown tubercle bacilli." Jpn Med Sci Biol 1970;23:327–33.

45. Amar C, Vilkas E. Isolement d'un phosphate d'arabinose à partir des parois de *Mycobacterium tuberculosis*, H37Ra. C R Seances Acad Sci Ser III Sci Vie 1973; D277:1949–51. (In French)

46. Miyamae M, Shigi M. Unpublished.

47. Sohler A, Romano AH, Nickerson WJ. Biochemistry of the Actinomycetales. III: Cell wall composition and the action of lysozyme upon cells and cell walls of the Actinomycetales. J Bacteriol 1958;75:283–90.

48. Beaman BL. Structural and biochemical alterations of *Nocardia asteroides* cell walls during its growth cycle. J Bacteriol 1975;123:1235–53.
49. Beaman BL, Kim KS, Salton MRJ, Barksdale L. Amino acids of the cell wall of *Nocardia rubra*. J Bacteriol 1971;108:941–3.
50. Wietzerbin-Falszpam J, Das BC, Gros C, et al. The amino acids of the cell wall of *Mycobacterium tuberculosis* var. *bouis*, strain BCG. Presence of a poly (L-glutamic acid). Eur J Biochem 1973;32:525–32.
51. Braun V, Bosch V. Sequence of the murine-lipoprotein and the attachment site of the lipid. Eur J Biochem 1972;28:51–69.

Activation of cellular networks and cytokine cascade with *Nocardia rubra* cell wall skeleton

Hatsuo Aoki

International Development Group, Fujisawa Pharmaceutical Co., Ltd., Osaka, Japan

Introduction

Nocardia rubra cell wall skeleton (N-CWS) is a potent reticuloendothelial and hematopoietic stimulant (1), showing antitumor and antiinfective effects in numerous experimental models (2,3). It has been used in combination with chemotherapeutic agents and has been demonstrated to have a beneficial effect in clinical trials of various cancers including small cell carcinoma (4), gastric cancer (5), and leukemia (6). Although precise mechanisms of action of N-CWS in vivo are complex and not fully understood, some effector cells, such as immune T cells and activated macrophages, appear to be involved in eradicating tumor cells. A number of antitumor cytokines have been described. Tumor necrosis factor (TNF), interleukin 1 (IL-1), and various types of interferon (IFN) have been reported as having a direct cytotoxic effect on certain tumor cells (7–9) as well as regulating immune responses, culminating in the development of T killer cells and/or activated macrophages (10). To understand better the immunotherapeutic activity of N-CWS, we have conducted a series of investigations to delineate its cytokine-inducing ability, with the use of simple in vitro systems.

Induction of interferons

Effect of N-CWS on interferon production in mouse tissue

In the 1st series of experiments, we examined the IFN-inducing activity of N-CWS in cell cultures derived from various mouse tissues, including spleen cells (SC), thymocytes, peritoneal resident cells (PRC), peritoneal exudative cells (PEC), bone marrow cells (BMC), and peripheral blood mononulear cells (11). PEC were harvested from the peritoneal cavities of C3H/HeN mice after intraperitoneal (ip) injection of 2 mL of sterile 3% Brewer's thioglycolate medium (TG). To induce IFN production, cells were cultured in the presence of N-CWS for 24 h at 37°C. The supernatants were obtained and measured for IFN activity by a conventional cytopathic effect (CPE)-reduction assay using L-929 cells and vesicular stomatitis virus (VSV) as the challenge virus. The sample titers were expressed in international units (IU)/mL in comparison with a World Health Organization reference IFN standard. Significant IFN production was observed in PEC, PRC, and BMC cultures after N-CWS treatment (Table 1). Marginal levels of IFN activity were occasionally detected in supernatants of SC cultures. Peripheral blood mononuclear cells or lymph node cells do not produce detectable levels of IFN after N-CWS treatment.

Characterization of N-CWS-induced IFN from BMC, PRC, and PEC

IFN produced in BMC, PRC, and PEC in response to N-CWS stimulation was characterized by pH stability and neutralization studies (Table 1). IFN produced in BMC and PRC culture did not show any significant loss of activity at pH 2, whereas the IFN activity in PEC cultures was partially lost under the same conditions. In neutralization studies, acid-stable IFN preparations obtained in BMC and PRC cultures were neutralized by anti-IFN-α/β serum, but were not affected by treatment with anti-IFN-γ serum. The IFN in PEC cultures was partially neutralized by the separate treatments with anti-IFN-α/β and anti-IFN-γ serum, and was completely neutralized by simultaneous treatment with the 2 antisera.

Enhanced interferon production in mixed cultures of SC and PEC

During the IFN induction study, we noticed that exposure of the mixture of PEC

Table 1 Characterization of N-CWS-induced IFN produced in cultures of BMC, PRC, TG-elicited PEC, and mixed cultures.

N-CWS-induced IFN preparation	IFN titer (U/mL) after neutralization by antiserum			
	Nontreated	Anti-IFN-α/β	Anti-IFN-γ	Anti-IFN-α/β + anti-IFN-γ
MBC	40	<4	41	
Resident PEC (PRC)	72	<4	78	<4
TG-elicited PEC	85	12	36	<4
TG-PEC + SC	215	70	33	<9
TG-Mϕ + SC	350	378	<9	
IFN-α/β	200	<4	200	
IFN-γ	235	210	<4	
IFN-α/β + IFN-γ	185	58	37	<4

Lymphocytes from various organs 2.5×10^6/mL or peritoneal cells 8.5×10^5/mL incubated in the presence of N-CWS 50 μg/mL for 24 h at 37°C. Supernatants treated with appropriate dilutions of antiserum for 1 h at 37°C. TG, thioglycolate medium; SC, spleen cells; Mϕ, macrophage.

and SC to N-CWS resulted in an enhanced production of IFN, which was partially neutralized by treatment with anti-IFN-α/β or anti-IFN-γ sera, respectively. Since TG-induced PEC were rich in macrophage exudate (macrophage, 90.3 $\pm$ 7.7%; lymphocyte, 3.9 $\pm$ 2.4%) it is probable that macrophages were involved in the enhancement of IFN production in this mixed-culture system. Macrophages were purified either by adhesion to dishes, with washing by jet pipeting of buffer over PEC monolayers, or by passage in tissue culture for 2 weeks. The latter method gave a macrophage culture virtually free of lymphocytes. IFN activity produced by the mixed culture of TG-macrophages and SC was acid labile and completely neutralized by anti-IFN-γ antiserum (Table 1). These data show that when TG-macrophages were used instead of TG-PEC in mixed culture, elevated amounts of INF-γ were produced, but there was no detectable production of IFN-α/β.

Cellular origin of INF-γ in TG-macrophage-SC mixed-culture system

To determine cell populations in SC, which are responsible for IFN-γ production, SC from normal mice or nude mice were passed through a nylon-wool column, and the nonadherent cells were mixed with purified TG-macrophages and incubated in the presence of N-CWS. A high titer of IFN-γ was produced in these cultures, suggesting that mature T cells were not involved in this type of IFN production. Elimination of T cells by treatment with anti-Thy1,2 serum and complement, and destruction of B cells with anti-IgG(G + A + M) serum plus complement showed no effect on IFN production. When the nylon-nonadherent cells were treated with antiasialo-GM$_1$ serum plus complement, IFN production was completely abolished as well as the natural killer (NK) activity. Thus, asialo-GM$_1$-positive NK-like cells play an important role in the production of IFN-γ in the mixed culture.

IFN-γ-producing cells and accessory cells

A mixture of TG-macrophages and SC was stimulated with N-CWS for production of IFN-γ, and the cells were stained by an indirect immunofluorescence technique (Fig 1). After 3 h of incubation, some lymphocytes had bright cytoplasmic fluorescence and the number of positively stained lymphocytes increased with time, whereas the macrophages were not stained with anti-IFN-γ serum in the test period up to 24 h.

When lymphocytes (SC) were separated from macrophage monolayers after incubation of the mixed culture with N-CWS, the cells were disrupted and the IFN titer of the supernatants was measured. Measurable IFN activity was detected in the supernatant of the disrupted SC cells but IFN activity was not detected in the supernatant of macrophages. These results demonstrate that NK-like cells in spleen produce IFN-γ, and that macrophages play a helper function.

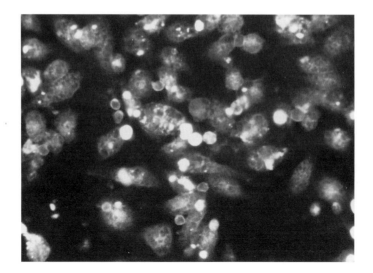

Fig 1 Immunofluorescent detection of cytoplasmic IFN-γ in lymphocytes of a TG-macrophage-SC mixed-culture system. Equal volumes (0.5 mL) of TG-macrophage 1.7 × 10⁶/mL and spleen cells 5 × 10⁵/mL placed in 24-well plates and cultured for 18 h in the presence of N-CWS 50 μg/mL. Cells fixed in 4% paraformaldehyde in 0.1M-phosphate buffer for 16 h at 4°C and treated with 0.5% Nonidet P-40 in phosphate-buffered saline for 20 min, washed, and stained with rabbit anti-mouse IFN-γ antiserum for 1 h, and then with fluorescein isothiocyanate-goat anti-rabbit immunoglobulin antiserum.

Induction of tumor necrosis factor

Production of cytotoxic factors by N-CWS-stimulated mouse macrophages in vitro

Spleen cells or macrophages derived from normal or TG-injected C3H/He mice were incubated with N-CWS, and the cell-free supernatants were tested in the standard TNF assay for their lytic activity on L-929 target cells (12). SC did not produce detectable amounts of cytotoxic factors in these experimental conditions and a low level of cytotoxin was present in the culture of PRC from normal mice. In contrast, plastic-adherent PEC (macrophage >98%) responded to N-CWS and produced a high titer of cytotoxic factor. Treatment of TG-PEC with specific toxins to macrophages, such as 2-chloroadenosine or silica particles, abrogated cytotoxin productivity, whereas treatment with anti-Thy1,2 antiserum plus complement did not affect the cytotoxin production. These data suggest the involvement of macrophages in this cytotoxin production. The onset of cytotoxin production was rapid (Fig 2); when TG-PEC were induced with 50 μg of N-CWS, the activity was detectable in the supernatant within 2 h and the level increased to a maximum at 9 h before declining rapidly to low levels.

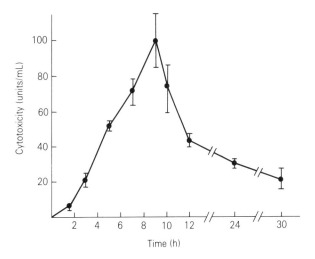

Fig 2 Kinetics of N-CWS-induced cytotoxin production from adherent thioglycolate-induced PEC. TG-PEC 8.5×10^5/well obtained from C3H/He mice 4 days after TG injection were allowed to adhere for 3 h, followed by vigorous pipetting to remove nonadherent cells. Subsequent monolayers cultured in the presence of N-CWS 10 μg/mL up to 30 h. Supernatant was collected at various intervals and assayed for cytotoxic activity on L-929 cells.

Physicochemical character of N-CWS-induced cytotoxins

N-CWS-induced cytotoxins were partially purified by DEAE-Sepharose chromatography. The cytotoxic activity of the preparations revealed both acid and base lability, with a maximum stability at pH 7.0 to 8.0. The cytotoxins are also heat labile and inactivated by trypsin or pronase digestion. The elution patterns of N-CWS cytotoxic factors from ion-exchange, gel filtration, and concanavalin A (Con-A)-affinity chromatography were compared with those of the cytotoxins in tumor necrosis serum (TNS) obtained from mice treated with BCG and lipopolysaccharide (LPS) (13). The N-CWS cytotoxic factors and the cytotoxins in TNS are heterogeneous with respect to charge, size, and expression of carbohydrate. Both preparations have a main peak of relative molecular mass (M_r) of 48 000, which showed almost identical elution patterns on Con-A-Sepharose columns. Thus the N-CWS cytotoxic factors seem to be similar or identical to TNF obtained from the serum of mice treated with the BCG-LPS combination.

Production of TNF-like cytotoxins by N-CWS-stimulated human peripheral blood lymphocytes

Fresh peripheral blood lymphocytes (PBL) from healthy donors were incubated for 16 h in the presence of 50 μg/mL of N-CWS, and were tested for cytotoxic activity on L-929 target cells. None of the PBL from any of the donors tested produced any cytotoxic activity spontaneously. In the presence of N-CWS they released a significant cytotoxic activity, although the levels of the activity were variable and were donor dependent (Table 2). Anti-human TNF antiserum neutralized completely the cytotoxic activity produced by N-CWS-treated human PBL, but anti-human-lymphotoxin antiserum showed no effect on the activity. Production of TNF by N-CWS-treated PBL was greatly diminished when they were treated with anti-Leu-M3 (anti-human macrophage/monocyte) antiserum but not when they were treated with anti-Leu-7 (anti-human K/NK cells), anti-Leu-11 (anti-human cytolytic NK cells), or anti-Leu-1 (anti-human pan-T cell) antiserum. Thus, the macrophage population of human PBL have been shown to produce TNF when cultured in the presence of N-CWS. For production to be stimulated, the human PBL do not require the presence of inflammatory stimuli such as thioglycolate in vitro, suggesting that the population of monocytes in human PBL are as functionally well differentiated as mice inflammatory macrophages.

Induction of IL-1

Induction of IL-1 production from macrophages by N-CWS

Peritoneal exudate macrophages (PEM) and peritoneal resident macrophages (PRM) of C3H/He mice were cultured in the presence of N-CWS and the super-

Table 2 Production of N-CWS cytotoxic factor from human PBL obtained from random donors.

Donor	Cytotoxic activity (units/mL)
A	30
B	36
C	78
D	20
E	15
F	35
G	12
H	9
I	24
J	16
K	37
L	18
M	20

Normal PBL 2.5×10^6 cells/well, separated by centrifugation on Ficoll-Hypaque, incubated at 37°C for 16 h in the presence of N-CWS 50 μg/mL. For each donor, did not release cytotoxic activity in the absence of N-CWS.

natants collected. Supernatant IL-1 activity of the supernatant was measured by a standard IL-1 assay for ability to promote proliferation of phytohemagglutinin (PHA)-stimulated thymocytes (14). Increased IL-1 levels in culture supernatant were observed at concentrations of N-CWS higher than 3 μg/mL. The production of IL-1 increased linearly and reached a peak at 48 h (Fig 3). In contrast to TNF or IFN-γ, IL-1 was produced by PRM as well as by PEM. Thus, the mechanism of increased IL-1 production seems to differ from that of TNF or IFN-γ.

IL-1-rich supernatants from N-CWS-stimulated macrophage culture were applied to Sephadex G-75 column chromatography. The main IL-1 activity of the supernatants was obtained at a position corresponding to an M_r of 17 000, which seems to be similar to the IL-1 activity produced by LPS-stimulated macrophages.

Control of N-CWS-augmented IL-1 production by cyclooxygenase products

When a low concentration (10^9–10^{10}M) of prostaglandin E_2 was added to the macrophage monolayers incubated with N-CWS, a significant suppression of IL-1 production was observed. Addition of a cyclooxygenase inhibitor, indomethacin, showed a dose-dependent augmentation of IL-1 production (Fig 4). The effects of a leukotriene product, LTB_4, and a lipoxygenase inhibitor on IL-1 production were also examined. Neither showed any effect on IL-1 production by N-CWS-stimulated macrophage cultures. These results indicate an involvement of cyclooxygenase but not lipoxygenase products in the production of IL-1 by activated macrophages.

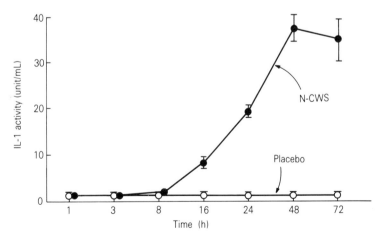

Fig 3 Kinetics of N-CWS-augmented IL-1 production by macrophages. Peritoneal cells plated into 24-well plates (10^6/well), allowed to adhere for 2 h and cultured for various times in the presence of N-CWS 10 μg/mL or a placebo. Supernatants collected and assayed for their comitogenic activity with PHA for thymocytes.

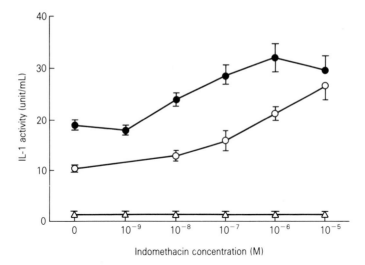

Fig 4 Augmentation by indomethacin of IL-1 production by N-CWS-stimulated macrophages. Peritoneal macrophages cultured in the presence of N-CWS 10 μg/mL and graded concentrations of indomethacin for 48 h. Supernatants were collected and assayed for IL-1 activity. ● LPS, ○ N-CWS, △ placebo.

Effect of N-CWS on other cytokines (colony-stimulating factors)

When a murine myeloid leukemia cell line, M1, was cultured in the presence of N-CWS, an augmentation of colony-stimulating factor activity (CSF) was detected in 1-day-old culture supernatant, and this increased gradually, reaching a maximum after 5 to 7 days (15). Also, N-CWS enhanced the differentiation of M1 cells with regard to characteristics specific for macrophages, such as phagocytosis, adhesion to plastic, and erythrocyte amboceptor rosette formation.

An enhancing effect of N-CWS on CSF production in conditioned medium of the lung of BALB/c mice has been reported (16). The lungs were removed from mice injected with 100 μg of N-CWS intraperitoneally 5 days before the experiment, then minced and incubated for 48 h. Significant CSF activity was detected in the culture supernatant, but was not observed with lung culture from non-treated mice. Serum CSF activity was also significantly enhanced after ip injection of N-CWS to mice.

Discussion

The immunotherapeutic potential of N-CWS is supported by the results of a number of clinical trials, as reported by Ogura and others in this volume, as well as by preclinical evaluations. Several effector cell populations, such as killer T cells, NK cells, and macrophages have been reported to be involved in N-CWS-induced resistance to transplanted or metastatic tumors, among which macrophages seem to play the most important role. To elucidate the mode of action of N-CWS, we have investigated its effect on the production of cytokines, which play an important part in immunological responses, especially in activation of macrophages for tumoricidal activity.

N-CWS was found to induce 2 distinct types of IFN in thioglycolate-elicited PEC cultures, IFN-α/β and IFN-γ. Macrophages and/or macrophage progenitor cells in the peritoneal cavity or bone marrow respond to N-CWS stimulation, and produce IFN-α/β. N-CWS is reported to increase CSF levels in mice sera in vivo and also to enhance CSF secretion by bone marrow and peritoneal cells (16). Thus, IFN-α/β, as well as CSF produced by peritoneal and/or bone marrow cells in N-CWS-treated mice, may help to enhance the generation of monocytes/macrophages. IFNs have been shown to possess a variety of biological activities. They are antiproliferative or cytostatic for many types of tumor cells (9) and activate effector cells (10) to become cytotoxic to malignant cells. IFNs are also reported to be differentiation factors, regulating expression of cell surface-associated antigens such as the major histocompatibility complex class 1 (17). IFN-β plays a role as an autocrine differentiation factor for the murine myeloid leukemia cell line, M1 (18).

Our findings indicate the need for synergic interaction between macrophages and NK cells for the N-CWS-stimulated production of IFN-γ. The simultaneous induction of more than 1 type of IFN may be significant. Weigent et al have presented evidence that IFN-γ and IFN-α/β synergically enhance NK cell activity (19). The potentiation of the antitumor effect of IFN-α/β by IFN-γ in vivo has also been reported (9). IFN-γ is also shown to synergize with other cytokines such as TNF, IL-1, and CSF to augment macrophage cytotoxicity against tumor cells (10).

While studying the effect of N-CWS on IFN production, we have observed that peritoneal macrophages produce a low titer of cytotoxic factor when cultured in the presence of N-CWS. Thioglycolate-elicited peritoneal cells produced a much higher titer of the cytotoxin under the same conditions, suggesting that inflammatory macrophages may be the effector cells. A number of papers have reported that macrophages produce growth inhibitory factors constitutively and/or after mitogen or alloantigen stimulation and, among these, TNF, IL-1, and IFN-β are biochemically well-characterized monokines. N-CWS-induced cytotoxin had the same or similar properties as those described for murine TNF, in temperature, pH and protease sensitivity, and elution patterns from ion-exchange, gel filtration, and Con-A affinity chromatography.

TNF is reported to be an important mediator of macrophage-dependent tumor cell killing. Urban et al (7) have found evidence that antibody to murine recombinant TNF blocks the tumoricidal effect of macrophages and that selection of a tumor cell line resistant to either macrophage cytotoxicity or recombinant TNF leads to simultaneous resistance to both macrophages and TNF, but not resistance to other tumoricidal mechanisms. The role of TNF is unlikely to be restricted to direct tumor cell killing.

Another important role TNF may play is to augment the production of CSFs. Munker et al (20) and Broudy et al (21) reported that TNF markedly stimulated fibroblasts, endothelial cells, and smooth muscle cells to release multilineage (granulocyte–macrophage) CSF (GM-CSF). GM-CSF is reported to stimulate peripheral blood monocytes in vitro to become cytotoxic for certain malignant cell lines, and this activity is synergistically enhanced by IFN-γ (22). Thus, in addition to its direct cytotoxic effect, TFN may exert an antitumor activity by stimulating a growth factor and/or a mediator involved in immune responses.

We found that fresh PBL from healthy donors did not produce a detectable level of TNF, but responded to N-CWS stimulation to release a high titer of the cytotoxin. Fresh human PBL did not require elicitation by inflammatory stimuli such as thioglycolate in vitro. In circulating human PBL, some populations of monocytes may be as functionally well differentiated as murine inflammatory macrophages as in the case of lymphocyte function-associated (LFA)-1 antigen, which appears involved in cell–cell interactions. Murine LFA-1 antigen can be induced on TG-elicited macrophages but not on resident counterparts. Human LFA-1 antigen is expressed at high density on native PBL and at low density on BMC (23).

We have shown that PRM and PEM responded to N-CWS stimulation to release IL-1. The characteristics of IL-1 produced by N-CWS-stimulated macrophages seemed identical to those of the standard preparation. It is especially interesting that IL-1 was produced not only from PEM, but also from PRM, because the functional activities of resident macrophages are much lower than those of exudate macrophages, in superoxide anion production in relation to killing microorganisms, and in induction of tumoricidal activity (24) or production of cytokines. Thus, the mechanism of the augmented IL-1 production may differ from that of the other functions. Fresh PBL from human donors responded to N-CWS stimulation to release a high titer of IL-1 in the medium.

IL-1 production by LPS stimulation is reported to be regulated by metabolites of arachidonic acid. In our experiment, prostaglandin E_2 suppressed IL-1 production by N-CWS-stimulated macrophages; a cyclooxygenase inhibitor, indomethacin, augmented IL-1 production. Neither lipoxygenase products nor lipoxygenase inhibitor had any effect on this system.

IL-1 plays important roles in immunological responses, promoting IL-2 and IFN generation and the proliferation of lymphocytes in response to antigenic stimuli. Recent studies have indicated that IL-1 is involved in the tumoricidal activity of lymphocytes (8). IL-1-treated monocytes exhibited a higher cytotoxicity for a target cell, A375, than did control monocytes. The promotion of monocyte toxicity by IL-1 was mediated by metabolites of arachidonic acid. Also IL-1 induced a concentration-dependent inhibition of the proliferation of several tumor cell lines such as human myeloid K562 and murine T-lymphoma Eb (8).

The development of recombinant DNA technology has made possible the large-scale production of a variety of cytokines such as TNF, IL-1, IL-2, and IFNs. However, purified recombinant cytokines alone have been observed to be less active than their crude natural counterparts in clinical situations. Synergistic activity between cytokines has been observed with combinations such as IFN-α/β

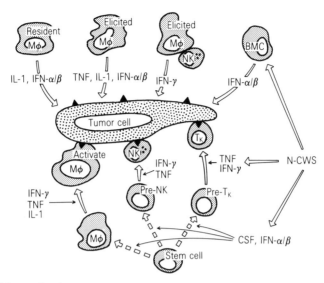

Fig 5 Possible mechanisms of antitumor effect of N-CWS.

plus IFN-γ, IFN-γ plus TNF, and TNF plus IL-1. This suggests the importance of combined therapy, rather than monotherapy, for each cytokine to exert its maximum efficacy in the treatment of cancer or infection.

The wide range of side effects observed with systemic administration of these cytokines is another problem to be solved. The systemic injection of IFN, TNF, or IL-1 causes adverse reactions in patients, resulting in fever, fatigue, or metabolic disorders. These cytokines are involved in cell-to-cell communications in human microenvironments such as autocrine or paracrine functions. Thus it may be desirable to induce or apply combinations of cytokines to the tumor or infection site without raising their concentrations in other organs or in the bloodstream.

We can currently conclude that immunotherapy with the use of N-CWS has a potential clinical relevance because of the ability of N-CWS to induce multiple species of cytokines simultaneously, especially from macrophages activated with invasive stimuli (Fig 5).

References

1. Fujitsu T, Sakuma S, Yoneda K, et al. Effect of *Nocardia rubra* cell wall skeleton on immune responses in mice and guinea pigs. Pharmacometrics 1986;31:757–65.
2. Yamawaki M, Azuma I, Saiki I, et al. Antitumor activity of squalene-treated cell-wall skeleton of *Nocardia rubra* in mice. Jpn J Cancer Res (Gann) 1978;69:619–26.
3. Mine Y, Yokota T, Nonoyama S, Kikuchi H. Protective effect of *Nocardia rubra* cell wall skeleton on experimental infection in normal and immunosuppressed mice.

Arzneimittelforschung 1986;10:1489–92.

4. Yamamura Y, Ogura T, Sakatani M, et al. Randomized controlled study of adjuvant immunotherapy with *Nocardia rubra* cell wall skeleton for inoperable lung cancer. Cancer Res 1983;43:5575–9.

5. Ochiai T, Sato H, Sato H, et al. Randomly controlled study of chemotherapy versus chemoimmunotherapy in postoperative gastric cancer patients. Cancer Res 1983;43:3001–7.

6. Ohno R, Nakamura H, Kodera Y, et al. Randomized controlled study of chemoimmunotherapy of acute myelogenous leukemia in adults with *Nocardia rubra* cell wall skeleton and irradiated allogenic AML cells. Cancer 1986;57:1483–8.

7. Urban JL, Shepard HM, Rothstein JL, et al. Tumor necrosis factor: a potent effector molecule for tumor cell killing by activated macrophages. Proc Natl Acad Sci USA 1986;83:5233–7.

8. Lovett D, Kozan B, Hadam M, et al. Macrophage cytotoxicity: interleukin 1 as a mediator of tumor cytostasis. J Immunol 1986;136:340–7.

9. Fleishman WR Jr, Kleyn KM, Baron S. Potentiation of antitumor effect of virus-induced interferon by mouse immune interferon preparation. J Natl Cancer Inst 1980;65:963–6.

10. Chen L, Suzuki Y, Wheelock EF. Interferon-γ synergizes with tumor necrosis factor and with interleukin 1 and requires the presence of both monokines to induce antitumor cytotoxic activity in macrophages. J Immunol 1987;139:4096–101.

11. Izumi S, Ueda H, Okuhara M, et al. Effect of *Nocardia rubra* cell wall skeleton on murine interferon production in vitro. Cancer Res 1986;46:1960–5.

12. Izumi S, Hirai O, Hayashi K, et al. Induction of a tumor necrosis factor-like activity by *Nocardia rubra* cell wall skeleton. Cancer Res 1987;47:1785–92.

13. Männel DN, Farer JJ, Murgenhagen SE. Separation of a serum-derived tumoricidal factor from a helper factor for plaque-forming cells. J Immunol 1980;124:1106–10.

14. Inamura N, Nakahara K, Kuroda Y, et al. Effect of *Nocardia rubra* cell wall skeleton on interleukin 1 production from mouse peritoneal macrophages. Int J Immunopharmacol (in press).

15. Maeda M, Ichikawa Y, Azuma I. Differentiation and production of colony-stimulating factor induced by immunostimulants in a leukemia cell line. J Cell Physiol 1980;105:33–8.

16. Ito M, Suzuki H, Nakano N, et al. Effect of *Nocardia rubra* cell-wall skeleton on colony-stimulating activity and myeloid colony formation. Jpn J Cancer Res (Gann) 1982;73:403–7.

17. Klyczek KK, Murasako DM, Blank KJ. Interferon-γ, interferon-$\alpha/-\beta$, and tumor necrosis factor differentially affect major histocompatibility complex class 1 expression in murine leukemia virus-induced tumor cell lines. J Immunol 1987;139:2641–8.

18. Onozaki K, Urawa H, Tamatani T, et al. Synergistic interactions of interleukin 1, interferon-β and tumor necrosis factor in terminally differentiating a mouse myeloid leukemia cell line (M1). J Immunol 1988;140:112–9.

19. Weigent DA, Lanfold MP, Fleishman WR JR, Stamton GJ. Potentiation of lymphocyte natural killing by mixtures of alpha or beta interferon with recombinant gamma interferon. Infect Immun 1983;40:35–8.

20. Munker R, Gasson J, Ogawa M, Koefler HP. Recombinant human TNF induces production of granulocyte-monocyte colony-stimulating factor. Nature 1986;234:79–82.

21. Broudy VC, Kaushansky K, Segal GM, et al. Tumor necrosis factor type α stimulates human endothelial cells to produce granulocyte/macrophage colony-

stimulating factor. Proc Natl Acad Sci USA 1986;83:7467–71.
22. Grabstein KH, Uradal DL, Tushinski RJ, et al. Induction of macrophage tumoricidal activity by granulocyte-macrophage colony-stimulating factor. Science 1986;232:506–8.
23. Krensky AM, Sanchez-Madrid F, Robbins E, et al. The functional significance, distribution and structure of LFA-1, LFA-2 and LFA-3: cell surface antigens associated with CTL-target interactions. J Immunol 1983;131:611–6.
24. Inamura N, Fujitsu T, Nakahara K, et al. Potentiation of tumoricidal properties of murine macrophages by *Nocardia rubra* cell wall skeleton. J Antibiot 1984;37:244–55.

Immunopharmacological effect of *Nocardia rubra* cell wall skeleton on host defense against cancer in an experimental system

Tomiya Masuno

3rd Department of Internal Medicine, Osaka University Medical School, Fukushima, Osaka, Japan

Introduction

Nocardia rubra cell wall skeleton (N-CWS) not only possesses a potent adjuvant activity on humoral or cellular immune responses, and a mitogenic activity on splenocytes or splenic T cells, but it also augments antitumor effector mechanisms in experimental animals and humans (Table 1) (1–59). Randomized controlled clinical studies have shown that treatment with N-CWS prolongs the survival time or the complete remission period of patients with lung cancer (47–49), gastric cancer (50,51), or leukemia (52,54). Strong evidence has been accumulating that activated macrophages play a crucial role as effector cells in host defense against malignant neoplasms (60–63). These findings suggest that macrophages activated with N-CWS are responsible for its therapeutic effects in cancer patients. The present review describes the mechanisms whereby N-CWS induces macrophage activation in animals, with special reference to its effects on the production of granulocyte-macrophage colony-forming units (GM-CFU), colony-stimulating factor (CSF), and macrophage activating factor (MAF).

Effect of N-CWS on production of GM-CFU and CSF in animals

It has been demonstrated that an ip injection of N-CWS induces peritoneal macrophage activation (9,11) and that an iv injection of N-CWS induces alveolar macrophage activation (16,17). Differentiation and proliferation of GM-CFU and CSF are essential factors for the induction of activated macrophages. Many reports have indicated that various bacteria and their components can increase the number of GM-CFU in the bone marrow and peripheral blood and can stimulate CSF production (64–66). Hayashi et al (32) have clarified the effect of N-CWS on GM-CFU in the murine bone marrow and CSF production by splenocytes in N-CWS-immunized mice.

Table 1 Recent reports on immunopharmacological effects of N-CWS.

	Reference no.
Adjuvant activity	1,2
Mitogenic activity	3–5
Cytotoxic T cell activation	6,7
Macrophage activation	
Peritoneal macrophages of animals in vivo	8–15
Alveolar macrophages of animals in vivo	16,17
Human macrophages in vivo	18
Macrophage activation in vitro	19–21
Natural killer cell activation	22,23
Polymorphonuclear cell activation	24,25
Enhancement of antibody production	26
Production of TNF-like factor	27
Production of interferon	28
Production of CSF or CSF-like factor	29–32
Antitumor effects	
Inhibition of carcinogenesis in animals	33–37
Tumor regression in animals	38–46
Clinical therapeutic effect against cancer	
Lung cancer	47–49
Gastric cancer	50,51
Leukemia	52–54
Maxillary sinus carcinoma	55,56
Brain tumor	57,58
Antiinfectious effect	59

Effect of N-CWS on GM-CFU in bone marrow in N-CWS-immunized mice

C3H/HeN mice were immunized with N-CWS by weekly sc injections of N-CWS for 3 weeks. Both N-CWS-immunized and normal control mice were injected ip with N-CWS and the number of GM-CFU in the femoral bone marrow was determined over time (Fig 1) (32). In control mice, an increase in GM-CFU was evident after ip injection of N-CWS, reaching a peak on day 1 and gradually decreasing to the level observed prior to the injection of N-CWS. In immunized mice, GM-CFU increases rapidly following ip injection of N-CWS, peaking on day 2 and gradually decreasing thereafter. These results suggest that N-CWS enhances the production of GM-CFU in the bone marrow, especially in N-CWS-immunized mice.

Augmentation of CSF production by N-CWS in N-CWS-immunized mice

CSF activity in the serum obtained from N-CWS-immunized and normal control mice was tested 1 h to 7 days after an ip injection of N-CWS. In both immunized

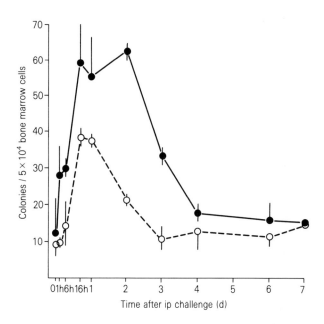

Fig 1 Chronological changes in number of GM-CFU in bone marrow. N-CWS-immu-nized (●) or age-matched control normal (○) mice injected ip with N-CWS 100 µg. Bone marrow cells obtained from 3 mice in each group harvested on designated days. Bone marrow cells (5×10^4) cultured in the presence of 10% (vol/vol) L-cell CM as exogenous CSF. Colony numbers counted after 7 days of culture. Each point represents mean ± SD of 3 mice. Reprinted, with permission, from Hayashi S, Masuno T, Hosoe S, et al (32).

and control mice, serum CSF activity increased as early as 6 h after the ip injection of N-CWS, and CSF activity in the serum of immunized mice was significantly higher than that of control mice.

Ito et al (31) have studied the in vitro effect of N-CWS on the generation of GM-CFU and the levels of CSF in the conditioned medium of the lung (LCM) and the serum of normal BALB/c mice. They found that intraperitoneal treatment of mice with N-CWS markedly enhanced the generation of GM-CFU. They have also shown that CSF levels in LCM as well as in the serum of mice injected ip with N-CWS were markedly higher than those of control mice.

These results suggest that a single injection of N-CWS into the peritoneal cavity of mice initially increases the CSF in the serum which in turn increases the number of GM-CFU in the bone marrow.

Interaction of adherent cells and nonadherent cells in CSF production by stimulation with N-CWS

Table 2 (32) shows the effect of cell fractionation and reconstitution on CSF production by N-CWS stimulation in vitro. When whole mononuclear leukocytes

Table 2 Effect of cell fractionation and reconstitution on CSF production by splenocytes.* Reprinted, with permission, from Hayashi S, Masuno T, Hosoe, et al (32).

Expt	Splenocyte donor	N-CWS	CSF activity (no. of colonies/10^5 bone marrow cells)[†] of medium conditioned with			
			WMNL	ADC	NADC	ADC-NADC
1						
	Control	−	0	ND	0	ND
	Control	+	6.2 ± 2.1[‡]	ND	5.0 ± 1.0	ND
	Immune	−	0.3 ± 0.6	ND	0.3 ± 0.6	ND
	Immune	+	34.0 ± 3.1[‡]	ND	2.3 ± 0.6	ND
2						
	Immune	−	0	0.3 ± 0.6	0	0
	Immune	+	45.0 ± 1.0	0.9 ± 4.4	8.0 ± 4.6	45.7 ± 6.8

*N-CWS-immunized and control splenocyte fractions cultured for 48 h with (+) and without (−) 10 μg N-CWS/mL.
[†]Values are means ± SD of triplicate cultures.
[‡]Significant at p < 0.001.
ND, not done.

(WMNL) or nonadherent cells (NADC) from N-CWS-immunized or control mice were cultured without N-CWS, no significant CSF could be detected in the culture supernatant. Immunized WMNL cultured with N-CWS produced significantly higher CSF activity than did the control WMNL. However, both control and immunized NADC alone, cultured with N-CWS, produced only a low titer of CSF (experiment 1, Table 2). On the other hand, CSF production returned to previous levels when immunized adherent cells (ADC) and immunized NADC were reconstituted and then cultured with N-CWS (experiment 2, Table 2). Greatly increased CSF production required interaction of NADC and ADC in the presence of N-CWS.

With mixed cultures of immunized NADC plus control or immunized ADC, production of CSF was significantly higher than that with control NADC plus control or immunized ADC, respectively (Table 3) (32). However, there was no significant difference between the CSF activities of the culture supernatant from immunized NADC mixed with immunized ADC and that of immunized NADC mixed with control ADC. These data suggest that the NADC of splenocytes are mainly responsible for the marked increase in CSF production that follows stimulation with N-CWS in N-CWS-immunized animals.

Analysis of CSF-producing cells by stimulation with N-CWS in N-CWS-immunized mice

A wide variety of cell types, such as fibroblasts (67) and tumor cell lines (68), can

Table 3 Effect of addition of ADC to NADC on CSF production.* Reprinted, with permission, from Hayashi S, Masuno T, Hosoe S, et al (32).

NADC donor	ADC donor	N-CWS	CSF activity of CM (no. of colonies/10^5 bone marrow cells)[†]
Control	Control	−	1.7 ± 0.6
Control	Control	+	12.0 ± 2.6[‡]
Control	Immune	−	0.7 ± 0.6
Control	Immune	+	13.3 ± 2.5[ǁ]
Immune	Control	−	2.0 ± 1.0
Immune	Control	+	39.0 ± 6.0[‡§]
Immune	Immune	−	1.3 ± 0.6
Immune	Immune	+	33.7 ± 1.2[§ǁ]

*ADC mixed with NADC cultured with (+) and without (−) N-CWS for 48 h. CSF activity of each conditioned medium (CM) tested.
[†]Values are means ± SD of triplicate cultures.
[‡]Significant at $p < 0.02$.
[§]Not significant.
[ǁ]Significant at $p < 0.001$.

produce CSF. With regard to immunocompetent cells, the following have been demonstrated to produce CSF: murine macrophages (69); a monocyte tumor cell line (70); human peripheral blood monocytes stimulated with lipopolysaccharide (71); and T or B lymphocytes stimulated with mitogens (72,73). Hayashi et al have investigated the CSF-producing cells by N-CWS-stimulation in N-CWS-immunized mice. When immunized ADC were cultured in the culture supernatant from immunized NADC that had been incubated with N-CWS, the ADC produced only low CSF activity (Table 4) (32). When immunized NADC were cultured in the culture supernatant prepared by incubation of immunized ADC with N-CWS, NADC produced markedly increased CSF activity. However, when N-CWS-immunized WMNL were treated with anti-Lyt1.1 or anti-Lyt2.1 monoclonal antibody plus complement and then cultured with N-CWS, the production of CSF from the cells significantly decreased. Moore et al (74) have demonstrated that Lyt1.1$^+$ and Lyt2.1$^+$ cells are CSF-producing cells. These findings demonstrate that immunized Lyt1.1$^+$ cells and Lyt2.1$^+$ cells are major producers of CSF, and that immunized ADC, and the culture supernatant of immunized ADC, help these cells to produce CSF.

Replacement of ADC by J774 cells or their culture supernatant

Fractionation of WMNL into ADC and NADC is not a complete method for purification of macrophages or T lymphocytes. We therefore investigated whether J774 cells, a macrophage-like cell line, or their culture supernatant could replace the function of ADC in CSF production by N-CWS stimulation. Im-

Table 4 CSF production by fractionated immunized splenocytes cultured in media conditioned with immunized splenocytes. Reprinted, with permission, from Hayashi S, Masuno T, Hosoe S, et al (32).

Cells	N-CWS	Culture medium*	CSF activity of CM (no. of colonies/10^5 bone marrow cells)[†]
None	−	NADC	0
None	−	NADC + N-CWS	6.0 ± 2.0
ADC	−	NADC	0.3 ± 0.6
ADC	−	NADC + N-CWS	2.0 ± 1.0
ADC	+	NADC	5.3 ± 3.1
ADC	+	NADC + N-CWS	7.3 ± 2.9
None	−	ADC	0.3 ± 0.6
None	−	ADC + N-CWS	11.7 ± 2.5
NADC	−	ADC + N-CWS	9.0 ± 4.6
NADC	+	ADC	19.3 ± 1.2
NADC	+	ADC + N-CWS	49.7 ± 10.3

*Cells adjusted to 1.25×10^6 cells/mL in RPMI 1640 medium plus 2% FCS and cultured for 48 h with (+) or without (−) N-CWS 10 μg/mL. Cell-free supernatant harvested was filtered to deplete the N-CWS particles. In each supernatant, ADC or NADC adjusted to 1.25×10^6 cells/mL cultured with or without N-CWS 10 μg/mL. CSF activity of each conditioned medium tested.
[†]Values are means ± SD of triplicate cultures.

munized NADC were cultured with various numbers of J774 cells in the presence of N-CWS. The CSF activity of the culture supernatant increased in proportion to the number of J774 cells that were added to immunized NADC. J774 cells alone produced no significant CSF activity, whereas CSF production by NADC was synergistically increased when NADC were cultured with N-CWS in the culture supernatant from J774 cells. These data suggest that J774 cells, or the culture supernatant of J774 cells, could be substituted for ADC.

Effect of N-CWS on CSF production and proliferation of M1 cells

The M1 cell line is one established from a spontaneous myeloid leukemia of an SL-strain mouse, and can be stimulated to differentiate into either macrophages or neutrophil granulocytes (75,76). Maeda et al (29) have examined whether several microorganism-associated immunostimulators induce differentiation of M1 cells. N-CWS, as well as *Mycobacterium tuberculosis* and *Mycobacterium bovis* BCG, enhanced the differentiation of M1 cells. However, *Propionibacterium acnes* and its cell wall skeleton had no effect on the induction of differentiation or growth of M1 cells. Maeda et al also examined whether immunostimulants cause M1 cells to produce CSF. When M1 cells were incubated with N-CWS, CSF activity was evident in 1-day-old culture fluid, increasing gradually, to reach a maximum after 5 to 7 days. In contrast, *P. acnes*-CWS did not stimulate CSF production by M1 cells. Also, N-CWS has been shown to stimulate murine splenocytes to produce D factors, which are distinct from CSF and induce differentiation of M1 cells into phagocytic cells. In summary, N-CWS increases CSF production which, in turn, induces proliferation and differentiation of GM-CFU in mice. And CSF, in the sera of immunized mice that have been challenged with an N-CWS ip injection, is mainly produced by N-CWS-immunized Lyt1.1[+] and Lyt2.1[+] T cells, with the help of macrophage or macrophage-derived humoral factor(s).

Effect of N-CWS on macrophages in vitro

Effect of N-CWS on mouse peritoneal macrophages in vitro

It has been shown that N-CWS augments CSF production and induces the proliferation and differentiation of macrophage progenitor cells. Interest is now focusing on the mechanism(s) of macrophage activation. Masuno et al (20) have studied the effect of N-CWS on murine macrophages in vitro to determine its mechanism of macrophage activation.

Whole peritoneal cells (WPC) from BALB/c mice were incubated with 0.05 to 50 μg/mL of oil-attached N-CWS (oil-N-CWS) for 3 days, and adherent peritoneal cells (APC) were measured for cytostatic activity against syngeneic Meth A fibrosarcoma cells (Table 5) (20). In vitro treatment of WPC with a placebo did not activate the cytostatic property of APC, whereas APC from the

Table 5 Dose-dependent activation of cytostatic property of peritoneal macrophages with oil-N-CWS in vitro. Reprinted, with permission, from Masuno T, Hayashi S, Ito M, et al (20).

Origin of effector APC	Concentration (μg/mL)	Cytostasis
WPC incubated in medium alone*	—	11.3 ± 0.7[†]
WPC incubated with oil-N-CWS placebo	—	13.6 ± 4.1
WPC incubated with oil-N-CWS	0.05	15.8 ± 6.5
	0.5	16.4 ± 0.0
	5.0	30.0 ± 2.2
	25.0	47.5 ± 0.2
	50.0	22.5 ± 2.8

*WPC (2×10^6) from normal BALB/c mice incubated in medium alone, or with oil-N-CWS placebo at a concentration corresponding to 25.0 μg/mL oil-N-CWS, or with 0.05 to 50.0 μg/mL oil-N-CWS for 3 days. After washing to remove nonadherent cells and immunomodulators, resulting adherent cells tested for cytostatic activity against syngeneic Meth A fibrosarcoma cells at an E:T ratio of 50:1.
[†]Mean ± SE of triplicate determinations.

WPC that were incubated with 5.0 to 50.0 μg/mL of oil-N-CWS augmented the cytostatic activity. The maximum cytostatic activity of the APC was obtained when incubated with 25.0 μg/mL of N-CWS.

Table 6 (20) shows the cytostatic activities of APC incubated with 25.0 μg/mL of N-CWS in the absence of nonadherent peritoneal cells (NAPC). The cytostatic activity of APC from WPC which had been treated with N-CWS increased in proportion to the effector to target cell (E:T) ratio. However, when APC were incubated with N-CWS in the absence of NAPC, there was no enhancement in cytostatic activity of APC at any E:T ratios. When APC were cultured with N-CWS-treated NAPC (N-CWS-NAPC) or with supernatant from N-CWS-NAPC, the cytostatic activity of APC was augmented (Table 7) (20). APC were activated with N-CWS in the presence but not in the absence of NAPC. Reconstitution of APC with N-CWS-NAPC or with N-CWS-NAPC supernatant induced potent antitumor activity. These results suggest that humoral factors released from peritoneal lymphocytes treated with N-CWS may play a crucial role in the in vitro macrophage activation by N-CWS. To determine the lymphocyte subpopulation that mediated APC activation in vitro, the effect of T cell depletion from WPC on APC activation in vitro was examined (Table 8) (20). APC, when prepared from WPC pretreated with anti-Thy1.2 antibody and complement, were not cytostatically activated with N-CWS. Pretreatment of WPC with anti-Thy1.2 antibody alone or with complement alone did not affect in vitro APC activation with N-CWS. These results indicate that in vitro activation of BALB/c peritoneal macrophages with N-CWS is mainly mediated by the humoral factor released from T lymphocytes.

Table 6 Cytostatic activity of peritoneal macrophages in vitro activated with oil-N-CWS tested at various E:T ratios. Reprinted, with permission, from Masuno T, Hayashi S, Ito M, et al (20).

Expt	Origin of effector APC	Cytostasis (%) at ET ratio		
		10:1	25:1	50:1
1	WPC incubated in medium alone*	$-1.3 \pm 1.4^\dagger$	8.5 ± 1.2	11.3 ± 0.7
	WPC incubated with oil-N-CWS placebo	7.8 ± 2.4	10.4 ± 2.6	13.6 ± 4.1
	WPC incubated with oil-N-CWS	9.0 ± 3.9	29.4 ± 1.1	47.5 ± 0.4
2	APC incubated in medium alone*	-4.2 ± 1.5	7.6 ± 0.6	14.7 ± 0.4
	APC incubated with oil-N-CWS placebo	3.3 ± 2.2	7.2 ± 5.4	11.8 ± 0.5
	APC incubated with oil-N-CWS	5.8 ± 1.6	6.5 ± 2.7	11.8 ± 0.7

*WPC (2×10^6) from normal BALB/c mice, or APC prepared from 2×10^6 WPC, incubated in medium alone, or with oil-N-CWS placebo at a concentration corresponding to 25.0 μg/mL oil-N-CWS, or with 25.0 μg/mL oil-N-CWS for 3 days. After washing to remove nonadherent cells and immunomodulators, resulting adherent cells tested for cytostatic activity against syngeneic Meth A fibrosarcoma cells at E:T ratios indicated.
†Mean ± SE of triplicate determinations.

Table 7 In vitro macrophage activation with N-CWS-NAPC or with N-CWS-NAPC supernatant. Reprinted, with permission, from Masuno T, Hayashi S, Ito M, et al (20).

Expt	Origin of effector APC	Cytostasis
1	APC incubated with N-NAPC*	$9.9 \pm 0.4^{\dagger}$
	APC incubated with placebo − NAPC	13.6 ± 1.0
	APC incubated with N-CWS-NAPC	28.8 ± 1.0
2	APC incubated in N-NAPC supernatant	14.6 ± 1.2
	APC incubated in placebo NAPC supernatant	13.1 ± 0.7
	APC incubated in N-CWS-NAPC supernatant	31.3 ± 4.0

*APC prepared from 2×10^6 WPC of normal BALB/c mice incubated with 5×10^5 N-NAPC, placebo-NAPC, or with N-CWS-NAPC, or in 100% N-NAPC supernatant, placebo-NAPC supernatant, or in N-CWS-NAPC supernatant for 3 days. After washing to remove nonadherent cells, resulting APC were tested for cytostatic activity against syngeneic Meth A fibrosarcoma cells at an E:T ratio of 50:1.
†Mean ± SE of triplicate determinations.

Table 8 Effects of T lymphocyte depletion on in vitro macrophage activation with oil-N-CWS. Reprinted, with permission, from Masuno T, Hayashi S, Ito M, et al (20).

Agent added to effector APC prepared from WPC*	N-CWS	Cytostasis
Medium alone	−	$14.5 \pm 0.3^{\dagger}$
Medium alone	+	47.5 ± 0.2
Anti-Thy1.2 antibody alone	+	43.7 ± 4.9
Complement alone	+	25.8 ± 1.2
Anti-Thy1.2 antibody + complement	+	8.0 ± 6.8

*WPC (2×10^6) of normal BALB/c mice treated with anti-Thy1.2 antibody alone, complement alone, or anti-Thy1.2 antibody and complement, and incubated with 25.0 μg/mL oil-N-CWS for 3 days. After washing to remove nonadherent cells and immunomodulators, resulting adherent cells tested for cytostatic activity against syngeneic Meth A fibrosarcoma cells at an E:T ratio of 50:1.
†Mean ± SE of triplicate determinations.

Effect of N-CWS on rat alveolar macrophages in vitro

Sone et al (19) investigated whether the direct interaction of N-CWS with rat alveolar macrophages (AM) can render them tumoricidal. AM from F344 rat incubated with various concentrations of N-CWS (0.001 to 50 μg/mL) for 24 h were tested for cytocidal activity against ^{125}I-labeled syngeneic MADB-100 or MADB-200 mammary adenocarcinoma cells (Fig 2) (19). Potent AM-mediated

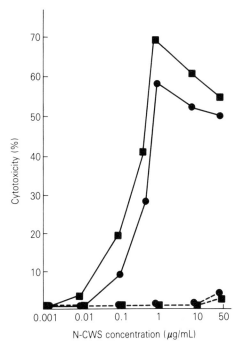

Fig 2 The dose-response curve of rat alveolar macrophages (AM) to N-CWS. 10^5 AM incubated for 24 h with N-CWS (——) or N-CWS placebo (- - -) at indicated concentrations and washed thoroughly prior to addition of 1×10 ^{125}I IUdR-labeled tumor cells. Cultures terminated at 72 h, and the adherent viable tumor cells were collected and counted. Results are expressed as the percent cytotoxicity of N-CWS-activated vs unstimulated AM (p < 0.005). MADB 100 (■—■) and MADB 200 (●—●) are types of mammary adenocarcinoma cells. Reprinted, with permission, from Sone S, Pollack VA, Fidler IJ (19).

cytotoxicity was evident when AM were pretreated with a concentration as low as $0.1 \, \mu g/mL$ of N-CWS, and maximal cytotoxicity was obtained when they were pretreated with $1.0 \, \mu g/mL$ of N-CWS.

AM treated with $1.0 \, \mu g/mL$ of N-CWS for 24 h and then washed and incubated in medium alone completely lost their tumoricidal properties after 96 h. However, a second in vitro exposure to N-CWS reactivated AM to their full tumoricidal potential.

These data suggest that rat AM obtained by pulmonary lavage can respond to direct activation by N-CWS to become tumoricidal in vitro.

Effect of N-CWS on MAF production by murine splenocytes

In vitro experiments have demonstrated that acquisition of nonspecific tumoricidal activity by murine macrophages results from a sequence of reactions

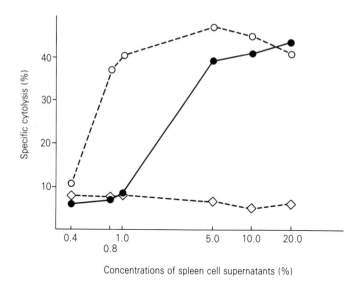

Concentrations of spleen cell supernatants (%)

Fig 3 Dose-dependent activation of peritoneal macrophages with N-CWS-SC supernatant. Adherent peritoneal cells (APC) from C3H/HeN mice given an ip injection of 1 mL 10% thioglycolate 4 days previously were incubated in 0.5% to 20% N-SC supernatant (◇), N-CWS-SC supernatant (●) or in Con A-SC supernatant (○) for 4 h. The cytolytic activity of the APC against FBL-3 leukemic cells was measured at an E:T ratio of 50:1. Reprinted, with permission, from Masuno T, Hayashi S, Ito M, et al (20).

involving at least 2 signals. The first signal is macrophage activating factor (MAF), which primes the macrophage and makes it sensitive to the effects of a second signal that triggers the development of cytocidal activity (77,78). It has been shown that interferon-γ (IFN-γ) displays MAF-like properties, including the quantitative ability to prime macrophages for nonspecific tumoricidal activity (79). N-CWS stimulates human pleural cells to produce IFN-γ in some cases with lung cancer or with mediastinal tumor (21). It was indicated that in vitro macrophage activation with N-CWS may depend on the humoral factor released from T lymphocytes stimulated with N-CWS. Masuno et al examined whether N-CWS could induce MAF from murine spleen cells. Spleen cells from C3H/HeN mice were incubated with 10 μg/mL of N-CWS, 2.5 μg/mL concanavalin A (Con A), or in medium alone for 48 h. The culture supernatants harvested were designated N-CWS-stimulated splenocyte supernatant, Con A-stimulated splenocyte supernatant, and normal splenocyte supernatant, respectively. C3H/HeN peritoneal macrophages were incubated with 0.4 to 20% of N-CWS-SC supernatant or Con A-SC supernatant for 4 h, and tested for cytocidal activity against ^{125}I-labeled syngeneic FBL-3 leukemic cells (Fig 3) (20). The cytolytic activity of peritoneal macrophages incubated with supernatants from N-CWS-SC or Con A-SC reached a plateau at a concentration of 5% and 1%, respectively, and the magnitude of maximum cytolytic activity of macrophages incubated with N-CWS-SC supernatant was equivalent to that with supernatant from Con A-SC. These results suggest that N-CWS can induce potent MAF from murine spleen cells.

In conclusion, N-CWS stimulates CSF-producing cells such as Lyt1.1$^+$ cells, Lyt2.1$^+$ cells, or lung parenchymal cells to produce CSF; N-CWS subsequently generates GM-CFU and differentiates them to macrophages. Finally, N-CWS renders tumoricidal the macrophages that are differentiated from GM-CFU by direct activation, or through MAF production, or through both.

References

1. Azuma I, Taniyama T, Yamawaki M, et al. Adjuvant and antitumor activities of *Nocardia rubra* cell-wall skeletons. Jpn J Cancer Res (Gann) 1976;67:733–6.
2. Fujitsu T, Sakuma S, Yoneda K, et al. Effect of *Nocardia rubra* cell wall skeleton (N-CWS) on immune responses in mice and guinea pigs. Pharmacometrics 1986;31:757–65.
3. Azuma I, Taniyama T, Yamawaki M, et al. Mitogenic activity of the cell walls of Mycobacteria, *Nocardia*, Corynebacteria and anaerobic coryneforms. Jpn J Microbiol 1976;20:263–71.
4. Ciorbaru R, Pett J-F, Lederer E, et al. Presence and subcellular localization of *Nocardia rubra* and *Nocardia opaca*: preparation of soluble mitogenic peptidoglycan fractions. Infect Immun 1976;13:1084–90.
5. Sugimura K, Uemiya M, Azuma I, et al. Macrophage dependency of T-lymphocyte mitogenesis by *Nocardia rubra* cell-wall skeleton. Microbiol Immunol 1977;21:525–30.
6. Yanagawa E, Yasumoto K, Ohta M, et al. Comparative study of *Mycobacterium bovis* BCG and *Nocardia rubra* with reference to T-cell dependency and independency. Jpn J Cancer Res (Gann) 1979;70:141–6.
7. Kawase I, Uemiya M, Yoshimoto T, et al. Effect of *Nocardia rubra* cell wall skeleton on T-cell-mediated cytotoxicity in mice bearing syngeneic sarcoma. Cancer Res 1981;41:660–6.
8. Masuno T, Ito M, Ogura T, et al. Activation of peritoneal macrophages by oil-attached cell-wall skeleton of BCG and *Nocardia rubra*. Jpn J Cancer Res (Gann) 1979;70:223–7.
9. Ogura T, Namba M, Hirao F, et al. Association of macrophage activation with antitumor effect on rat syngeneic fibrosarcoma by *Nocardia rubra* cell wall skeleton. Cancer Res 1979;39:4706–12.
10. Ito M, Iizuka H, Masuno T, et al. Killing of tumor cells in vitro by macrophages from mice given injection of squalene-treated cell wall skeleton of *Nocardia rubra*. Cancer Res 1981;41:2925–30.
11. Ogura T, Shinzato O, Sakatani M, et al. Analysis of therapeutic effect in experimental chemoimmunotherapy for rat ascites tumor. Cancer Immunol Immunother 1982;14:67–72.
12. Ito M, Suzuki H, Nakano N, et al. Superoxide anion and hydrogen peroxide release by macrophages from mice treated with *Nocardia rubra* cell-wall skeleton: inhibition of macrophage cytotoxicity by a protease inhibitor but not by superoxide dismutase and catalase. Jpn J Cancer Res (Gann) 1983;74:128–36.

13. Inamura N, Fujitsu T, Nakahara K, et al. Potentiation of tumoricidal properties of murine macrophages by *Nocardia rubra* cell wall skeleton (N-CWS). J Antibiot 1984;37:244–52.
14. Kagawa K, Yamashita T, Tsubura E, Yamamura Y. Inhibition of pulmonary metastasis by *Nocardia rubra* cell wall skeleton, with special reference to macrophage activation. Cancer Res 1984;44:665–70.
15. Mine Y, Watanabe Y, Tawara S, et al. In vivo activation of functional properties in mouse peritoneal macrophages by *Nocardia rubra* cell wall skeleton. Arzneimiltelforschung 1986;36:1651–5.
16. Sone S, Fidler IJ. Activation of rat alveolar macrophages to the tumoricidal state in the presence of progressively growing pulmonary metastases. Cancer Res 1981;412:2401–6.
17. Sone S, Fidler IJ. In situ activation of tumoricidal properties in rat alveolar macrophages and rejection of experimental lung metastases by intravenous injections of *Nocardia rubra* cell wall skeleton. Cancer Immunol Immunother 1982;12:203–9.
18. Yanagawa E, Yasumoto K, Manabe H, et al. Cytostatic activity of peripheral blood monocytes against bronchogenic carcinoma cells in patients with lung cancer. Jpn J Cancer Res (Gann) 1979;70:533–9.
19. Sone S, Pollack VA, Fidler IJ. Direct activation of tumoricidal properties in rat alveolar macrophages by *Nocardia rubra* cell wall skeleton. Cancer Immunol Immunother 1980;9:227–32.
20. Masuno T, Hayashi S, Ito M, et al. Mechanism(s) of in vitro macrophage activation with *Nocardia rubra* cell wall skeleton: the effects on macrophage activating factor production by lymphocytes. Cancer Immunol Immunother 1986;22:132–8.
21. Sakatani M, Ogura T, Masuno T, et al. Effect of *Nocardia rubra* cell wall skeleton on augmentation of cytotoxicity function in human pleural macrophages. Cancer Immunol Immunother 1987;25:119–25.
22. Saijyo N, Ozaki A, Beppu Y, et al. In vivo and in vitro effects of *Nocardia rubra* cell wall skeleton on natural killer activity in mice. Jpn J Cancer Res (Gann) 1983;74:137–42.
23. Yamakido M, Ishioka S, Onari K, et al. Changes in natural killer cell, antibody-dependent cell-mediated cytotoxicity and interferon activities with administration of *Nocardia rubra* cell wall skeleton to subjects with high risk of lung cancer. Jpn J Cancer Res (Gann) 1983;74:896–901.
24. Shimizu E, Saijyo N, Shibuya M, et al. The analysis of cytostatic activity of human peripheral blood granulocytes and its augmentation with *Nocardia rubra* cell wall skeleton (N-CWS). Cancer Res Clin Oncol 1983;106:139–45.
25. Morikawa K, Takeda R, Yamazaki M, Mizuno D. Induction of tumoricidal activity of polymorphonuclear leukocytes by a linear β-1,3-D-glucan and other immunomodulators in murine cells. Cancer Res 1985;45:1496–501.
26. Yamakido M, Matsuzaka S, Yanagida J, et al. Effect of N-CWS injection against influenza virus infection in the retired workers of the Okunojima poison gas factory. Hiroshima J Med Sci 1984;33:547–51.
27. Izumi S, Hirai O, Hayashi K, et al. Induction of a tumor necrosis factor-like activity by *Nocardia rubra* cell wall skeleton. Cancer Res 1987;47:1785–92.
28. Izumi S, Ueda H, Okuhara M, et al. Effect of *Nocardia rubra* cell wall skeleton on murine interferon production in vitro. Cancer Res 1986;46:1960–5.
29. Maeda M, Ichikawa Y, Azuma I. Differentiation and production of colony-stimulating factor induced by immunostimulants in a leukemia cell line. J Cell

Physiol 1980;105:33-8.

30. Yamamoto Y, Tomida M, Hozumi M, Azuma I. Enhancement by immunostimulants of the production by mouse spleen cells of factor(s) stimulating differentiation of mouse myeloid leukemic cells. Jpn J Cancer Res (Gann) 1981;72:828-33.

31. Ito M, Suzuki H, Nakano N, et al. Effect of *Nocardia rubra* cell-wall skeleton on colony-stimulating activity and myeloid colony formation. Jpn J Cancer Res (Gann) 1982;73:403-7.

32. Hayashi S, Masuno T, Hosoe S, et al. Augmented production of colony-stimulating factor in C3H/HeN mice immunized with *Nocardia rubra* cell wall skeleton. Infect Immun 1986;52:128-33.

33. Nagasawa H, Yanai R, Azuma I. Suppression by *Nocardia rubra* cell wall skeleton of mammary DNA synthesis, plasma prolactin level, and spontaneous mammary tumorigenesis in mice. Cancer Res 1978;38:2160-2.

34. Namba M, Yoshimoto T, Ogura T, et al. Effect of *Nocardia rubra* cell-wall skeleton on the induction of lung cancer in ACI/N rats. Jpn J Cancer Res (Gann) 1979;70:55-62.

35. Nagasawa H, Yanai R, Azuma I. Inhibitory effect of *Nocardia rubra* cell wall skeleton on carcinogen-induced mammary tumorigenesis in rats. Eur J Cancer 1980;16:389-93.

36. Hirao F, Sakatani M, Nishikawa H, et al. Effect of *Nocardia rubra* cell-wall skeleton on the induction of lung cancer and amyloidosis by 3-methylcholanthrene in rabbits. Jpn J Cancer Res (Gann) 1980;71:398-401.

37. Inoue T, Yoshimoto T, Ogura T, et al. Effect of *Nocardia rubra* cell-wall skeleton treatment on tumor formation in two-stage chemical carcinogenesis of mouse skin. Cancer Immunol Immunother 1981;11:207-10.

38. Tokuzen R, Okabe M, Nakahara W, et al. Effect of *Nocardia* and *Mycobacterium* cell-wall skeleton on autochthonous tumor grafts. Jpn J Cancer Res (Gann) 1975;66:433-5.

39. Tokuzen R, Okabe M, Nakahara W, et al. Suppression of autochthonous tumors by mixed implantation with *Nocardia rubra* cell-wall skeleton and related bacterial fractions. Jpn J Cancer Res (Gann) 1978;69:19-24.

40. Azuma I, Yamawaki M, Yasumoto K, Yamamura Y. Antitumor activity of *Nocardia* cell wall skeleton preparations in transplantable tumors in syngeneic mice and patients with malignant pleurisy. Cancer Immunol Immunother 1978;4:95-100.

41. Yamawaki M, Azuma I, Saiki I, et al. Antitumor activity of squalene-treated cell-wall skeleton of *Nocardia rubra* in mice. Jpn J Cancer Res (Gann) 1978;69:619-26.

42. Pimm MV, Baldwin RB, Lederer E. Suppression of an ascitic rat hepatoma with cord factor and *Nocardia* cell-wall skeleton in squalene emulsions. Eur J Cancer 1980;16:1645-7.

43. Terashima H, Yasumoto K, Yanagawa E, et al. Combined treatment of syngeneic murine tumors and xenotransplanted human lung cancer by immunotherapy and radiotherapy. Jpn J Cancer Res (Gann) 1981;72:363-9.

44. Nagano N, Yasumoto K, Tanaka K, et al. Successful regional immunotherapy with cell-wall skeletons of BCG and *Nocardia rubra* against autochthonous rat tumors. Jpn J Cancer Res (Gann) 1982;73:613-7.

45. Ichinose Y, Yasumoto K, Tanaka K, et al. Combined treatment of autochthonous 3-methylcholanthrene-induced murine tumors by immunotherapy and radiotherapy. Jpn J Cancer Res (Gann) 1983;74:143-7.

46. Haraguchi S, Kurakata S, Matsuo T, Yoshida TO. Strain differences in antitumor ac-

tivity of an immunopotentiator, *Nocardia rubra* cell-wall skeleton, in B10 congenic and recombinant mice. Jpn J Cancer Res (Gann) 1985;76:400-13.

47. Yamamura Y, Ogura T, Sakatani M, et al. Randomized controlled study of adjuvant immunotherapy with *Nocardia rubra* cell wall skeleton for inoperable lung cancer. Cancer Res 1983;43:5575-9.

48. Yasumoto K, Yamamura Y. Randomized clinical trial of nonspecific immunotherapy with cell-wall skeleton of *Nocardia rubra*. Biomed Pharmacother 1984;38:48-54.

49. Yasumoto K, Yaita H, Ohta M, et al. Randomly controlled study of chemotherapy versus chemoimmunotherapy in postoperative lung cancer patients. Cancer Res 1985;45:1414-7.

50. Koyama S, Ozaki A, Iwasaki Y, et al. Randomized controlled study of postoperative adjuvant immunochemotherapy with *Nocardia rubra* cell wall skeleton (N-CWS) and tegafur for gastric carcinoma. Cancer Immunol Immunother 1986;22:148-54.

51. Ochiai T, Sato H, Sato H, et al. Randomly controlled study of chemotherapy versus chemoimmunotherapy in postoperative gastric cancer patients. Cancer Res 1983;43:3001-7.

52. Araki K, Kawano F, Matsuzaki H, et al. Chemoimmunotherapy for acute nonlymphocytic leukemia with BCG- and/or *Nocardia rubra* cell-wall skeleton (CWS). I: Clinical efficacy. Kumamoto Med J 1983;36:15-27.

53. Kawano F, Araki K, Eto T, et al. Chemoimmunotherapy for acute nonlymphocytic leukemia with BCG- and/or *Nocardia rubra* cell-wall skeleton (CWS). II: Analysis of the mechanisms of immunological destruction of tumor cells. Kumamoto Med J 1983;36:29-38.

54. Ohno R, Nakamura H, Kodera Y, et al. Randomized controlled study of chemoimmunotherapy of acute myelogenous leukemia (AML) in adults with *Nocardia rubra* cell-wall skeleton and irradiated allogeneic AML cells. Cancer 1986;57:1483-8.

55. Sakai S, Murata M, Sasaki R, et al. Combined therapy for maxillary sinus carcinoma with special reference to cryosurgery. Rhinology 1983;21:179-84.

56. Sakai S, Hohki A, Fuchihata H, Tanaka Y. Multidisciplinary treatment of maxillary sinus carcinoma. Cancer 1983;52:1360-4.

57. Ha K, Tawa A, Ikeda T, et al. Intrapleural therapy of malignant pleurisy in patients with neuroblastoma. Med Pediatr Oncol 1981;9:355-9.

58. Yoshida J, Kobayashi T, Kageyama N. Multimodality treatment of malignant glioma—Effect of chemotherapy with ACNU and immunotherapy with N-CWS. Neurol Med Chir 1984;24:19-26.

59. Mine Y, Yokota Y, Nonoyama S, Kikuchi H. Protective effect of *Nocardia rubra* cell wall skeleton on experimental infection in normal and immunosuppressed mice. Arzneimiltelforschung 1986;36:1489-92.

60. Hibbs JB, Lambert LH, Remington JS. Possible role of macrophage-mediated nonspecific cytotoxicity in tumour resistance. Nature 1972;235:48-50.

61. Evans R, Alexander P. Cooperation of immune lymphoid cells with macrophages in tumour immunity. Nature 1981;228:620-2.

62. Keller RC. The cytostatic and cytocidal effects of macrophages: are they really specific for tumor cells? In: Pick E, ed. Lymphokines 3. New York: Academic Press; 1981:283.

63. Fidler IJ, Barnes Z, Fogler WE, et al. Involvement of macrophages in the eradication of established metastases following intravenous injection of lyposomes containing macrophage activators. Cancer Res 1982;42:496-501.

64. Foster RS Jr. Effect of *Corynebacterium parvum* on the proliferative rate of

162

granulocyte-macrophage progenitor cells and the toxicity of chemotherapy. Cancer Res 1978;38:2666–72.

65. Hiraoka A, Yamagishi M, Ohkubo T, et al. Effect of streptococcal preparation, OK-432, on murine hematopoietic stem cells. Acta Haematol Jpn 1981;44:860–3.

66. Ladish S, Poplack DG, Bull JM. Acceleration of myeloid recovery from cyclophosphamide-induced leukopenia by pretreatment with *Bacillus* Calmette-Guérin. Cancer Res 1978;38:1049–51.

67. Koury MJ, Pragnell IB. Retrovirus-induced granulocyte-macrophage colony-stimulating activity in fibroblast. Nature 1982;299:638–40.

68. Yamada T, Hirohashi S, Shimosato Y, et al. Giant cell carcinoma of the lung producing colony-stimulating factor in vitro and in vivo. Jpn J Cancer Res (Gann) 1985;76:967–76.

69. Eaves AC, Bruce WR. In vitro production of colony-stimulating activity. I: Exposure of mouse peritoneal cells to endotoxin. Cell Tissue Kinet 1974;7:19–30.

70. Ralph P, Broxmyer HE, Nakomz I. Immunostimulants induce granulocyte/macrophage colony-stimulating activity and block proliferation in monocyte tumor cell line. J Exp Med 1977;146:611–6.

71. Cline MJ, Rothman B, Golde DW. Effect of endotoxin on the production of colony-stimulating factor by human monocytes and macrophages. J Cell Physiol 1974;84:193–6.

72. Kees U, Kaltmann B, Marcucci F, et al. Frequency and activity of immune interferon (IFN-γ) and colony-stimulating factor-producing human peripheral blood T lymphocytes. J Immunol 1984;14:368–73.

73. Parker JW, Metcalf D. Production of colony-stimulating factor in mitogen-stimulated lymphocyte cultures. J Immunol 1974;112:502–12.

74. Moore RN, Hoffeld JT, Farrar JJ, et al. Role of colony-stimulating factors as primary regulators of macrophage functions. In: Pick E, ed. Lymphokines 3. New York: Academic Press; 1981:124.

75. Ichikawa Y. Differentiation of a cell line of myeloid leukemia. J Cell Physiol 1969;74:223–34.

76. Ichikawa Y. Further studies on the differentiation of a cell line of myeloid leukemia. J Cell Physiol 1970;76:175–84.

77. Ruco LP, Meltzer MS. Macrophage activation for tumor cytotoxicity: tumoricidal activity by macrophages from C3H/HeJ mice requires at least 2 activation stimuli. Cell Immunol 1978;41:35–51.

78. Meltzer MA. Tumor cytotoxicity by lymphokine-activated macrophages: development of macrophage tumoricidal activity requires a sequence of reactions. In: Pick E, ed. Lymphokines 3. New York: Academic Press; 1981:319.

79. Schreiber RD, Pace JL, Russel SW, et al. Macrophage-activating factor produced by a T cell hybridoma: physicochemical and biosynthetic resemblance to γ-interferon. J Immunol 1983;131:826–32.

Experimental immunotherapy with *Nocardia rubra* cell wall skeleton in tumor-bearing animals

Ichiro Kawase

3rd Department of Internal Medicine, Osaka University Medical School, Osaka, Japan

Introduction

In the 1970s, experimental and clinical immunotherapy for malignancies using live BCG revealed several problems associated with differences between strains of the microorganisms in terms of their antitumor activities and with hazards related to the use of viable organisms (1,2). To overcome these problems, more specific and nonliving bacterial products were needed for clinical use.

Azuma et al (3,4) demonstrated that the cell wall skeleton (CWS) of *Mycobacterium bovis* BCG (BCG-CWS), consisting of the complex of mycolic acid-arabinogalactan-mucopeptide, is the minimal component essential for developing adjuvant activity on immune responses. BCG-CWS in an oil-attached form was tested for its antitumor activity and found to be as effective for both animal (5,6) and human cancers (7–9) as live BCG. In clinical trials, however, oil-attached BCG-CWS was also associated with severe complications, such as ulceration at the injection site and high fever. One further problem to be considered was the large number of pathogenic organisms necessary for the preparation of BCG-CWS in a large enough amount for clinical use.

Azuma et al (10) screened a wide variety of non- or poorly pathogenic, mycobacteria-related organisms and found that the CWS of *Nocardia rubra* (N-CWS), possessing potent adjuvant activities on T cell-mediated immune responses, exhibits apparent antitumor effects comparable to those of BCG-CWS when tested by a tumor growth suppression test. Based on this finding, the antitumor activities of N-CWS and its usefulness in antitumor immunotherapy were further investigated using a variety of animal tumor models, including syngeneic murine tumors and autografts of spontaneously arising or chemically induced murine and rat tumors (11–13). In these studies, N-CWS (prepared as an oil-attached form using squalene, a metabolizable intermediate in the biosynthesis of cholesterol) was found to be useful as an immunotherapeutic agent because of its low toxicity, good stability but high antitumor activity (14).

Antitumor activity of squalene-treated N-CWS in experimental immunotherapy

The antitumor activity of squalene-treated N-CWS was investigated in therapeutic experiments using syngeneic murine and rat tumors. Ogura et al (15) demonstrated the antitumor effect of repeated injections against a rat ascitic fibrosarcoma. ACI/N rats inoculated ip with 10^4–10^6 AMC-60 syngeneic fibrosarcoma cells were given ip injections of 100 or 500 μg of N-CWS repeatedly at 5-day intervals from day 1 after tumor inoculation. As shown in Table 1, treatment with N-CWS significantly prolonged the survival period of rats bearing AMC-60 ascitic tumor when the tumor cell challenge was 10^4 cells. Pimm et al (16) also investigated the effect of single or repeated ip injections of N-CWS on the survival period of rats bearing D23As ascitic hepatoma. Rats inoculated ip with 10^4 D23As tumor cells were given an ip injection of 500 μg of N-CWS once or 3 times at 4-day intervals from the day of tumor inoculation. N-CWS prolonged the survival period of tumor-bearing rats, and the prolongation of the survival period was further augmented by repeating the injection of N-CWS.

The immunotherapeutic effect of squalene-treated N-CWS on murine solid tumors has been also demonstrated. Kawase et al (17) investigated the effect of interlesional injections of N-CWS on survival of mice bearing MC104 syngeneic fibrosarcoma. C57BL/6N mice inoculated sc with 10^6 fibrosarcoma cells were given intratumoral injections of 50 μg of N-CWS twice, 2 and 7 days after tumor

Table 1 Immunotherapeutic effect of N-CWS for rats bearing ascites tumor. Reprinted, with permission, from Ogura T, Namba M, Hirao F, et al (15).

Experiment	Tumor cell inoculation	CWS injection Dose (μg)	CWS injection Frequency	No. of rats	No. of survivors on day 20	30	40	50	Log-rank test (p)
A		0		10	0	0			
	1×10^4	100	8	10	7	5	4	3	<0.05
		500	8	9	9	6	5	5	<0.01
B	1×10^4	0		9	8	0			
		500	8	9	8	6	4	4	<0.05
C		0		10	7	0			
	1×10^5	50	8	10	6	0			NS
		250	8	10	7	5	4	3	NS
D	1×10^5	0		10	6	0			
		500	8	10	6	3	3	3	NS
E	1×10^5	0		10	8	0			
		400	8	10	8	5	4	4	NS

Rats inoculated ip with tumor cells on day 0. Treatment with N-CWS initiated on day 1 and repeated at 5-day intervals. All survivors killed on days 51 to 55. NS, not significant.

inoculation. Mice given the same amount of squalene served as controls. Figure 1 shows the survival rate of mice in the nontreated controls, squalene-treated controls, and N-CWS group. Two intratumoral injections of N-CWS significantly improved the survival rate, whereas treatment with squalene alone produced no effect on survival.

Haraguchi et al (18) tested N-CWS on virus-induced tumors in order to investigate genetic control in the development of the antitumor effect of N-CWS, using B10 congenic and recombinant mice. In their report, weekly intratumoral injections of N-CWS initiated 1 week after tumor inoculation were shown to the effective in B10 but not in B10.A mice, and the antitumor effect in B10 mice was further augmented by the presensitization of mice with N-CWS. They further demonstrated that N-CWS exhibited a marked antitumor effect, not only in B10 (H-2^b) but also in B10.A (5R) (H-2^{i5}) strains, and a moderate effect in B10.BR (H-2^k) strain, but no apparent effect in either B10.D2 (H-2^d) or B10.A (H-2^a) strains. The H-2 gene region (KAESD) in the B10 strain is (bbbbb), while those of B10.A (5R), B10.BR, B10.D2, and B10.A strains are (bbkdd), (kkkkk), (ddddd), and (kkkdd), respectively. They speculated that at least 1 gene controlling the manifestation of the antitumor effect of N-CWS is present in the H-2 region.

The combined use of squalene-treated N-CWS with chemotherapeutic agents or with irradiation was investigated in animal tumor models. Ogura et al (19) tested chemoimmunotherapy for a rat ascitic tumor using N-CWS and mitomycin C (MMC). ACI/N rats inoculated ip with 10^4 AMC-60 fibrosarcoma cells were given an ip injection of 100 or 200 μg of MMC 3 days after tumor inculation. Injection of 500 μg ip of N-CWS was initiated 3 or 5 days after tumor inoculation and repeated 8 times at 5- or 6-day intervals. As shown in Table 2, the

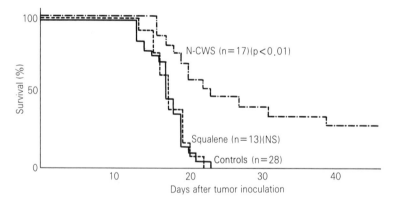

Fig 1 Effect of intralesional injection N-CWS on survival of mice bearing MC104 fibrosarcoma. C57BL/6N mice were given sc inoculations of 10^6 MC104 tumor cells into the dorsum of the hind foot on day 0 and given 50 μg of squalene (------) or N-CWS (–··–··) intratumorally on days 2 and 7. Control mice bearing MC104 tumor (——) were given no treatment. NS, not significant. Reprinted, with permission, from Kawase I, Uemiya M, Yoshimoto T, et al (17).

Table 2 Chemoimmunotherapy with MMC and N-CWS in tumor-bearing rats. Reprinted, with permission, from Ogura T, Shinzato O, Sakitani M, et al (19).

Treatment (ip) in rats*	Total no. of rats	Survival (d)						Tumor-free rats†	Mean survival (days)‡	Mann-Whitney U-test
		20	30	40	50	60	70			
Experiment I										
A None (control)	10	8	0					0	26	
B MMC 100 µg	10	10	5	4	4	4	4	4	48	A/B NS
C MMC 100 µg +CWS 500 µg (day 5)	10	10	10	9	8	8	8	6	72	A/C p<0.001 B/C p<0.05
Experiment II										
A None (control)	14	11	2	1	0			0	24	
B MMC 100 µg	14	14	9	8	5	5	5	4	49	A/B p<0.01
C MMC 100 µg +CWS 500 µg (day 5)	14	14	13	11	8	8	6		65	A/C p<0.01 B/C p<0.05
Experiment III										
A None (control)	10	9	1	0				0	25	
B MMC 200 µg	10	10	7	6	5	5	4	4	54	A/B p<0.05
C MMC 200 µg +CWS 500 µg (day 5)	10	10	10	10	9	8	6	6	70	A/C p<0.01 B/C NS
D MMC 200 µg +CWS 500 µg (day 3)	10	10	8	8	8	7	7	5	67	A/D p<0.01 B/D NS

*All rats inoculated with 1×10^4 tumor cells on day 0 and MMC given once on day 3. Injection of CWS initiated on day 5 (day 3 in experiment III-D) and administered 8 times at 5- or 6-day intervals.
†All survivors killed for autopsy on day 80.
‡Mean survival days of all rats in a group.
NS, not significant.

combined therapy with N-CWS and MMC resulted in a significant prolongation of the survival period compared with that of rats treated with MMC alone, when the chemotherapy was insufficient.

Ichinose et al (20) tested N-CWS in combination with irradiation against chemically induced autochthonous tumors. Fibrosarcomas were induced by im injection of 3-methylcholanthrene (MCA) in the hind leg in C57BL/6 mice. The tumors were irradiated at 2000 rad when they grew to 1 and 2 cm in diameter in experiments I and II, respectively, and the mice were given weekly sc injections of 100 µg of N-CWS into the ipsilateral footpad from the day of irradiation. In both experiments, the combination therapy with irradiation and N-CWS resulted in a more potent suppression of tumor growth than that obtained by irradiation or N-CWS alone (Fig 2).

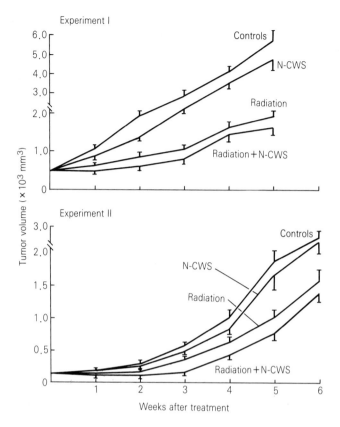

Fig 2 Growth suppression of autochthonous MCA-induced tumors by local irradiation and/or regional N-CWS injections (20). Bars, SE. Reprinted, with permission, from Ichinose Y, Yasumoto K, Tanaka K, et al (20).

Effects of N-CWS on experimental metastases

The antimetastatic activity of N-CWS has been observed in 2 different experimental systems. One is the antimetastic effect correspondingly seen with the local effect of N-CWS on primary tumors. The other is that obtained by stimulating the target organ of tumor metastases with N-CWS. In the report from Ogura et al (15), the effect of intralesional injections of N-CWS on tumor metastases was also investigated. AMC-60 fibrosarcoma inoculated im often metastasizes to the lung and the draining lymph nodes. ACI/N rats inoculated im with 2×10^6 AMC-60 tumor cells into the hind leg were given intratumoral injections of 100 μg of N-CWS 6 or 9 times at 5-day intervals from day 5 after tumor inoculation. As shown in Table 3, the treatment resulted not only in complete regression of the primary tumors in 6 of 21 rats but also in significant inhibition of tumor metastases to the lung and the draining lymph nodes.

Table 3 Treatment with repeated injections of N-CWS for rats bearing solid tumors. Reprinted, with permission, from Ogura T, Namba M, Hirao F, et al (15).

Treatment	Total no. of rats	Primary tumor bearer	None	Lung or DLN	DLN and kidney	DLN and lung	Lung and kidney	DLN, lung, and kidney	Total no. of metas- tases	Fisher test (p)
Experiment A*										
None (control)	10	10	2	6	0	2	0	0	8	
CWS 100 µg, 6 it inj†	10	7	8	0	0	2	0	0	2	0.023
Experiment B‡										
None (control)	12	12	0	5	0	2	1	4	12	
CWS 100 µg, 9 it inj†	11	8	5	0	0	4	0	2	6	0.014
CWS 100 µg, 9 iv inj‡	11	9	2	3	1	1	2	2	9	NS

*Rats inoculated with 2×10^6 tumor cells and killed on day 35.
†Treatment with N-CWS initiated 5 days after tumor inoculation and repeated at 5-day intervals.
‡Rats inoculated with 5×10^6 tumor cells and killed on day 55.
DLN, draining lymph node (isolateral paraaortic lumbar node); NS, not significant.

Similar results were shown by Ichinose et al (20). C57BL/6 mice bearing autochthonous fibrosarcomas induced by an MCA injection were treated with local irradiation (2000 rad) and repeated injections of N-CWS to the peripheral site of the tumors. This combined therapy completely prevented the occurrence of pulmonary metastases, and simultaneously augmented suppression of primary tumor growth (Table 4).

Stimulation of the metastatic target organ with N-CWS has also been reported to be effective against tumor metastases. Kagawa et al (21) investigated the effect of iv injection of N-CWS on tumor metastasis to the lung. C57BL/6 mice were inoculated sc with Lewis lung carcinoma 3LL, a tumor line possessing a high ability to metastasize to the lung, into the hind footpads, and the tumor-bearing legs were amputated 10 days after tumor inoculation. As shown in Table 5, 3 iv injections of N-CWS 2.5 mg/kg resulted in the apparent inhibition of pulmonary metastases when the treatment was repeated at 2-day intervals from the day of tumor resection. The inhibition of pulmonary metastases of 3LL tumor by N-CWS became more apparent when chemotherapy was successfully combined. The combined therapy with an ip injection of cyclophosphamide (CY) on the day of tumor resection and 3 iv injections of N-CWS after surgery produced a marked inhibition of pulmonary metastases, resulting in the apparent prolongation of the survival period (Table 6).

Table 4 Suppression of pulmonary metastases in mice bearing autochthonous MCA-induced tumors by combined treatment with local irradiation and regional N-CWS injections. Reprinted, with permission, from Ichinose Y, Yasumoto K, Tanaka K, et al (20).

Group	No. of mice sacrificed	Average primary tumor volume (mm³ ± SE)	No. of mice with pulmonary metastases (%)	No. of pulmonary metastases/mouse
Control	21	4327 ± 536	5(23.8)	10,7,2,2,1
N-CWS	23	3770 ± 466	4(17.4)	17,3,2,1
Radiation	32	3665 ± 350	7(21.9)	3,1,1,1,1,1,1
Radiation +N-CWS	27	3573 ± 351	0(0)*	

Mice in the control and N-CWS groups sacrificed at the 7th week after initial treatment and those in the irradiation and irradiation + N-CWS groups sacrificed at the 9th week. *Significantly different from control (p < 0.01), N-CWS (p < 0.05), and irradiation control (p < 0.01).

Table 5 Effect of time and route of N-CWS on its inhibition of pulmonary metastases. Reprinted, with permission, from Kagawa K, Yamashita T, Tsubura E, Yamamura Y (21).

Experimental group*	N-CWS Dose (mg/kg)	Route	Days of injection	Pulmonary metastases No. of surface nodules	Incidence[†]
Untreated				33.3 ± 6.4[‡](38)[§] 62–12[‖]	10/10
N-CWS	2.5	iv	3, 5, 7	19.8 ± 4.1 (28) 36–3	10/10
	2.5	iv	10,12,14	11.8 ± 3.4 (6) 28–1[¶]	10/10
Untreated				36.8 ± 4.5 (42) 62–12	10/10
N-CWS	2.5	ip	10,12,14	48.3 ± 8.3 (56) 79–5	10/10

*Inocula of 10^6 tumor cells injected sc into a footpad. The implanted tumor removed on day 10 after tumor inoculation. In experiment 1, a dose of 2.5 mg of N-CWS per kg injected iv 3 times before or after removal of the implanted tumor.
[†]Number of mice with pulmonary metatases/number of mice tested.
[‡]Mean ±SE.
[§]Number in parentheses, median number of pulmonary metastases.
[‖]Range of the number of surface nodules.
[¶]p < 0.01 (Student's *t*-test); p < 0.025 (Mann-Whitney U-test) compared with untreated group.

Antitumor mechanisms of N-CWS

Tumor growth suppression resulting from local treatment with bacterial immunoadjuvants has been suggested to be mediated mainly by macrophages. This theory is based on the findings that the granulomatous reaction is predominantly

Table 6 Combined effect of N-CWS (mg/kg) and cyclophosphamide (CY) (mg/kg) on pulmonary metastases. Reprinted, with permission, from Kagawa K, Yamashita T, Tsubura E, Yamamura Y (21).

Experimental group*	CY (ip)		N-CWS (iv)		Pulmonary metastases		Survival time	
	Dose	Days of injection	Dose	Days of injection	No. of surface nodules	Incidence†	Days	%
Untreated					31.0 ± 5.0§(27)‖ 64–15¶	10/10	22.4 ± 0.7	100
N-CWS			2.5	10,12,14	18.1 ± 2.0 (19) 32–3#	10/10	24.1 ± 0.6	118
CY	50	10			4.8 ± 1.9 (3) 19–0**	8/10	29.9 ± 1.0**	134
N-CWS + CY	50	10	2.5	10,12,14	1.9 ± 1.0 (1) 10–0††	6/10	34.0 ± 1.4††,‡‡	>185

*Inocula of 10^6 tumor cells injected sc into a footpad. Implanted tumor removed on day 10 after tumor implantation.

†Number of mice with pulmonary metastases/number of mice tested.

‡Survival time of treated group as a percentage of that of the control.

§Mean ± SE.

‖Numbers in parentheses: median number of pulmonary metastases.

¶Range of the number of surface nodules.

#$p < 0.05$ compared with untreated group.

**$p < 0.01$ compared with untreated group.

††$p < 0.001$ compared with untreated group.

‡‡$p < 0.05$ compared with CY.

seen in the regressing tumor mass injected with the adjuvants (22) and that macrophages induced by the adjuvants in normal animals exhibit significant antitumor activity in vitro and in vivo (23,24). N-CWS, as well as BCG-CWS, has also been shown to be able to activate macrophage-nonspecific cytotoxicity to syngeneic and allogeneic tumor cells in mice (25,26). Several investigators have demonstrated direct and indirect data indicating that macrophages act as major effector cells in the tumor growth suppression induced by N-CWS. A report by Ogura et al (15), demonstrating the prolongation of survival period of ACI/N rats bearing AMC-60 ascitic fibrosarcoma by ip injections of N-CWS, showed that rat peritoneal cells induced by ip injection of N-CWS exhibited a potent cytolytic activity against AMC-60 tumor cells in 24-h [^{125}I]iododeoxyuridine-release assay and that the cytotoxicity was mainly mediated by adherent but not by nonadherent cells (Fig 3).

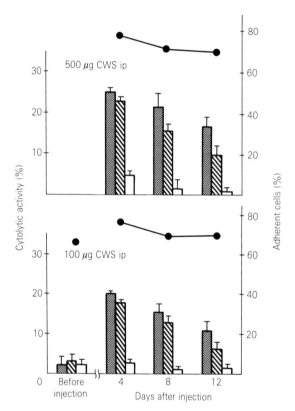

Fig 3 Induction of cytolytic activity for AMC-60 tumor cells after a single ip injection of N-CWS. Radiolabeled tumor cells (1 × 10⁴ cells) cultured with 10⁶ whole PEC (▨) and resulting fractions of macrophages (▨) and nonadherent PEC (▢). Each column, mean of data from 3 or 4 rats; bars, ± SE; each point, percentage of adherent cells (macrophages) in whole PEC. Difference between groups given injections of 100 μg and 500 μg in cytolytic activity significant on day 4 at p<0.05. Reprinted, with permission, from Ogura T, Namba M, Hirao F, et al (15).

The major role of activated macrophages in N-CWS-induced inhibition of pulmonary metastases was reported by Kagawa et al (21). Their study demonstrated that iv injection of N-CWS after the resection of 3LL tumor resulted in the potent inhibition of pulmonary metastases of the tumor, and that lung macrophages obtained from mice given iv injections of N-CWS exhibited a high cytotoxicity against 3LL tumor cells in 48-h [³H]thymidine-release assay, whether the donor mice were normal or were mice bearing micrometastases of 3LL tumor in the lung (Fig 4).

Although N-CWS has been shown to activate macrophages directly (27), the antitumor mechanisms of N-CWS cannot be ascribed only to the direct activation of macrophages. N-CWS exhibits poor antitumor effects in athymic nude mice, compared with those shown in normal mice (11), suggesting that mature T cells may be involved in the antitumor mechanisms of N-CWS. Mechanisms other than macrophage-mediated cytotoxicity may also play an important role in N-CWS-induced antitumor effects: there is no apparent correlation between the ability to generate activated macrophages in response to N-CWS and the degree of antitumor effects induced by N-CWS in B10 congenic and recombinant mice (18). N-CWS has been shown to be mitogenic to T cells (28), and Haraguchi et al (18) have demonstrated that strain differences in the development of antitumor effects of N-CWS show a good correlation with those in the mitogenic respon-

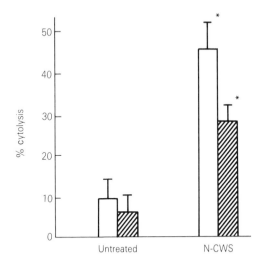

Fig 4 Cytolytic activity of lung macrophages activated with N-CWS. Lung macrophages from normal mice collected 5 days after iv injection of 10 mg of N-CWS per kg. Those from mice with pulmonary metastases collected after iv injection of 2.5 mg of N-CWS per kg 3 times after removal of the implanted tumor. ☐ Lung macrophages from normal mice; ▨ lung macrophages from mice with pulmonary metastases. The ratio of effector cells to 3LL target cells was 10:1. Columns, mean of 3 experiments; bars, SD; *p<0.01 compared with the untreated group by Student's *t*-test. Reprinted, with permission, from Kagawa K, Yamashita T, Tsubara E, Yamamura Y (21).

siveness of spleen cells to N-CWS. In several strains of mice, indeed, their presensitization with N-CWS before tumor challenge often results in the apparent augmentation of the antitumor effects of the following therapy with N-CWS (12,18). There have been increasing data indicating that N-CWS stimulates T cells to produce a variety of cytokines, including interferons (IFNs), colony-stimulating factor (CSF), and macrophage-activating factor (MAF), and that the presensitization of T cells with N-CWS enhances the cytokine production by T cells in response to N-CWS (29–32). These cytokines may increase macrophage progenitors, accelerate macrophage activation, and induce cytotoxic effector cells other than macrophages such as natural killer (NK) or killer (K) cells. Therefore, nonspecific antitumor mechanisms of N-CWS may consist not only of the direct activation of macrophages, but also of the cytokine-mediated activation of macrophages and, probably to a lesser extent, the activation of NK or K cells.

Tumor-specific cytotoxicity mediated by T cells, on the other hand, has been shown to be induced at the early stage of tumor growth when the tumors possess high antigenicity (33). N-CWS has been reported to act as adjuvant on T cell-mediated immune responses (10,14). These findings strongly suggest that tumor-specific, T cell-mediated cytotoxicity may be augmented by N-CWS against highly antigenic tumors. Kawase et al (17) proved this possibility using a murine syngeneic tumor. Spleen and draining lymph node cells obtained from C57BL/6N mice bearing MC104, a highly antigenic fibrosarcoma, exhibited T cell-mediated cytotoxicity specifically against MC104 tumor cells at the early stage of tumor growth (1 week after tumor inoculation), and the cytotoxicity was dramatically depressed 2 weeks after tumor inoculation. Two intratumoral injections of 50 μg of N-CWS on days 2 and 7 after tumor inoculation resulted not only in the apparent inhibition of tumor growth, but also in a marked elevation of the cytotoxicity of draining lymph node cells but not of spleen cells (Table 7). They further demonstrated that the intralesional injections of N-CWS also enhanced the immigration of T cells into both the tumor masses and the draining lymph nodes. These findings suggest that antitumor cytotoxicity mediated by T cells can be augmented by N-CWS, and may play a role in the development of the antitumor effects of N-CWS when tumors possess apparent antigenicity.

Discussion

The antitumor efficacy of experimental immunotherapy with N-CWS has been described. In therapeutic experiments using syngeneic and autochthonous tumors of mice and rats, N-CWS was shown to be able to suppress tumor growth resulting in the apparent prolongation of the survival period, either when used alone or when used as an adjuvant for chemotherapy and radiotherapy. In these studies, however, the antitumor effects were achieved only when N-CWS was repeatedly administered near or into the growing tumors or into the peritoneal cavities of animals bearing ascitic tumors. These results are consistent with the finding that activation of macrophages by N-CWS is mainly observed at the site

Table 7 Effect of intratumor injection of N-CWS on antitumor cytotoxicity of spleen and draining popliteal lymph node (DPLN) cells activated in vitro from mice bearing MC104 fibrosarcoma. Reprinted, with permission, from Kawase I, Uemiya M, Yoshimoto T, et al (17).

Experimental group*	No. of experiments	Tumor diameter (mm)	Specific cytolysis (%)	
			Spleen cells	DPLN cells
Control	5	7.2 ± 0.3[†]	-44.3 ± 9.8	-12.1 ± 4.6
Squalene	5	5.6 ± 0.5	-30.0 ± 9.9	-12.0 ± 7.5
N-CWS	5	3.0 ± 0.3	-17.0 ± 7.5	37.6 ± 7.0
p (Student's *t*-test)				
Control vs squalene		<0.02	NS	NS
Squalene vs N-CWS		<0.001	NS	<0.001
Control vs N-CWS		<0.001	NS	<0.001

*C57BL/6N mice given sc inoculations of 10^6 MC104 tumor cells into the dorsum of the hind foot on day 0, and 2 intratumoral injections of $50 \mu g$ of N-CWS on days 2 and 7. On day 14, spleen and DPLN cells obtained and activated in vitro with MMC-treated MC104 tumor cells for 5 days. Cytotoxicity against MC104 tumor cells determined by 4-h ^{51}Cr-release assay at an effector to target cell ratio of 100:1.
[†]Mean $\pm$ SE.
NS, not significant.

of N-CWS injection (26). Therefore, the repeated, intralesional injection would be the most successful administration protocol for N-CWS to exhibit apparent antitumor effects against locally growing tumors or malignant pleural effusion and ascites. It has been suggested that iv injection of N-CWS is effective for the prevention of pulmonary metastases of tumors, from the study by Kagawa et al (21) demonstrating that the growth of pulmonary metastatic foci can be successfully inhibited by repeated iv injections of N-CWS. Clinical studies of iv injection of N-CWS are needed, following careful investigation of the side effects resulting from iv administration of N-CWS.

There has been increasing evidence that N-CWS not only directly activates macrophages but also stimulates some part of T cells to produce a variety of cytokines, resulting in the further activation of macrophages or other cytotoxic effector cells, and that N-CWS can also augment the generation of cytotoxic T cells against highly antigenic tumors. Therefore, it seems possible that the antitumor activities of N-CWS are expressed as final events of the stimulation of the host's defense mechanisms, consisting of T and non-T cells, and macrophages, even though the main effector cells may be macrophages.

References

1. Hersh EH, Gutterman JU, Mavlight GM. BCG as an adjuvant immunotherapy for

neoplasia. Annu Rev Med 1977;28:489–515.

2. Willmott N, Pimm MW, Baldwin RW. Quantitative comparison of BCG strains and preparations in immunotherapy of a rat sarcoma. J Natl Cancer Inst 1979;63:787–95.

3. Azuma I, Ribi EE, Meyer TJ, Zbar B. Biologically active components from mycobacterial cell walls. I: Isolation and composition of cell wall skeleton and component P3. J Natl Cancer Inst 1974;52:95–101.

4. Taniyama T, Azuma I, Aladin AA, Yamamura Y. Effect of cell-wall skeleton of *Mycobacterium bovis* BCG on cell-mediated cytotoxicity in tumor-bearing mice. Jpn J Cancer Res (Gann) 1975;66:705–9.

5. Azuma I, Taniyama T, Hirao F, Yamamura Y. Antitumor activity of cell-wall skeletons and peptidoglycolipids of mycobacteria and related microorganisms in mice and rabbits. Jpn J Cancer Res (Gann) 1974;65:493–505.

6. Yoshimoto T, Azuma I, Sakatani M, et al. Effect of oil-attached BCG cell-wall skeleton on the induction of pleural fibrosarcoma in mice. Jpn J Cancer Res (Gann) 1976;67:441–5.

7. Yamamura Y, Ogura T, Yoshimoto T, et al. Successful treatment of patients with malignant pleural effusion with BCG cell-wall skeleton. Jpn J Cancer Res (Gann) 1976;67:669–77.

8. Yamamura Y, Yoshizaki K, Azuma I, et al. Immunotherapy of human malignant melanoma with oil-attached BCG cell-wall skeleton. Jpn J Cancer Res (Gann) 1975;66:355–63.

9. Yasumoto K, Manabe H, Ueno M, et al. Immunotherapy of human lung cancer with BCG cell-wall skeleton. Jpn J Cancer Res (Gann) 1976;67:787–95.

10. Azuma I, Taniyama T, Yamawaki M, et al. Adjuvant and antitumor activities of *Nocardia* cell-wall skeletons. Jpn J Cancer Res (Gann) 1976;67:733–6.

11. Yanagawa Y, Yasumoto K, Ohta M, et al. Comparative study on antitumor effect of cell-wall skeleton of *Mycobacterium bovis* BCG and *Nocardia rubra*, with reference to T-cell dependency and independency. Jpn J Cancer Res (Gann) 1979;70:141–6.

12. Tokuzen R, Okabe M, Nakahara W, et al. Suppression of autochthonous tumors by mixed implantation with *Nocardia rubra* cell-well skeleton and related bacterial fractions. Jpn J Cancer Res (Gann) 1987;69:19–24.

13. Nagano N, Yasumoto K, Tanaka K, et al. Successful regional immunotherapy with cell-wall skeletons of BCG and *Nocardia rubra* against autochthonous rat tumors. Jpn J Cancer Res (Gann) 1982;73:613–7.

14. Yamawaki M, Azuma I, Saiki I, et al. Antitumor activity of squalene-treated cell-wall skeleton of *Nocardia rubra* in mice. Jpn J Cancer Res (Gann) 1978;69:619–26.

15. Ogura T, Namba M, Hirao F, et al. Association of macrophage activation with antitumor effect on rat syngeneic fibrosarcoma by *Nocardia rubra* cell wall skeleton. Cancer Res 1979;39:4706–12.

16. Pimm MV, Baldwin RW, Lederer E. Suppression of an ascitic rat hepatoma with cord factor and *Nocardia* cell wall skeleton in squalene emulsions. Eur J Cancer 1980;16:1645–7.

17. Kawase I, Uemiya M, Yoshimoto T, et al. Effect of *Nocardia rubra* cell wall skeleton on T-cell-mediated cytotoxicity in mice bearing syngeneic sarcoma. Cancer Res 1981;41:660–6.

18. Haraguchi S, Kurakata S, Matsuo T, Yoshida TO. Strain differences in the antitumor activity on an immunopotentiator, *Nocardia rubra* cell-wall skeleton, in B10 congenic and recombinant mice. Jpn J Cancer Res (Gann) 1985;76:400–13.

176

19. Ogura T, Shinzato O, Sakatani M, et al. Analysis of therapeutic effect in experimental chemoimmunotherapy for rat ascites tumor. Cancer Immunol Immunother 1982: 14:67–72.

20. Ichinose Y, Yasumoto K, Tanaka K, et al. Combined treatment of autochthonous 3-methylcholanthrene-induced murine tumors by immunotherapy and radiotherapy. Jpn J Cancer Res (Gann) 1983;74:143–7.

21. Kagawa K, Yamashita T, Tsubura E, Yamamura Y. Inhibition of pulmonary metastases by *Nocardia rubra* cell wall skeleton, with special reference to macrophage activation. Cancer Res 1984;44:665–70.

22. Hanna MG Jr, Zbar B, Rapp HJ. Histopathology of tumor regression after intralesional injections of *Mycobacterium bovis*. I: Tumor growth and metastasis. J Natl Cancer Inst 1972;48:1441–55.

23. Cleveland RP, Meltzer MS, Zbar B. Tumor cytotoxicity in vitro by macrophages from mice injected with *Mycobacterium bovis*, strain BCG. J Natl Cancer Inst 1974;52:1887–95.

24. Olivotto M, Bomford R. In vitro inhibition of cell growth and DNA synthesis by peritoneal and lung macrophages from mice injected with *Corynebacterium parvum*. Int J Cancer 1974;13:478–88.

25. Masuno T, Ito M, Ogura T, et al. Activation of peritoneal macrophages by oil-attached cell-wall skeleton of BCG and *Nocardia rubra*. Jpn J Cancer Res (Gann) 1979;70:223–7.

26. Ito M, Iizuka H, Masuno T, et al. Killing of tumor cells in vitro by macrophages from mice given injections of squalene-treated cell wall skeleton of *Nocardia rubra*. Cancer Res 1981;41:2925–30.

27. Sone S, Pollack LA, Fidler IJ. Direct activation of tumoricidal properties in rat alveolar macrophages by *Nocardia rubra* cell wall skeleton. Cancer Immunol Immunother 1980;9:227–32.

28. Sugimura K, Uemiya M, Azuma I, et al. Macrophage dependency of T-lymphocyte mitogenesis by *Nocardia rubra* cell-wall skeleton. Microbiol Immunol 1977;21:525–30.

29. Masuno T, Hayashi S, Ito M, et al. Mechanism(s) of in vitro macrophage activation with *Nocardia rubra* cell wall skeleton: The effect on macrophage activating factor production by lymphocytes. Cancer Immunol Immunother 1986;22:132–8.

30. Hayashi S, Masuno T, Hosoe S, et al. Augmented production of colony-stimulating factor in C3H/HeN mice immunized with *Nocardia rubra* cell wall skeleton. Infect Immun 1986;52:128–33.

31. Sakatani M, Ogura T, Masuno T, et al. Effect of *Nocardia rubra* cell wall skeleton on augmentation of cytotoxicity function in human pleural macrophages. Cancer Immunol Immunother 1987;25:119–25.

32. Izumi S, Ueda H, Okuhara M, et al. Effect of *Nocardia rubra* cell wall skeleton on murine interferon production in vitro. Cancer Res 1986;46:1960–5.

33. Takei F, Levy JG, Kilburn DG. In vitro induction of cytotoxicity against syngeneic mastocytoma and its suppression by spleen and thymus cells from tumor-bearing mice. J Immunol 1976;116:288–93.

Prevention of carcinogenesis with BCG cell wall skeleton and *Nocardia rubra* cell wall skeleton in experimental models

Takahiko Yoshimoto,[1] Manabu Namba,[2] Fumio Hirao[1]

[1]*Section of Internal Medicine, Nishinomiya Municipal Central Hospital, Nishinomiya,* [2]*Namba-Iin, Takarazuka, Japan*

Introduction

Recent studies (1–5), have reported that BCG cell-wall skeleton (BCG-CWS) and *Nocardia rubra*-CWS (N-CWS) have potent adjuvant activities and are as effective as living BCG for the suppression and regression of transplantable tumors in various animals. On the other hand, living BCG and its preparations are known to reduce the incidence of tumors (6–13).

In previous work, we established the method of induction of lung cancers by repeated intratracheal instillation of chemical carcinogens in rabbits (14–16), rats (17), and mice (18). We also established the method of inducing pleural fibrosarcomas in mice (19). In this study, we investigated the effects of BCG-CWS on the induction of pleural fibrosarcoma in mice (19) and lung cancer in rabbits (20), and the effects of N-CWS on the induction of lung cancer in rabbits (21), rats (17), and mice. We also studied the effect of BCG-CWS administration and thymectomy on carcinogenesis and amyloidgenesis in a rabbit model (20).

Materials and methods

Preparation of oil-attached BCG-CWS and N-CWS

The cells of *Mycobacterium bovis* BCG (strain 1173 P2) were grown on Sauton's synthetic liquid medium as a pellicle culture at 37°C for 10 to 14 days. The preparation of CWS from the cells of *M. bovis* BCG and oil-attached BCG-CWS for injection has been described previously (2,22). The cells of *N. rubra* were cultured on medium containing 1% peptone and 0.5% yeast extract (Difco), pH 7.0, and shaken at 30°C for 5 days. Oil-attached N-CWS was prepared by the same method (2,22).

178

Induction of pleural fibrosarcomas in mice and injection of BCG-CWS

Eight-week-old ddO albino mice used in these experiments were supplied from the Central Breeding Laboratory of Experimental Animals of Osaka University. After grinding 50 mg of 3-methylcholanthrene (3-MCA, Wako Chemical Co., Osaka) for about 0.5 h in a mullite mortar, 5 mL of sterile olive oil was added to the powder and triturated well for 10 min to avoid formation of large clumps. A suspension of 1 mg of 3-MCA in 0.1 mL of olive oil was injected substernally using a tuberculin syringe fitted with an 18-gauge needle, under light ether anesthesia.

One week after injection of the carcinogen, the oil-attached BCG-CWS, prepared as described previously (2), was administered every week for 10 weeks. In the experimental group, 100 μg of BCG-CWS suspended in 0.1 mL of 0.2% Tween 80 saline solution was injected subcutaneously into right and left lateral portions of the back of a mouse. In the control group, 0.1 mL of saline solution was injected subcutaneously.

Induction of lung cancer in rabbits and injection of BCG-CWS

Details for the procedure for experimental lung cancer have been described previously (14–16). 3-MCA and 4-nitroquinoline 1-oxide (4-NQO) were used as chemical carcinogens. Normal rabbit plasma or distilled water was used as a vehicle for chemical carcinogens. As shown in Table 1, 6 experimental groups (A–F) were designated. Rabbits in groups A, C, D, E, and F were approximately 100 days old and weighed 2–2.5 kg, male and female, and those in group B were approximately 30 days old, weighing 0.8–1.0 kg, male and female.

Rabbits in all the groups received intrabronchial instillation of a mixture of 40 mg of 3-MCA and 0.4 mg of 4-NQO suspended in 0.5 mL rabbit plasma or distilled water, using a specially made bronchoscope. To protect rabbits from infection, oxytetracycline hydrochloride (50 mg/kg body weight) was given at the same time as the carcinogens. Administration of carcinogens was continued in the rabbits throughout the experiments unless the rabbits became severely ill or died. Rabbits in group B were thymectomized when about 30 days old and instillation of carcinogens was started 1 month later. Instillation of carcinogens was repeated every 30 to 40 days in all rabbits. Rabbits in group C received an iv injection of 5 mg of oil-attached BCG-CWS in 1 mL of 0.85% NaCl solution containing 0.2% Tween 80 at the same time as the first administration of carcinogens. Rabbits in groups D and F received an iv injection of 5 mg of oil-attached BCG-CWS at the start of the experiment and 2 mg of oil-attached BCG-CWS every 30 to 40 days.

Induction of lung cancer in rats and injection of N-CWS

Ten-week-old male inbred ACI/N rats, obtained from Fuji Animal Farm, Tokyo, were used in this experiment. All the ACI/N rats received 15 weekly intratracheal instillations of a suspension of 3 mg benzo[a]pyrene with 3 mg ferric oxide. Rats in the control group received no further treatment and those in the N-CWS treated group received 7 injections of 100 μg of N-CWS at 2-week intervals after the 10th instillation of the carcinogen. N-CWS was injected subcutaneously into bilateral portion of the back of the rat. Animals were checked daily, and allowed to die spontaneously or killed when moribund. The surviving rats were killed 56 weeks after the first instillation of carcinogen. Autopsies were performed on all the animals.

Induction of lung cancer in rabbits and injection of N-CWS

Details of the procedure for inducing experimental lung cancer have also been described previously (14–16). 3-MCA was used as a chemical carcinogen, with sterile distilled water as a vehicle. The outbred albino rabbits used were approximately 3 months old, male and female, and weighed about 2.6–3.0 kg. Rabbits in all groups received an intrabronchial instillation of 40 mg of 3-MCA suspended in 0.4 mL of distilled water, using a specially designed bronchoscope. Instillation of the carcinogen was repeated every 10 days. Administration of the carcinogen was continued unless the rabbits became severely ill or died.

As shown in Table 1, the rabbits were tentatively classified into 6 groups (groups A–F), according to survival time after the initiation of the experiment. Controls (groups A, C, and E) used were the same as in previous experiments (16). Rabbits in groups B, D, and F received an iv injection of 2 mg of oil-attached N-CWS in 1 mL of 0.85% NaCl solution containing 0.2% Tween 80 every 30 days. The injection of N-CWS was started from the first administration of carcinogen.

Induction of lung cancer in mice and injection of N-CWS

Ten-week-old male C56BL/6 mice were supplied from the Funabashi Animal Farm, Kyoto. All the mice received 8 weekly intratracheal instillations of a suspension of 0.5 mg benzo[a]pyrene with 0.5 mg of charcoal powder, according a method previously described (23). Mice in the control group received no further treatment; those in the N-CWS-treated group received 2 iv injections and 10 sc injections of 100 μg of N-CWS weekly after the 8th instillation of the carcinogen. Animals were checked daily, and allowed to die spontaneously or killed when moribund.

Histologic examinations

Autopsies and histologic examinations were performed on animals that died or became severely ill during the course of the experiment. For histologic examinations, each organ was fixed in 10% formalin and sections of these materials were stained with hematoxylin and eosin (H and E) as a routine method, periodic acid-Schiff (PAS), van Gieson's stains, and silver impregnation, when necessary. For the study of amyloidosis, sections were stained by the PAS method, Congo red, azan-Mallory, van Gieson's, and thioflavine T for fluorescence.

Results

Effect of oil-attached BCG-CWS on induction of pleural fibrosarcomas in mice

As shown in Fig 1, in the group that received 100 μg of oil-attached BCG-CWS subcutaneously every week for 10 weeks, the incidence of pleural fibrosarcoma was 39%, compared with 67% in the control group. In the group treated with BCG-CWS, the first tumor found at autopsy was recorded on the 89th day after the 3-MCA injection, compared with the 100th day in the control group. Histologically, pleural fibrosarcomas found in the BCG-CWS-treated group were not very different from those in the control group. The incidence of pulmonary adenoma in the BCG-CWS-treated group (3/18) was almost the same as that in the control group (2/18).

Effect of oil-attached BCG-CWS and thymectomy on incidence of lung cancer and amyloidosis induced by chemical carcinogens in rabbits

As shown in Table 1, intrabronchial instillation of 40 mg 3-MCA and 0.4 mg 4-NQO was performed every 30 to 40 days and lung cancer appeared in 17 out of 36 (47.2%) of the rabbits that survived more than 300 days (group A), but no lung cancer was seen in the animals given an iv injection of 5 mg of BCG-CWS at the time of the first carcinogen instillation and then iv injections of 2 mg of BCG-CWS every 30 to 40 days at the time of each carcinogen instillation (group D).

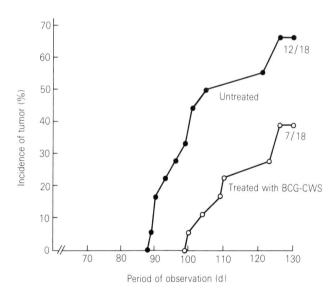

Fig 1 Cumulative incidence of pleural fibrosarcoma in male ddO mice either treated with BCG-CWS or untreated. Reprinted, with permission, from Yoshimoto T, Azuma I, Sakatani M (19).

Table 1 Effect of oil-attached BCG-CWS and thymectomy on the incidence of lung cancer and amyloidosis caused by instillation of chemical carcinogens. Reprinted, with permission, from Hirao F, Nishikawa H, Yasaki S, et al (20).

Group	Type of rabbit used	Injection iv (mg) of oil-attached BCG-CWS	Survival period (d)	Incidence (%)		
				Lung cancer	Amyloidosis	Lung cancer + amyloidosis
A	Normal	NT	<300	17/36 (47.2)	9/36 (25.0)	3/36 (8.3)
B	Thymec-tomized	NT	<300	32/40 (80.0)	11/40 (27.5)	4/40 (10.0)
C	Normal	5*	<300	5/10 (50.0)	4/10 (40.0)	1/10 (10.0)
D	Normal	5* + 2†	<300	0/20 (0)	6/20 (30.0)	0/20 (0)
E	Normal	NT	200–300	7/25 (28.0)	4/25 (16.0)	0/25 (0)
F	Normal	5* + 2†	200–300	0/24 (0)	0/24 (0)	0/24 (0)

* × 1.
†Every 30–40 days.
A=control 1; E=control 2.
NT, no treatment.

However, in animals given only a single iv injection at the time of the first administration of carcinogen, there was no difference in the incidence of lung cancer between BCG-CWS-treated animals in group C and those in group A (control 1).

In group E (control 2), lung cancer developed in 7 out of 25 animals (28%) within 200 to 300 days of the experimental period, but there was no induction of lung cancer in animals in group F, which received an iv injection of BCG-CWS every 30–40 days and the animals survived for 200 to 300 days. There was no death or case of granuloma in the lung and liver that could be considered to be caused by the iv injection of BCG-CWS.

In thymectomized rabbits (group B) given carcinogens every 30–40 days over an experimental period of more than 300 days, there was a high lung cancer rate of 32 out of 40 rabbits (80%) when compared with 17 out of 36 (47.2%) in nonthymectomized rabbits (group A). There were no marked differences in the appearance of amyloidosis between the thymectomized and BCG-CWS-administered rabbits and the controls. Amyloidosis was involved most frequently in the kidneys and then in the spleen and liver, in decreasing order of frequency.

Effect of N-CWS on induction of lung cancer in rats

As shown in Fig 2, in the N-CWS-treated group, the first tumor was detected at autopsy in the 31st week of the experiment, compared with the 15th week in the control group. The cumulative incidence of lung cancer was 71.4% (45 of 63 animals) in the control group. In contrast, it was only 48.0% (12 of 25) in the N-

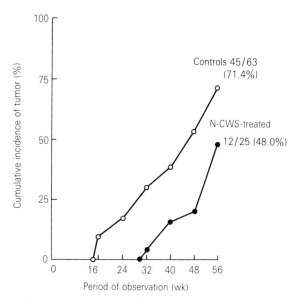

Fig 2 Effect of N-CWS on the incidence of lung cancers in ACI/N rats. Reprinted, with permission, from Namba N, Yoshimoto T, Ogura T, et al (17).

CWS-treated group. Statistical analysis of tumor incidence between the 2 groups gives a χ^2 value of 4.3, indicating a significant difference at the 5% level. Thus, repeated sc injections of N-CWS significantly reduced the incidence of lung cancers and prolonged the latent period of tumor induction.

Effect of N-CWS on induction of lung cancer and amyloidosis by 3-MCA in rabbits

As shown in Table 2, intrabronchial instillation of 40 mg of 3-MCA every 10 days induced lung cancers in 21 out of 40 (52.5%) rabbits that survived for more than 300 days (group E). As shown in Table 2, 14 rabbits among the 21 bearing lung cancers in group E (approximately 66.7%) showed metastases and/or invasion of neighboring tissue.

In contrast, lung cancer could be detected in only 3 rabbits in group F, which consisted of rabbits that had received intrabronchial instillation of 3-MCA every 10 days and iv injection of N-CWS every 30 days for more than 300 days. The lung cancers in these 3 rabbits were histologically identified as a squamous cell carcinoma and 2 adenocarcinomas; they were localized and showed no indication of metastases or invasion into tissues adjacent to the lung.

In groups A and C, lung cancer developed in 3 out of 18 rabbits (16.7%) that survived for more than 100 days but died within 300 days. On the other hand, there was no induction of lung cancer in groups B and D, which received an iv in-

Table 2 Effect of oil-attached N-CWS on the incidence of lung cancer and amyloidosis caused by instillation of 3-MCA. Reprinted, with permission, from Hirao F, Sakatani M, Nishikawa H, et al (21).

Group	Intravenous injection of oil-attached N-GWS	Survival period (d)	Incidence (%)			
			Lung cancer	Adeno-matous hyperplasia	Adenoma	Amyloidosis
A	No treatment	100–200	1/7* (14.3)	3/7 (42.9)	1/7 (14.3)	0/7 (0)
B	2 mg (every 30 d)	100–200	0/8 (0)	2/8 (25.0)	1/8 (12.5)	2/8 (25.0)
C	No treatment	200–300	2/11† (18.2)	5/11 (45.5)	2/11 (18.2)	0/11 (0)
D	2 mg (every 30 d)	200–300	0/7 (0)	0/7 (0)	3/7 (42.9)	1/7 (14.3)
E	No treatment	<300	21/40‡ (52.5)	9/40 (22.5)	6/40 (15.0)	5/40 (12.5)
F	2 mg (every 30 d)	<300	3/31# (9.7)	3/31 (9.7)	2/31 (6.5)	15/31**

*Adenocarcinoma; †1 squamous cell carcinoma, 1 adenocarcinoma; ‡10 squamous cell carcinomas, 6 adenocarcinomas, 3 adenosquamous carcinomas, 1 pleomorphic carcinoma, 1 sarcoma; ¶1 squamous cell carcinoma, 2 adenocarcinomas.
#$p < 0.001$ vs group E; **$p < 0.005$ vs group E.

jection of N-CWS every 30 days and survived for 100 to 300 days. Thus, the repeated iv injections of N-CWS significantly depressed the incidence of lung cancers. No differences were observed in tumor induction and prevention between male and female rabbits. No death appeared to be attribttable to iv injection of N-CWS.

The histological types and incidence of lung cancer are shown in Table 2. In addition to lung cancers, various benign pathological changes were observed (eg, proliferation of atypical squamous epithelium of the bronchioli, adenomatous hyperplasia, and adenoma), but only the major pathological changes are recorded in Table 2. Histological criteria have been defined previously (15,16). No remarkable difference was observed between N-CWS-administered rabbits and controls as regards the incidence of adenomatous hyperplasia and adenoma. Changes were observed in the lung periphery, mainly in the terminal bronchioli and alveoli.

In this experiment, amyloidosis was seen in both the controls and the N-CWS-administered rabbits, and its incidence was higher in the N-CWS-administered groups than in the control groups, as shown in Table 2. Amyloidosis was involved most frequently in the kidneys and then in the spleen and liver, in decreasing order of frequency.

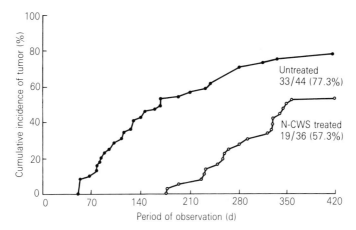

Fig 3   Cumulative incidence of squamous cell carcinoma in the lung of C57BL/6 mice either treated with N-CWS or untreated.

Effect of N-CWS on induction of lung cancer in mice

As shown in Fig 3, in the group that received 2 iv injections and 10 sc injections of 100 μg of N-CWS weekly, the incidence of squamous cell carcinoma was 52.7%, compared with 77.3% in the control group. The latent period of lung cancer induction was prolonged in the mice treated with N-CWS.

Discussion

In the present work, we studied the effects of BCG-CWS and N-CWS on carcinogenesis in experimental animals. As shown in Fig 1, we demonstrated that sc administration of BCG-CWS prolonged the latent period of pleural fibrosarcoma induction and reduced the incidence of the tumor in ddO mice. We also attempted, by the administration of oil-attached BCG-CWS, to prevent the induction of lung cancer and amyloidosis in rabbits by chemical carcinogens. As shown in Table 1, in rabbits that received an iv injection of 5 mg of oil-attached BCG-CWS at the start of experiment (group C), the incidence of lung cancer was about 50%, a figure almost identical to that for rabbits in group A (control 1). However, no lung cancer occurred in rabbits that received 5 mg of oil-attached BCG-CWS every 30 to 40 days; these rabbits survived more than 300 days (group D) and from 200 to 300 days (group F) after the initial instillation of carcinogens. It is interesting that the lung cancer incidence in thymectomized rabbits was much higher than in nonthymectomized controls (group A). In the present experiment, administration of BCG-CWS and thymectomy did not affect the occurrence of amyloidosis due to chemical carcinogens.

On the other hand, repeated injections of N-CWS prolonged the latent period of lung cancer induction and significantly reduced the cumulative incidence of lung cancers in rats and mice, as shown in Figs 2 and 3. As shown in Table 2, repeated iv administration of oil-attached N-CWS prevented the induction of lung cancer by intrabronchial instillations of 3-MCA in rabbits. Amyloidosis was seen after administration of 3-MCA, and the incidence was higher in the N-CWS-administered rabbits than in the controls.

A preventive effect against chemical carcinogenesis has been confirmed by some investigators with BCG (9–12) and its preparations such as cord factor (6), methanol-extracted residue (MER) (7), and cell wall (13). On the possible mechanism of the effect, Old et al (9) first suggested that the success of BCG was directly related to the enhancement of the immunological surveillance mechanism of the host by BCG. This seems to be supported by the observation that BCG was effective as long as the host was able to mount a strong cell-mediated response to PPD and the tumor was immunogenic (11). Another study (24) reported that activated alveolar macrophage, which was capable of destroying target tumor cells in vitro, is also important. Nagasawa et al (25) showed that spontaneous mammary tumorigenesis in mice was inhibited by injections of of N-CWS, and that the treatment also reduced normal mammary gland DNA synthesis and prolactin levels in the circulation, both of which are primary factors for mammary tumorigenesis. They also showed (26) that both the incidence and progression of DMBA-induced mammary tumors in rats were markedly suppressed by injections of N-CWS.

The mechanism of the prevention of lung cancer development in animals is not thoroughly elucidated but the above results suggest that the continuous stimulation of the immune response of the host by iv injection of oil-attached BCG-CWS and N-CWS may affect the incidence of lung cancer caused by the instillation of carcinogens. From the analysis of immunopotentiation with N-CWS, it appears that the prophylactic effect of N-CWS on chemical carcinogenesis possibly relates to the immunopotentiation (2–5) induced by repeated injections of N-CWS, although the details of the mechanism responsible for this effect are undetermined. The exact mechanism by which amyloidosis develops may not be simple, but a complex combination of various factors. It however appears that the concomitant use of chemical carcinogens and BCG-CWS is an effective method for the creation of an experimental model of amyloidosis without lung cancer.

References

1. Yamamura Y, Azuma I, Taniyama T, et al. Suppression of tumor growth and regression of established tumor in mice with oil-attached mycobacterial fractions. Jpn J Cancer Res (Gann) 1974;65:179–81.
2. Azuma I, Taniyama T, Hirao F, Yamamura Y. Antitumor activity of cell-wall skeletons and peptidoglycolipids of mycobacteria and microorganisms. Jpn J Cancer Res (Gann) 1974;65:493–505.

3. Azuma I, Taniyama T, Yamawaki M, et al. Adjuvant and antitumor activities of *Nocardia* cell-wall skeletons. Jpn J Cancer Res (Gann) 1976;67:733–6.

4. Azuma I, Yamawaki M, Yasumoto K, Yamamura Y. Antitumor activity of *Nocardia* cell-wall skeletons in mice, and patients with malignant pleurisy. Cancer Immunol Immunother 1978;4:95–100.

5. Tokuzen R, Okabe M, Nakahara W, et al. Suppression of autochthonous tumors by mixed implantation with *Nocardia rubra* cell-wall skeleton and related bacterial fractions. Jpn J Cancer Res (Gann) 1978;69:19–24.

6. Bekierkunst A, Levij IS, Yarkoni E. Suppression of urethan-induced lung adenomas in mice treated with trehalose-6,6-dimycolate (cord factor) and living Bacillus Calmette Guérin. Science 1971;174:1240–2.

7. Lavrin DH, Rosenberg SA, Connor RJ, Terry WD. Immunoprophylaxis of methylcholanthrene-induced tumors in mice with Bacillus Calmette-Guérin and methanol-extracted residue. Cancer Res 1973;33:472–7.

8. Nilsson A, Révész L, Stjernswärd J. Suppression of strontium-90-induced development of bone tumors by infection with Bacillus Calmette-Guérin (BCG). Radiat Res 1965;26:378–82.

9. Old LJ, Benacerraf B, Clarke DA, et al. The role of the reticuloendothelial system in the host reaction to neoplasia. Cancer Res 1961;21:1281–1300.

10. Piessens WF, Hermann R, Legros N, Henson J-C. Effect of Bacillus Calmette-Guérin on mammary tumor formation and cellular immunity in dimethylbenz(a)anthracene-treated rats. Cancer Res 1971;31:1061–5.

11. Schinitsky MR, Hyman LR, Blazkovec AA, Burkholder PM. Bacillus Calmette-Guérin vaccination and skin tumor promotion with croton oil in mice. Cancer Res 1973;33:659–63.

12. Tokunaga T, Yasumoto S, Nakamura RM, Kataoka T. Immunotherapeutic and immunoprophylactic effects of BCG on 3-methyl-cholanthrene-induced autochthonous tumor in Swiss mice. J Natl Cancer Inst 1974;53:459–63.

13. Zwilling BS, Springer ST, Kaufman DG. Effect of systemic administration of BCG cell walls on bronchogenic carcinoma in hamsters. J Natl Cancer Inst 1977;58:1473–7.

14. Hirao F, Fujisawa T, Tsubura E, et al. Experimental lung cancer in rabbits induced by chemical carcinogens. Jpn J Cancer Res (Gann) 1968;59:497–505.

15. Hirao F, Fujisawa T, Tsubura E, Yamamura Y. Experimental lung cancer of the lung in rabbits induced by chemical carcinogens. Cancer Res 1972;32:1209–17.

16. Hirao F, Yamamura Y. Comparison of lung cancer and amyloidosis in rabbits induced by chemical carcinogens. Jpn J Cancer Res (Gann) 1975;66:49–55.

17. Namba N, Yoshimoto T, Ogura T, et al. Effect of *Nocardia rubra* cell-wall skeleton on the induction of lung cancer in ACI/N rats. Jpn J Cancer Res (Gann) 1979; 70:55–62.

18. Yoshimoto T, Inoue T, Iizuka H, et al. Differential induction of squamous cell carcinomas and adenocarcinomas in mouse lung by intratracheal instillation of benzo[a]pyrene and charcoal powder. Cancer Res 1980;40:4301–7.

19. Yoshimoto T, Azuma I, Sakatani M. Effect of oil-attached BCG cell-wall skeleton on the induction of pleural fibrosarcomas in mice. Jpn J Cancer Res (Gann) 1976; 67:441–5.

20. Hirao F, Nishikawa H, Yasaki S, et al. Effect of oil-attached BCG cell-wall skeleton and thymectomy on the incidence of lung cancer and amyloidosis induced by chemical carcinogens in rabbits. Jpn J Cancer Res (Gann) 1978;69:453–9.

21. Hirao F, Sakatani M, Nishikawa H, et al. Effect of *Nocardia rubra* cell-wall skeleton

on the induction of lung cancer and amyloidosis by 3-methylcholanthrene in rabbits. Jpn J Cancer Res (Gann) 1980;71:398–401.

22. Azuma I, Ribi EE, Meyer TJ, Zbar B. Biologically active components from mycobacterial cell walls. I. Isolation and composition of cell wall skeleton and components P₃. J Natl Cancer Inst 1974;52:95–101.

23. Yoshimoto T, Hirao F, Sakatani M, et al. Induction of squamous cell carcinoma in the lung of C57BL/6 in mice by intratracheal instillation of benzo[a]pyrene with charcoal powder. Jpn J Cancer Res (Gann) 1977;68:343–52.

24. Zwilling BS, Campolito LB. Destruction of tumor cells by BCG-activated alveolar macrophages. J Immunol 1977;119:838–41.

25. Nagasawa H, Yanai R, Azuma I. Suppression by *Nocardia rubra* cell wall skeleton of mammary DNA synthesis, plasma prolactin level, and spontaneous mammary tumorigenesis in mice. Cancer Res 1978;38:2160–2.

26. Nagasawa H, Yanai R, Azuma I. Inhibitory effect of *Nocardia rubra* cell wall skeleton on carcinogen induced mammary tumorigenesis in rats. Eur J Cancer 1980; 16:389–93.

Immunological rationale for immunotherapy of lung cancer and clinical effect of surgical adjuvant immunotherapy with *Nocardia rubra* cell wall skeleton

Kosei Yasumoto, Hisashi Nakahashi

Respiratory Disease Center, Matsuyama Red Cross Hospital, Matsuyama, Japan

Introduction

Adequate surgical treatment for stage I lung cancer can achieve a 5-year survival rate of around 60%. However, the remaining 40% of patients will die from recurrence of the disease. This means that even if the lung cancer is completely resected, there will be a subclinical level of remnant disease in about 40% of patients (1). Therefore we have tried to develop a surgical adjuvant therapy for lung cancer. Radiotherapy, chemotherapy, and immunotherapy have been used for such purposes for a long time. However, radiation therapy may be effective only in patients with Pancoast's tumor, when applied preoperatively (2). The response rate to chemotherapy of non-small cell lung cancer has increased to over 30%, however no chemotherapeutic regimen has yet been able to improve the survival rate of postoperative lung cancer patients. In the field of cancer immunotherapy, on the other hand, many promising results have been obtained (3–5), although some others have been disappointing (6–8). Therefore, we would like to discuss, from our results, whether an immune response against lung cancer exists in lung cancer patients, and whether immunotherapy could be applied as an adjuvant to surgery for lung cancer.

Immunological response of lung cancer patients

Host defense mechanisms against lung cancer may include specific killer T cells, activated macrophages, natural killer (NK) cells, lymphokine-activated killer (LAK) cells, and K cells (antibody-dependent cell-mediated cytotoxicity) at the effector phase. The sites for such effector mechanisms to operate may be in primary lung cancer tissue, the pleural space, the alveolar space, regional lymph nodes, and peripheral blood. According to our previous reports (9–20), such effector mechanisms operate at all 5 sites, but perhaps most notably in the pleural space and in primary lung cancer tissue. From our own data, we shall review here antitumor effector mechanisms in the pleural space and in lung cancer tissue.

Host defense mechanisms in the pleural space (15,18)

The pleural cavity was irrigated with 1 L of saline immediately after thoracotomy, and the saline was collected and centrifuged at 1000 rpm for 15 min to allow cell pellets to be obtained. Plastic adherent cells were recovered as pleural cavity macrophages (PCM) and nonadherent cells as pleural cavity lymphocytes (PCL). The antitumor activity of PCM was assessed by the inhibition of DNA synthesis by allogeneic lung cancer cell lines, QG-56 and QG-90 (cytostatic activity). As shown in Table 1, the cytostatic activity of PCM was not affected by an advance of metastasis to regional lymph nodes or by an increase in tumor size. However, the cytostatic activity of PCM was markedly augmented when the pleural invasion of the lung cancer was limited to the visceral pleura, although the activity was low when pleural invasion was absent or if it extended beyond the visceral pleura.

Antitumor activity of PCL was assessed by a 4-h ^{51}Cr-release assay of autologous tumor (AT) cells, QG-56 cells, or K562 cells. PCL did not exert any cytolytic activity against these target cells. This must mean that there are neither specific killer T cells, NK cells, nor LAK cells in the pleural cavity of lung cancer patients (Table 2).

Table 1 Cytostatic activity of PCM according to prognostic factors. Reprinted, with permission, from Nagashima A, Yasumoto K, Nakahashi H, et al (18).

Prognostic observation (n)	% cytostatic activity against	
	QG-56	QG-90
Tumor size		
≦30 mm (23)	49 ± 7*	29 ± 11
>30 mm (52)	49 ± 5	46 ± 4
Lymph node metastasis		
N0 (43)	54 ± 5	46 ± 6
N1 (7)	49 ± 13	37 ± 9
N2 (25)	39 ± 9	34 ± 6
Pleural invasion		
Grade 0 (30)	40 ± 5†	29 ± 7†
Grade 1 (19)	76 ± 6	73 ± 6
Grade 2 (15)	36 ± 14‡	40 ± 9§

*Mean ± SEM; †significantly different from grade 1 ($p < 0.001$); ‡significantly different from grade 1 ($p < 0.05$); §significantly different from grade 1 ($p < 0.01$).

Table 2 Cytolytic activity of lymphocytes from different sites against various targets.

Effector lymphocyte (n)	% cytolytic activity against		
	Autologous tumor	QG-56	K562
Tumor infiltrating lymphocyte (12)	0.7 ± 1.8	0.6 ± 1.2	−0.8 ± 1.1
Pleural cavity lymphocyte (19)	−1.3 ± 2.1	−1.2 ± 1.0	2.8 ± 3.2
Alveolar lymphocyte			
Tumor-bearing segment (17)	0.1 ± 1.8	0.3 ± 0.8	−1.8 ± 0.9
Nontumor-bearing segment (16)	0.2 ± 2.1	−0.2 ± 2.4	−1.4 ± 0.8
Regional lymph node lymphocyte			
Hilar node (26)	5.2 ± 1.0	5.3 ± 0.8	2.8 ± 1.2
Mediastinal node (29)	6.2 ± 1.0	6.8 ± 0.6	6.8 ± 2.5
PBL (48)	5.2 ± 1.0	10.4 ± 1.5	31.8 ± 3.3

Table 3 Cytostatic activity of TAM according to prognostic factors. Reprinted, with permission, from Takeo S, Yasumoto K, Nagashima A, et al (16).

Prognostic factor (n)	Cytostatic activity (%)
Tumor size	
T1 (9)	47 ± 7*
T2 (28)	28 ± 6
T3 (7)	13 ± 13
Lymph node metastasis	
N0 (27)	31 ± 5
N1 (5)	25 ± 16
N2 (12)	29 ± 11

*Mean ± SEM.

Host defense mechanisms in lung cancer tissue (16,20)

Lung cancer tissue (thumb fingertip size) was obtained aseptically from surgical specimens immediately upon their removal. Tumor-associated macrophages (TAM), tumor-infiltrating lymphocytes (TIL), and AT cells were obtained from the specimens by the method reported previously.

As shown in Table 3, the cytostatic activity of TAM showed a tendency to decline as the tumor size increased, but it was relatively constant with metastasis to regional lymph nodes. The correlation between cytostatic activity of TAM and prognosis was investigated in patients who were subjected to curative resection of lung cancer. Although 10 of 17 (58.3%) patients with less than 30% cytostatic activity had recurrent disease following surgical treatment, only 3 of 19 (15.8%) patients with more than 30% cytostatic activity showed recurrence. There was a significant difference between these 2 groups (p<0.025) (Fig 1).

Antitumor activity of TIL was assessed against the 3 targets by the method used in the assessment of antitumor activity of PCL. TIL did not exert any cytolytic activity against these 3 targets (Table 2).

Production of macrophage activating factor by cocultivation of PCL or TIL with AT (18,20)

Thus, PCL and TIL did not exert any antitumor activity, at least at the effector phase. Therefore, we further investigated whether PCL and TIL work as helper cells or not. The stimulating cells used in this cocultivation to obtain supernatants (macrophage activating factor [MAF] sources) were AT, QG-56, and autologous normal lung (ANL) cells as a control. PCL or TIL (1 × 10⁶/mL) and these stimulating cells (2 × 10⁵/mL) were cocultivated for 72 h. The supernatant fluids were used as MAF sources. Peritoneal exudate cells (PEC) from normal guinea pigs were used as indicator cells. PEC (2 × 10⁵/mL) was placed in each well of a microtest plate (0.1 mL/well) and incubated for 2 h.

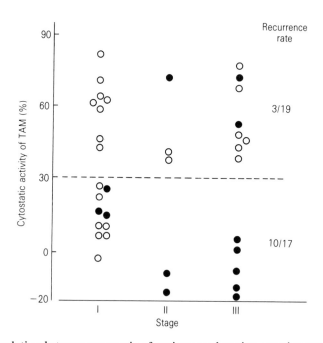

Fig 1 Correlation between prognosis of patients undergoing curative resection of lung cancer and cytostatic activity of TAM: ○ patients in remission; ● patients with recurrence. p<0.025. Reprinted, with permission, from Takeo S, Yasumoto K, Nagashima A, et al (16).

Each well was washed 3 times to remove nonadherent cells. Then, cocultured supernatants (0.1 mL), diluted 1/8 with fresh medium, were added to each well. After a 4-h incubation, each well was washed twice and QG-56 target cells (1 × 10 ^{3}/well) were added. Cytostatic activity was estimated as described before.

As shown in Fig 2, cytostatic activities of guinea pig PEC pretreated with supernatants obtained from coculture of PCL with QG-56 or ANL were below 20%. However, cytostatic activity of guinea pig PEC pretreated with that obtained from coculture of PCL with AT exceeded 20% in 9 of 17 patients. This means that MAF was produced by coculture of PCL with AT. Similar results were obtained in the experiments using TIL.

Correlation between MAF production of PCL or TIL and cytostatic activity of PCM or TAM (18,20)

Figure 3 shows the correlation between cytostatic activity of PCM and the degree of MAF activity of the supernatant in individual patients. A significant positive correlation (p < 0.01) was observed between MAF activity induced by PCL and the cytostatic activity of PCM. A similar correlation was observed between MAF

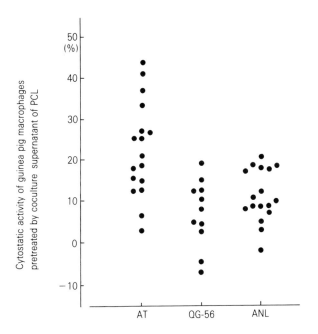

Fig 2 Effect of coculture supernatants of PCL with AT, QG-56, and ANL on cytostatic activity of guinea pig macrophages. The supernatant of PCL and AT rendered macrophages more cytostatic as compared with the supernatant of PCL and QG-56, or PCL and ANL. Reprinted, with permission, from Nagashima A, Yasumoto K, Nakahashi H, et al (18).

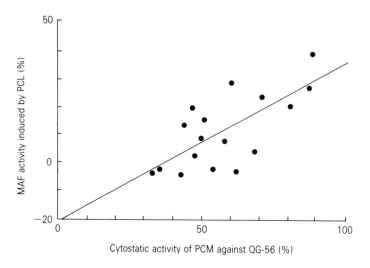

Fig 3 Correlation between cytostatic activity of PCM against QG-56 and degree of MAF activity of the coculture supernatant of PCL and AT. R = 0.703; $y = 0.566x - 21.1$; p<0.01. Reprinted, with permission, from Nagashima A, Yasumoto K, Nakahashi H, et al (18).

activity induced by coculture of TIL with AT and the cytostatic activity of TAM.

Our results show that lung cancer patients can respond to autologous cancer cells immunologically, and can produce MAF, at least in the pleural cavity and lung cancer tissue. Moreover, the final effector cells to attack cancer cells seem to be macrophages activated by the MAF produced by interaction of lymphocytes and autologous tumor cells. These results provide us with a rationale for applying immunotherapy against lung cancer.

Immunotherapy of lung cancer

Azuma et al (21) reported that BCG cell wall skeleton (BCG-CWS) was as active as live BCG when applied as an immunotherapeutic agent for many kinds of animal tumor systems. Therefore, immunotherapy with BCG-CWS was administered to lung cancer patients, and a clinical effect of improved patient survival was observed, especially in stages I and II (22–24). However, some limitations of the BCG-CWS treatment were also revealed in advanced stages of lung cancer. On the basis of these data, Azuma et al (25) sought more potent and less toxic immunoadjuvants. During these studies, the cell wall skeleton of *Nocardia rubra* (N-CWS) was shown to have many advantages over BCG-CWS as an immunotherapeutic agent for cancer therapy (26). We have therefore used N-CWS to apply postoperative adjuvant immunotherapy against lung cancer in a randomized fashion (27).

N-CWS treatment design and patients

All patients under 75 years of age who had been subjected to a surgical operation for lung cancer were eligible. All patients were given 1 course of chemotherapy following surgery according to the histological type of lung cancer, as reported previously (27). Patients who had been subjected to a palliative operation were also given radiotherapy (4000 to 6000 rad) to the residual tumor and the mediastinum. After completion of these conventional forms of therapy, patients were randomly allocated to N-CWS treatment or to no further treatment (control), by an envelope method.

First, N-CWS 300 μg suspended in 10 mL of 0.9% NaCl solution was instilled with a 19-gauge needle into the affected side of the intrapleural space, as induction therapy. Then 200 μg of N-CWS was serially injected intradermally into the forearm with a 26-gauge needle, as a maintenance therapy. The interval between each injection was 2 weeks until 20 weeks had passed, and thereafter injections were 4 weekly. The maintenance intradermal injection of N-CWS was continued until recurrence, or for 5 years. The control group was given no further treatment until recurrence.

In total, 119 patients were entered into this trial and randomly assigned to the control group (64 patients) and the N-CWS group (55 patients). Evaluable patients were 64 in the control group and the 52 in N-CWS group.

Clinical effect of N-CWS treatment

In this trial, survival time and remission duration were chosen as suitable evaluation end-points. Relapse was diagnosed by the appearance of new metastatic lesions or by increases in the size of tumors that had been treated previously.

Survival curves were compared in all patients subjected to surgery. Four-year survival rates were 54.0% in the control group and 57.2% in the N-CWS group. Seventy-five percent survival periods were 19 months in the control and 29 months in the N-CWS group. However, the difference in survival curves was not statistically significant.

The patients were divided into the curative operation group and the palliative operation group. In the curative operation group, there were 47 control patients and 37 N-CWS-treated patients, with 4-year survival rates of 63.4% and 81.2%, respectively. The difference was statistically significant ($p < 0.05$), as shown in Fig 4. No significant difference was observed in the palliative operation group, as shown in Fig 5. These operable patients were divided into stage I + II and stage III + V. Four-year survival rates of stage I + II patients were 68.8% and 81.5%, respectively, in the control and the N-CWS groups ($p < 0.10$), although no significant difference after N-CWS treatment was observed in the patients at stages III and IV.

Remission curves were compared in all patients subjected to surgery, as shown in Fig 6. Four-year remission rates were 28.7% and 52.0%, respectively, in the control and the N-CWS groups. The difference was statistically significant ($p < 0.01$). Therefore, N-CWS treatment effectively prolonged remission in all

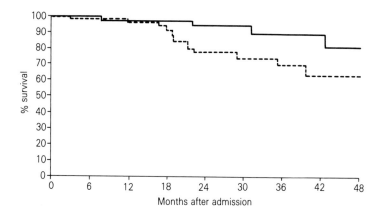

Fig 4 Survival curves of patients undergoing curative operation. —— N-CWS patients (n = 37, 4 died); ----- control patients (n = 47, 14 died); $Z_0 = 2.037$ (p<0.05); $\chi_0^2 = 4.146$ (p<0.05). Reprinted, with permission, from Yasumoto K, Yaita H, Ohta M, et al (27).

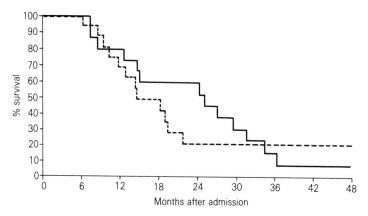

Fig 5 Survival curves of patients undergoing palliative operation. —— N-CWS patients (n = 15, 14 died); ---- control patients (n = 17, 12 died); $Z_0 = 0.816$ (NS); $\chi_0^2 = 0.013$ (NS). Reprinted, with permission, from Yasumoto K, Yaita H, Ohta M, et al (27).

patients subjected to surgery. However, it was effective in terms of the survival period only in patients who had undergone curative operations.

Differences in the mode of recurrence were compared in the curative operation group. The mode of recurrence was classified as local recurrence (including metastasis to the ipsilateral mediastinal lymph nodes) and distant metastasis. As shown in Table 4, recurrence was observed in 23 of 47 control patients (43.9%).

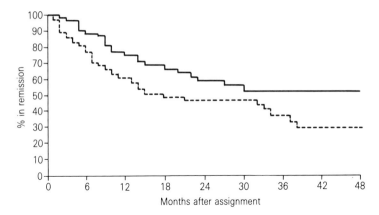

Fig 6 Remission curves of patients with operable lung cancer. —— N-CWS patients (n = 52, 22 recurred); ----- control patients (n = 64, 38 recurred); $Z_0 = 2.078$ (p < 0.05); $\chi_0^2 = 3.984$ (p < 0.05). Reprinted, with permission, from Yasumoto K, Yaita H, Ohta M, et al (27).

Table 4 Comparison of mode of recurrence in curative operation group. Reprinted, with permission, from Yasumoto K, Yaita H, Ohta M, et al (27).

Group	No. of patients	Patients with site of recurrence		Patients in remission (%)
		Local (%)	Distant (%)	
Control	47	7 (14.9)	16 (34.0)	24 (52.2)
N-CWS	37	0*	7 (18.9)	30 (81.1)†

*p < 0.05 by Fisher's exact test; †p < 0.05 by χ^2 test.

The 23 recurrences included 7 local (14.9%) and 16 distant metastases (34.0%). In contrast, recurrence was observed in only 7 of 37 patients (13.9%) in the N-CWS group and all 7 recurrences were distant metastases. These results suggest that N-CWS treatment can suppress not only local recurrence but also distant metastasis in the curative operation group. Such a difference in mode of recurrence was not observed in the palliative operation group.

Thus, adjuvant immunotherapy with N-CWS is effective in patients with operable lung cancer. However, it is effective only in patients subjected to curative resection in terms of survival rate. This is consistent with the results reported by McKneally et al (3) and Fujisawa et al (5). McKneally et al reported that a single intrapleural injection of live BCG was effective only in stage I resectable lung cancer, but not in stages II and III. Fujisawa et al reported that postoperative adjuvant immunotherapy with transfer factor was effective in stage I + II patients but not in stage III. These results may mean that immunotherapy, regardless of the type, can eradicate only minimal residual disease after surgery.

Acknowledgment

An oil-attached form of N-CWS was kindly provided by Fujisawa Pharmaceutical Co, Ltd., Osaka, Japan.

References

1. Matthews MJ, Kanhouwa S, Pickren J, Robinette D. Frequency of residual and metastatic tumor in patients undergoing curative surgical resection for lung cancer. Cancer Chemother Rep 1973;4:63-7.
2. Paulson DL. The survival rate in superior sulcus tumors treated by presurgical irradiation. JAMA 1966;4:342.
3. McKneally MF, Maver C, Lininger L, et al. Four-year follow-up on the Albany experience with intrapleural BCG in lung cancer. J Thorac Cardiovasc Surg 1981;81:485-92.
4. Watanabe Y, Iwa T. Clinical value of immunotherapy for lung cancer by the streptococcal preparation, OK-432. Cancer 1984;53:248-53.
5. Fujisawa T, Yamaguchi Y, Kimura H, et al. Adjuvant immunotherapy of primary resected lung cancer with transfer factor. Cancer 1984;54:663-9.
6. Edwards FR, Whitewell F. Use of BCG as an immunostimulant in the surgical treatment of carcinoma of lung—a five year follow-up report. Thorax 1978;33:250-2.
7. Mountain CF, Gail MH. Surgical adjuvant intrapleural BCG treatment for stage I non-small cell lung cancer. Preliminary report of the National Cancer Institute Lung Cancer Study Group. J Thorac Cardiovasc Surg 1981;82:649-57.
8. Ludwig Lung Cancer Study Group. Adverse effect of intrapleural *Corynebacterium parvum* as adjuvant therapy in resected stage I and II non-small cell carcinoma of the lung. J Thorac Cardiovasc Surg 1985;89:842-7.
9. Yasumoto K, Ohta M, Nomoto K. Cytotoxic activity of lymphocytes to bronchogenic carcinoma cells in patients with lung cancer. Jpn J Cancer Res (Gann) 1976;67:505-11.
10. Manabe H, Yasumoto K, Ohta M, et al. Effect of anticancer therapy on lymphocyte cytotoxicity in lung cancer patients. Jpn J Cancer Res (Gann) 1977;68:477-82.
11. Toyohira K, Yasumoto K, Manabe H, et al. Effect of radiotherapy on lymphocyte cytotoxicity against allogeneic lung cancer cells in patients with bronchogenic carcinoma. Jpn J Cancer Res (Gann) 1979;70:9-14.
12. Yanagawa E, Yasumoto K, Manabe H, et al. Cytostatic activity of peripheral blood monocytes against bronchogenic carcinoma cells in patients with lung cancer. Jpn J Cancer Res (Gann) 1979;70:533-9.
13. Yagawa K, Kaku M, Manabe H, et al. Superoxide assay-leukocyte adherence inhibition test and a soluble factor which stimulates the adherence of macrophages. Cancer Res 1980;40:4791-5.
14. Yasumoto K, Manabe H, Nomoto K, et al. Antibody specific for lung cancer cells detected in sera of patients with bronchogenic carcinoma. Jpn J Cancer Res Cancer Res (Gann) 1983;74:595-601.
15. Nakahashi H, Yasumoto K, Nagashima A, et al. Antitumor activity of macrophages in lung cancer patients with special reference to location of macrophages. Cancer Res 1984;44:5906-9.
16. Takeo S, Yasumoto K, Nagashima A, et al. Role of tumor-associated macrophages

in lung cancer. Cancer Res 1986;46:3179–82.

17. Kuda T, Yasumoto K, Yano T, et al. Role of antitumor activity of alveolar macrophages in lung cancer patients. Cancer Res 1987;47:2199–202.

18. Nagashima A, Yasumoto K, Nakahashi H, et al. Antitumor activity of pleural cavity macrophages and its regulation by pleural cavity lymphocytes in patients with lung cancer. Cancer Res 1987;47:5497–500.

19. Yaita H, Yasumoto K, Nagashima A, et al. Antitumor activity of regional lymph node lymphocytes in patients with lung cancer. J Surg Oncol (in press).

20. Yasumoto K, Takeo S, Yano T, et al. Role of tumor-infiltrating lymphocytes in host defence mechanisms against lung cancer. J Surg Oncol (in press).

21. Azuma I, Taniyama T, Hirao F, et al. Antitumor activity of cell-wall skeletons and peptidoglycolipids of Mycobacteria and related microorganisms in mice and rabbits. Jpn J Cancer Res (Gann) 1974;65:493–505.

22. Yasumoto K, Manabe H, Ueno M, et al. Immunotherapy of human lung cancer with BCG-cell-wall skeleton. Gann 1976;67:787–95.

23. Yasumoto K, Manabe H, Ohta M, et al. Immunotherapy of lung cancer and carcinomatous pleuritis. Gann Monogr Cancer Res 1978;21:129–41.

24. Yasumoto K, Manabe H, Yanagawa E, et al. Nonspecific adjuvant immunotherapy of lung cancer with cell wall skeleton of *Mycobacterium bovis* Bacillus Calmette-Guérin. Cancer Res 1979;39:3262–7.

25. Azuma I, Yamawaki M, Yasumoto K, Yamamura Y. Antitumor activity of *Nocardia* cell-wall skeleton preparations in transplantable tumors in syngeneic mice and patients with malignant pleurisy. Cancer Immunol Immunother 1978;4:95–100.

26. Yamamura Y, Yasumoto K, Ogura T, Azuma I. *Nocardia rubra* cell-wall skeleton in the therapy of animal and human cancer. In: Hersh EM, ed. Augmenting agent in cancer therapy. New York: Academic Press; 1981:71–90.

27. Yasumoto K, Yaita H, Ohta M, et al. Randomly controlled study of chemotherapy versus chemoimmunotherapy in postoperative lung cancer patients. Cancer Res 1985;45:1413–7.

Clinical application of *Nocardia rubra* cell wall skeleton in inoperable lung cancers

Takeshi Ogura,[1] Mitsunori Sakatani[2]

[1]*Third Department of Internal Medicine, Tokushima,* [2]*Department of Internal Medicine, National Kinki-Chuo Hospital for Chest Diseases, Osaka, Japan*

Introduction

Various immunomodulators have been introduced into the multidisciplinary treatment of cancer patients, especially in Japan. In general, no direct cytotoxicity to cancer cells is shown by these agents, and their clinical benefits have been determined mainly by the statistical evaluation of patient survival period in randomized controlled studies (1,2). In this paper, clinical studies are reviewed on the treatment of inoperable lung cancer patients with *Nocardia rubra* cell wall skeleton (N-CWS). A possible role for N-CWS in inducing therapeutic effects is discussed.

Methods and results

Immunotherapeutic effects of N-CWS in patients with lung cancer

Randomized controlled studies of inoperable lung cancers, with or without cancerous pleural effusions, have been done with patients who entered Osaka University Hospital and its affiliated institutions—Osaka Habikino Hospital, Kinki Central Hospital, Toneyama Hospital, and Osaka Center for Adult Diseases (3). Briefly, patients without pleural effusions were classified into 16 groups according to a combination of 4 histological types and 4 clinical stages, and they were treated according to a prescribed protocol of conventional therapy with irradiation and/or anticancer drugs. After that, in each of the 16 groups patients who were still in performance status (PS) 0 to 3 were randomly allocated into a control or an N-CWS treatment group. Patients in the N-CWS group were given local injections, at a dose of 400 to 600 μg, of N-CWS as an induction therapy into the tumor tissue or into the corresponding bronchial submucosal tissue under fiberoptic bronchoscopy.

Patients with histologically proven cancerous pleural effusions were randomly allocated into a control or an N-CWS treatment group immediately after registration. Patients in the N-CWS group were treated locally with 40 mg of doxorubicin and with 400 µg of N-CWS at weekly intervals; patients in the control group were given doxorubicin alone. All patients with cancerous pleural effusions received 3 to 5 local treatments by tubal thoracostomy.

In both trials, for those with and those without cancerous pleural effusions, all patients in the N-CWS group were injected intradermally with an additional 100 to 200 µg of N-CWS as a maintenance therapy at monthly intervals for as long a period as practicable.

The eligibility of all patients to enter these trials was checked by senior investigators and an independent controller. Subsequently, it was confirmed that 108 and 118 patients without effusions were eligible, and that 33 and 35 patients with cancerous effusions were also eligible in the control and N-CWS groups, respectively. After statistical analysis for patients' clinical characteristics, including response rate for initial conventional therapy in control and N-CWS groups, it was shown that both groups were completely comparable for statistical evaluation by the generalized Wilcoxon test of survival rate curves calculated by the method of Kaplan and Meier.

In patients without effusions, survival rate curves for all the eligible patients and for the patients in stages III and IV were not significantly different between the control and the N-CWS groups (Fig 1). Histologically, however, the survival period of the patients with small cell lung cancer in stages III and IV was significantly prolonged by the N-CWS treatment.

In the patients with cancerous pleurisy, the effects of local and systemic treat-

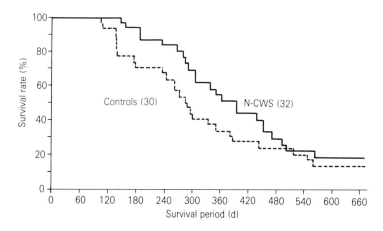

Fig 1 Effect of N-CWS immunotherapy on survival period of small cell lung cancer in stages III and IV. Response rates (complete response + partial response) were 73.3% and 75.0% in the control and the N-CWS group, respectively, indicating no statistically significant difference between the 2 groups (p = 0.0377). Reprinted, with permission, from Yamamura Y, Ogura T, Sakatani M, et al (3).

ment were statistically evaluated. Significant increases were observed in the local responses (Table 1) and in the survival rate (Fig 2).

During the maintenance therapy with repeated intradermal injections of N-CWS, considerable numbers of patients showed skin reaction such as ulceration, induration, or swelling. Thus, we analyzed the patient survival curve according to positivity of skin reaction and found a significant correlation between patient survival curve and skin reaction (Fig 3).

N-CWS immunotherapy for cancerous pleurisy of patients with pulmonary adenocarcinoma was conducted independently by a group from the National Cancer Center Hospital in Tokyo, and a similar clinical benefit of local instillations of an anticancer drug and N-CWS was demonstrated in a randomized controlled study (4).

Table 1 Local response to intrapleural instillations of N-CWS with anticancer drugs in patients with cancerous pleurisy.

Treatment	No. of patients		
	CR*	PR†	CR + PR‡
Adriamycin	8/33	12/33	60.1%
Adriamycin + N-CWS	14/33	16/33	85.7%

*CR, complete response (complete disappearance of tumor cells and a notable decrease of effusions for 4 weeks); †PR, partial response (complete disappearance of tumor cells and notable decrease of effusions for 4 weeks); ‡the total of CR and PR was significantly increased by N-CWS immunotherapy. $p < 0.05$; $\chi^2 = 4.287$; $Z = 2.161$.

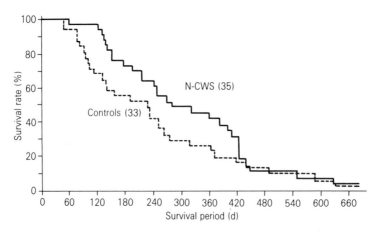

Fig 2 Effects of N-CWS immunotherapy on survival period in patients with cancerous pleurisy. Patient survival period was significantly increased by N-CWS immunotherapy ($p > 0.05$). Reprinted, with permission, from Yamamura Y, Ogura T, Sakatani M, et al (3).

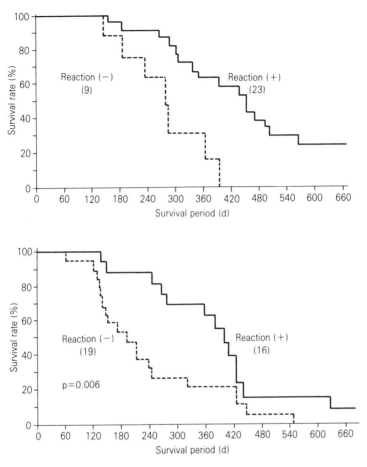

Fig 3 Analysis of survival period according to skin reaction induced by intradermal injections as maintenance therapy. In small-cell lung cancer (upper) and cancerous pleurisy (lower) the survival periods were remarkably prolonged in patients showing a positive (+) skin reaction to N-CWS. Numbers of patients are shown in parentheses.

Effector mechanism of N-CWS in cancer treatment

Many previous reports have demonstrated the prolongation of patient survival period by the use of an immunomodulator in a randomized controlled fashion. In such circumstances, the patient survival rate is modified by various factors, and studying the effector mechanism against cancer may help to evaluate the immunomodulator. However, there is little information about the effector mechanism(s) in cancer patients under immunotherapy. Thus, the following study was conducted to evaluate the mode of action of N-CWS in local immunotherapy for cancerous pleurisy (5).

First, the effect of intrapleural instillation of N-CWS on macrophage cytostatic activity was assessed in 6 cases. In this study, pleural effusions were harvested into heparinized glass bottles before and 5 to 7 days after intrapleural instillation of N-CWS. Mononuclear cells (MNC) were separated by Ficoll-Hypaque density gradient centrifugation. MNC (1×10^5) were incubated for 2 h in a microtest plate (96 wells), washed to remove nonadherent cells, and assayed for cytostatic activity for 1×10^4 allogeneic adenocarcinoma cells (PC-9). Cytostatic activity was expressed as percent inhibition of [^{3}H]thymidine incorporation into the tumor cells during an additional 6-h culture. As shown in Table 2, the intrapleural instillation of N-CWS markedly augmented the cytostatic activity of pleural macrophages.

To assess the induction of macrophage cytostatic activity, MNC (1×10^5) from 21 pleural effusions and 22 pleural washings at surgical operation were incubated with medium alone or with N-CWS at a concentration of 10 μg/mL for 24 h. The MNC were then washed and assayed for cytostatic activity. Cytostatic activity was markedly augmented in many cases (Fig 4).

Although the data are not shown here, the cytostatic activity was considerably decreased when nonadherent cells, mainly T cells, were depleted from MNC by washing out or by the SRBC-rosetting method before culture with N-CWS, indicating participation of a macrophage activating factor (MAF) produced during the culture with N-CWS. To elucidate the details of the underlying mechanism, we incubated nonadherent MNC (2×10^5), treated with complement alone or with complement and OKT3 monoclonal antibody, with N-CWS (10 μg/mL) for 24 h, and the resulting culture supernatants were assayed for MAF activity, which was expressed as the cytostatic activity of 2×10 freshly prepared macrophages incubated with the culture supernatant for 24 h. Although the number of cases is limited, MAF activity produced from N-CWS-incubated nonadherent cells was found to be significantly less by removing the OKT3$^+$ cells (Table 3).

We also examined the interferon (IFN) activity of the culture supernatant by a

Table 2 Augmentation of macrophage cytostatic activity after intrapleural instillation of N-CWS. Reprinted, with permission, from Sakatani M, Ogura T, Masuno T, et al (5).

Patient no.	Cytostatic activity (%) of macrophages prepared from pleural effusions		
	Before treatment	After treatment	Increase
1	21.0	48.2	27.2
2	3.0	64.3	61.3
3	-1.3	39.4	40.7
4	-2.8	17.5	20.3
5	21.2	74.6	53.4
6	0.4	36.0	35.6
Mean $\pm$ SEM	6.9 ± 4.6	46.7 ± 8.4	39.8 ± 6.3

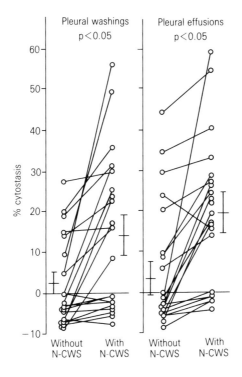

Fig 4 Cytostatic activity of human pleural macrophages treated with N-CWS in vitro. MNC (1×10^5) were incubated with or without $10 \, \mu g/mL$ of N-CWS for 24 h, washed, and tested for cytostatic activity against PC-9 adenocarcinoma cells (1×10^4). Bars indicate means ± SEM. Reprinted, with permission, from Sakatani M, Ogura T, Masuno T, et al (5).

virus plaque reduction assay that used human amniotic FL-WISH cells and vesicular stomatitis virus. IFN activity was detected in only 9 of 14 supernatants showing MAF activity, ranging from 64 to 512 U/mL (Table 4). The supernatants without MAF activity showed no significant IFN activity. Heat and acid stability studies in which samples of the culture supernatants were incubated for 30 min at 56°C, or were dialyzed in 0.1 M glycine-HCl buffer for 24 h revealed that the IFN activitiy in all 10 cases was not stable at all, while the MAF activity was notably reduced in only 2 cases.

Discussion and conclusions

In the adjuvant immunotherapies described here, N-CWS was administered locally as an induction therapy and then intradermally as a maintenance therapy. The design of this therapeutic regimen was based on previous results of clinical and

Table 3 Effect of OKT3 monoclonal antibody plus complement on the production of MAF from pleural nonadherent cells incubated with N-CWS. Reprinted, with permission, from Sakatani M, Ogura T, Masuno T, et al (5).

Case no.	Increase in cytostatic activity (%) of macrophages		
	No treatment	Complement	OKT3 + complement
37	11.3	10.3	1.2
38	31.1	22.4	−0.7
39	25.4	26.7	6.7

Table 4 MAF and IFN activities in supernatants of MNC cultured with N-CWS. Reprinted, with permission, from Sakatani M, Ogura T, Masuno T, et al (5).

Case no.	MNC culture			Treatment of supernatant		
	Without N-CWS	With N-CWS		Incubation at 56°C		Dialysis at pH 2
	MAF*	MAF	IFN†	MAF	IFN	IFN
9	NT	31.3	<4	28.9	<4	<4
10	NT	20.6	64	22.6	<4	<4
11	NT	20.5	256	2.8	<4	<4
12	NT	3.1	<4	NT	<4	<4
13	NT	26.7	512	39.4	<4	<4
14	NT	40.1	<4	NT	<4	<4
15	NT	3.2	<4	NT	<4	<4
16	NT	61.6	<4	NT	<4	<4
17	8.1	35.2	128	28.8	<4	NT
18	5.9	30.7	64	19.8	<4	NT
19	8.8	14.6	<4	8.8	<4	NT
20	5.0	18.6	64	13.9	<4	NT
21	6.6	15.0	32	10.6	<4	NT
22	7.3	62.9	32	39.3	<4	NT
23	NT	11.3	64	NT	<4	NT
24	NT	NT	64	NT	<4	NT
25	NT	11.0	<4	NT	<4	NT

*MAF activity quantitated as cytostatic activity (%) of macrophages incubated with test supernatant.
†Values are U/mL.
NT, not tested.

experimental immunotherapy (6–8) and phase I studies (9). We were able to demonstrate a significantly prolonged survival period in small cell lung cancer patients treated with N CWS (3). Furthermore, in patients with cancerous pleurisy who were treated with N-CWS, the therapeutic benefits—eradication of tumor cells and pleural effusions in the pleural cavity—have been observed independently in 2 randomized controlled studies (3,4). Similar therapeutic effects have been observed in another trial with OK432 (10).

There have been conflicting reports on prolongation of survival period by adjuvant immunotherapy (1,2), but our experimental studies have provided evidence that the CWS of BCG and *N. rubra*, when administered locally into rat ascites tumors, can activate macrophages and increase the survival period as well as eradicate ascites tumors (7,8). Thus, the studies conducted to elucidate the effector mechanisms in cancerous pleurisy focused on macrophage activation. It was clearly demonstrated that macrophages activated by locally administered N-CWS play an important role in producing the therapeutic effects of N-CWS.

With repeated intradermal injections of N-CWS, an unexpected significant increase in survival period was observed for patients with a positive skin reaction to intradermal N-CWS, compared with those who showed a negative skin reaction. Although the underlying mechanism has not yet been elucidated, a specific activation of the effector mechanism, as observed in association with repeated injections of N-CWS (11–13), may contribute to this phenomenon.

References

1. Ogura T. Randomized controlled trials with immunostimulants for cancer patients in Japan. In: Azuma I, Jollès G, eds. Immunomodulators: Now and tommorrow. Tokyo/Berlin: Japan Scientific Societies Press/Springer; 1987:155–66.
2. Ogura T. Present status of cancer immunotherapy for lung cancer. In: Fukunishi R, Mantz JM, Yamada M, et al, eds. Approaches to cancer therapy research in France and Japan. Oxford: Pergamon Press; 1987:129–34.
3. Yamamura Y, Ogura T, Sakatani M, et al. Randomized controlled study of adjuvant immunotherapy with *Nocardia rubra* cell wall skeleton for inoperable lung cancer. Cancer Res 1983;43:5575–9.
4. Saijo N, Eguchi K, Tominaga K, et al. Effect of *Nocardia rubra* cell wall skeleton against pleuritis carcinomatosa in adenocarcinoma of the lung. Jpn J Cancer Chemother 1983;10:290–5.
5. Sakatani M, Ogura T, Masuno T, et al. Effect of *Nocardia rubra* cell wall skeleton on augmentation of cytotoxicity function in human pleural macrophages. Cancer Immunol Immunother 1987;25:119–25.
6. Yamamura Y, Sakatani M, Ogura T, Azuma I. Adjuvant immunotherapy of lung cancer with BCG cell wall skeleton (BCG-CWS). Cancer 1979;43:1314–9.
7. Ogura T, Namba M, Hirao F, et al. Association of macrophage activation with antitumor effect on rat syngeneic fibrosarcoma by *Nocardia rubra* cell wall skeleton. Cancer Res 1979;34:4706–12.
8. Ogura T, Shinzato S, Sakatani M, et al. Analysis of therapeutic effect in experimental chemoimmunotherapy for rat ascites tumor. Cancer Immunol Immunother 1982;14:67–72.
9. Yamamura Y, Ogura T, Hirao F, et al. Phase I study with cell wall skeleton of *Nocardia rubra*. Cancer Treat Rep 1981;65:707–9.
10. Urata A, Nishimura M, Ohta K. Randomized controlled study of OK432 in the treatment of cancerous pleurisy. Jpn J Cancer Chemother 1983;10:1497–503.
11. Yamakido M, Yanagida J, Ishioka S, et al. Effect of *Nocardia rubra* cell wall

skeleton on interleukin 2 production and lymphocyte proliferation in former poison gas factory workers. Jpn J Cancer Res 1986;77:406–12.

12. Hayashi S, Masuno T, Hosoe S, et al. Augmented production of colony-stimulation factor in C3H/HeN mice immunized with *Nocardia rubra* cell wall skeleton. Infect Immun 1986;52:128–33.

13. Yokota S, Shirasaka T, Nishikawa H, et al. Augmentative effect of *Nocardia rubra* cell wall skeleton (N-CWS) on lymphokine-activated killer (LAK) cell induction. Cancer Immunol Immunother 1988;26:11–7.

Long-term results of *Nocardia rubra* cell wall skeleton immunotherapy in gastric cancer patients

Takenori Ochiai, Kaichi Isono

Department of Surgery, Chiba University School of Medicine, Chiba, Japan

Introduction

Nonspecific immunotherapy has received much attention as a new modality of treatment of cancer in the past decade (1,2). Enthusiasm for this kind of therapy seems now to have diminished in the USA, however nonspecific immunotherapy is widely applied clinically in Japan. In order to answer the crucial question as to whether or not nonspecific immunotherapy actually exists, we have performed 2 series of randomized clinical trials of nonspecific immunotherapy (3,4). Gastric cancer was chosen as the disease for study because it exists among a large proportion of people in Japan, and therefore its clinicopathologic features, definition of cancer stages, and patients' prognoses have been extensively studied by the Japanese Research Society for Gastric Cancer.

BCG cell wall skeleton (BCG-CWS) and *Nocardia rubra* cell wall skeleton (N-CWS) were first prepared, and their antitumor, adjuvant, and mitogenic activities were described by Azuma et al (5,6). This paper describes the long-term effects of N-CWS immunotherapy, compared with chemotherapy, in gastric cancer patients.

Patients and methods

A clinical trial of N-CWS was carried out at the Department of Surgery, Chiba University School of Medicine, and the surgical departments of its 14 affiliated hospitals. All surgeons at all the participating institutions were trained at the Department of Surgery, Chiba University, and operate under the same practical principles with closely similar procedures. The study was directed by an independent controller who was responsible for random allocation of therapy regimens, sealing of the randomly allocated key codes in envelopes, preservation of the key codes, and integrity in determining patient eligibility for inclusion in the evaluation and analysis of data.

The subjects were consecutive patients with gastric carcinoma, who underwent gastrectomy at the participant institutions during the 19-month period from September 1, 1979, until March 31, 1981.

After the patients had undergone gastrectomy, they were classified into 12 levels of disease, by macroscopic stage of gastric cancer and degree of surgical curability at the time of operation, according to the General Rules for Gastric Cancer Study of the Japanese Research Society for Gastric Cancer (1981). They were randomly allocated in each level to the chemotherapy or immunotherapy group, according to the randomization of therapy regimens arranged in advance by the controller.

After a specimen had been examined microscopically, the patients were classified by histologic stage of cancer and radicality of surgical intervention into curative and noncurative resection cases. The effect of immunotherapy was assessed between the groups on the basis of histologic curability.

The immunotherapeutic agent used in this study, N-CWS, was suspended in physiological saline and injected intradermally into the upper arm in a dose of 400 μg. N-CWS therapy was usually started within the 1st postoperative week, and given weekly for the 1st month. Subsequently, the patient received monthly injections for as long a period as deemed practicable.

The dosage regimen employed for anticancer chemotherapy in this study is shown in Fig 1. Patients received intravenous injections of mitomycin-C (MMC) during surgery and on the following day. Patients were then given combination chemotherapy consisting of MMC, 5-fluorouracil (5-FU), and cytarabine (MFC) chemotherapy for 10 weeks, beginning 1 month after surgery. Immediately after completion of MFC therapy, oral tegafur was instituted at a daily dose of 600 mg. A single iv injection of MMC 10 mg was combined with tegafur therapy trimonthly during the 1st year and at 6-month intervals thereafter.

Results

A total of 302 patients were entered into the study: 143 in the chemotherapy

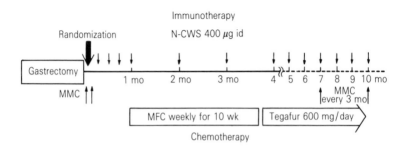

Fig 1 Schedule of immunotherapy and chemotherapy in controlled trial on N-CWS in gastric cancer. Reprinted, with permission, from Ochiai T, Sato H, Hayashi R, et al (4).

group and 159 in the immunotherapy group. Of these, 258 were evaluable, 118 in the chemotherapy group and 140 in the immunotherapy group. Forty-four patients were excluded from analysis, 25 from the chemotherapy group and 19 from the immunotherapy group. Nine exclusions from analysis were patients who dropped out of the study: 3 from the chemotherapy group and 6 from the immunotherapy group.

After histologic examination of the specimens, 90 patients from the chemotherapy group and 97 patients from the immunotherapy group were designated curative resection cases, and 28 from the chemotherapy and 43 from the immunotherapy group noncurative resection cases, respectively.

The curative and noncurative resection cases in both groups were analyzed with respect to various background factors to test intergroup statistical differences. No significant difference was noted between the chemotherapy and immunotherapy groups with respect to any of these factors.

The frequency of N-CWS injections ranged from 2 to 35 (mean 16.5) in the 140 patients of the immunotherapy group.

The patients who had undergone noncurative resection were surveyed for survival as of January 1, 1987, with continuing observation periods of between 6 and 8 years. Patient survival in the N-CWS group was significantly longer than that of the control group. None of the patients survived as long as 5 years in the control group; however 5-year survival in the N-CWS-treated group was 21.8% (Fig 2).

Discussion

There is a discrepancy in evaluation of the clinical effectiveness of nonspecific immunotherapy between the USA and Japan. From the results of our series of ran-

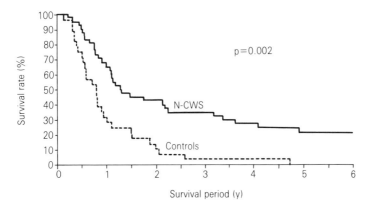

Fig 2 Survival rate in patients with noncurative resection of gastric cancer treated with N-CWS + chemotherapy (n = 43) vs controls (chemotherapy alone, n = 28).

domized clinical trials, we have concluded that nonspecific immunotherapy in postoperative gastric cancer patients is effective if an appropriate immunotherapeutic agent is applied. Several possible explanations may be offered for our positive results, the first of which is that we chose gastric cancer as our disease of study. Gastric cancer has a poorer prognosis than cancers of other organs. A poor prognostic cancer in advanced stages seems to be a good choice to test the effect of immunotherapy. The second explanation for our positive results is the schedule of postoperative adjuvant therapy in our trial. Immunotherapy was combined with chemotherapy in our trial, and the chemotherapeutic regimen was sufficient as anticancer treatment. Combination of immunotherapy with sufficient chemotherapy seems to be a good schedule for better survival.

The most important factor in our positive results is the choice of immunotherapeutic agents. On the basis of our understanding of the immunological mechanisms of BCG-CWS and N-CWS, we were able to produce positive results. We can therefore conclude that nonspecific immunotherapy with N-CWS is effective in postoperative gastric cancer patients.

References

1. Mathé G, Amiel JL, Schwarzenberg L, et al. Active immunotherapy for acute lymphoblastic leukemia. Lancet 1969;i:697–9.
2. Eilber FR, Morton DL, Holmes EC, et al. Adjuvant immunotherapy with BCG in the treatment of regional lymphnode metastasis for malignant melanoma. N Engl J Med 1976;294:237–40.
3. Ochiai T, Sato H, Hayashi R, et al. Postoperative adjuvant chemotherapy of gastric cancer with BCG-CWS. Cancer Immunol Immunother 1983;14:167–71.
4. Ochiai T, Sato H, Hayashi R, et al. Randomly controlled study of chemotherapy versus chemoimmunotherapy in postoperative gastric cancer patients. Cancer Res 1983;43:3001–7.
5. Azuma I, Taniyama T, Hirao F, Yamamura Y. Antitumor activity of cell-wall skeletons and peptidoglycolipids of mycobacteria and related microorganisms. Jpn J Cancer Res (Gann) 1974;65:493–505.
6. Azuma I, Yamawaki M, Yasumoto K, Yamamura Y. Antitumor activity of *Nocardia* cell-wall skeleton preparations in transplantable tumors in syngeneic mice and patients with malignant pleurisy. Cancer Immunol Immunother 1978;4:95–100.

Clinical application of *Nocardia rubra* cell wall skeleton for immunotherapy of gastric carcinoma based on the function of effector T cells against tumors

Shohei Koyama, Tsugio Ebihara

Department of Internal Medicine, Institute of Clinical Medicine, University of Tsukuba, Ibaraki, Japan

Introduction

Although the use of adjuvant immunotherapy has been extensively investigated in gastric cancer patients in Japan, there have been few reports on prolongation of survival in such patients (1–3). This report focuses on the clinical application of *Nocardia rubra* cell wall skeleton (N-CWS), developed by Yamamura and Azuma (4–6), for gastric carcinoma based on the concept of the function of the effector T cells against tumor cells.

Patients and methods

Patients

Patients admitted to the randomized, controlled study had undergone gastrectomy for gastric cancer between September 1979 and March 1983. The criteria for patient selection were as follows: a) macroscopically curative or relatively noncurative resection; b) no previous treatment for cancer; c) age under 75 years; and d) free of serious cardiac, renal, liver, or pulmonary complications and having a systemic condition good enough to tolerate the study protocol. Stratification and allocation of the patients, registration of patients, and operation procedure and pathological examination have been described previously (3).

Chemotherapy and immunotherapy

The protocol comprised 2 treatment groups, with and without N-CWS. In both groups, tegafur was administered as chemotherapy at a daily dose of 400 to

800 mg, starting 24–29 days after surgical operation. The duration schedule of chemotherapy has been described previously (3). In the immunochemotherapy group, a lyophilized preparation formulated with N-CWS (donated by Fujisawa Pharmaceutical Co., Ltd., Osaka) was used. The 400 μg of N-CWS suspended in sterile 0.85% NaCl solution was injected intradermally into the upper arm of patients within the 2nd postoperative week, and was given weekly for the 1st month. Subsequently, the patients received a monthly injection for as long a period as deemed practicable.

Preparation of peripheral blood lymphocytes

Peripheral blood lymphocytes (PBL) from 20 patients with advanced gastric cancer were isolated from venous blood by Ficoll-Hypaque density gradient centrifugation. Of 20 patients with gastric carcinoma, 10 had a nonresectable carcinoma owing to systemic metastasis.

Cell culture with recombinant interleukin 2 or recombinant interleukin 2 plus recombinant interferon-γ or T cell growth factor

Approximately 2×10^6 PBL were placed in tissue culture flasks (No. 163371, Nunk, Denmark) with RPMI-1640 medium supplemented with 10% fetal calf serum, 100 mg/mL kanamycin, and 100 U/mL recombinant interleukin 2 (rIL-2, Shionogi Co., Ltd, Osaka), or 100 U/mL rIL-2 plus 100 U/mL recombinant interferon-γ (rIFN-γ, Toray Co., Ltd, Osaka), or 50% T cell growth factor (TCGF) preparations. TCGF preparations were obtained from 48-h tissue culture medium with 0.08% phytohemagglutinin-P (Difco, Detroit)-stimulated human spleen cells, as described previously (7). All cultures were maintained for 14 days in 5% CO_2 in air at 37°C and fed 3 times per week by changing the culture medium.

Two-color flow cytometric analysis

FITC-conjugated anti-Leu 2a(CD8), anti-Leu 3a(CD4), anti-HLA-DR, and anti-Leu 7, and phycoerythrin(PE)-conjugated anti-Leu 15(CD11), anti-Leu 8, anti-Leu 2a(CD8), anti-Leu 11(CD16), and anti-IL-2R(CD25) were provided by Becton Dickinson Co. (Mountain View, California). Freshly isolated PBL, or rIL-2, or rIL-2 plus rIFNγ or TCGF-activated PBL were stained with fluorochrome-conjugated MAb for 30 min at 4°C and washed twice, as described previously (7,8). The cells were analyzed by flow cytometry (FACS-IV analyzer, Becton Dickinson Co., Mountain View, California).

Assay for killer cell activities

Killer cell activities of the cell population were tested against human natural killer (NK)-sensitive K562 cells and NK-resistant Daudi cells. Cytolytic activities of cultured lymphoid cells and PBL on tumor targets were examined by a standard 4-h ^{51}Cr-release, according to the formula:

$$\% \text{ of specific lysis} = \frac{\text{Experimental release} - \text{Spontaneous release}}{\text{Maximum release} - \text{Spontaneous release}} \times 100.$$

Spontaneous release determined from target cells incubated in culture medium was always 5% or less of maximum release.

Assay for suppressive activity of TCGF-activated PBL from patients with a cytotoxic reaction

This assay was performed according to a method described previously (9–11). To standardize results and permit evaluation of the degree of suppression, the following formula was used: % suppression $= (1 - \Delta\%^a/\Delta\%^b) \times 100$, where $\Delta\%^a$ is change in $\Delta\%$ of cytotoxicity after the addition of a suppressor cell source, and $\Delta\%^b$ is change in $\Delta\%$ of cytotoxicity of target cells admixed with effector cells without cells from a suppressor cell source.

Results

As shown in Table 1, PBL from normal healthy controls had the highest cytolytic activity against K562 cells. However, PBL from patients with resectable or nonresectable carcinoma showed significantly decreased killer cell activities compared with those from normal individuals (p<0.01). None of the freshly prepared PBL from each of the 3 experimental groups expressed any significant cytotoxicity against Daudi tumor cells. Human PBL cultured with rIL-2 or rIL-2 plus rIFN-γ or TCGF for 14 days acquired killer cell activity against K562 cells and Daudi cells (Table 1). In other words, the rIL-2-activated PBL from normal

Table 1 Cytolytic activities against K562 and Daudi cells of effector cells from normal healthy controls and gastric cancer (resectable and nonresectable) patients.

Subjects*	Target	PBL culture alone†	PBL cultured with		
			rIL-2	rIL-2 + rIFN-γ	TCGF
Normal	K562	22.6 ± 1.5††	43.0 ± 0.8	38.3 ± 1.5	24.6 ± 1.8
	Daudi	1.4 ± 0.2	40.0 ± 1.2	36.4 ± 1.9	9.5 ± 1.8
Cancer	K562	10.3 ± 1.1	39.1 ± 1.6	37.3 ± 0.7	20.1 ± 2.6
(resectable)	Daudi	0.8 ± 0.1	36.7 ± 1.9	34.1 ± 0.9	9.4 ± 2.2
Cancer	K562	8.4 ± 1.7	33.9 ± 2.2	40.4 ± 2.9	18.7 ± 2.1
(nonresectable)	Daudi	0.4 ± 0.1	18.9 ± 1.6	38.1 ± 1.5	5.3 ± 1.7

*Each experimental group consisted of 10 patients.
†Freshly prepared PBL.
††Target cell : effector cell ratio 1:10. Mean ± SE of 10 cases.

controls and gastric cancer patients had significantly higher lytic activity against K562 and Daudi cells than did the freshly prepared PBL from each group (p<0.01). However, the lymphokine-activated killer (LAK) cell activity against Daudi cells in rIL-2-activated PBL from patients with nonresectable carcinoma decreased significantly compared with that of patients with resectable carcinoma and of normal healthy controls (p<0.01). Depressed LAK cell activity was restored by additional culture with exogeneous rIFN-γ (Table 1). The LAK cell activity of TCGF-activated PBL from the 3 experimental groups was significantly decreased compared with that of rIL-2-activated PBL (p<0.001). In particular, LAK cells from patients with nonresectable carcinoma showed much lower cytolytic activity against Daudi cells.

To investigate the mechanisms of lower levels of LAK cell activity in TCGF-activated PBL, the suppressor cell activity of these cells was examined. This assay method was carried out by the inhibition of those cytotoxic actions clearly directed at the effector process carried out by rIL-2-activated PBL (LAK cells). Figure 1 shows the presence of suppressor cell activity of TCGF-activated PBL from a patient with nonresectable carcinoma. The high cytotoxicity of the LAK cells was decreased in proportion to the increased number of TCGF-activated

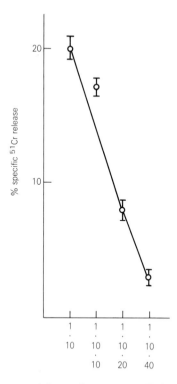

Fig 1 Suppression of cytotoxicity against tumor cells by TCGF-activated PBL from patients with nonresectable carcinoma. Killer cell activity linearly decreased with the increasing addition of the suppressor cell source.

PBL as the suppressor cell source was added. The TCGF-activated PBL with the suppressive activity were designated as lymphokine-activated suppressor (LAS) cells.

LAS cell function of TCGF-activated PBL from the 3 experimental groups is summarized in Fig 2. Of 10 patients with resectable carcinoma, 4 showed a significant depression of LAK cell activity by TCGF-activated PBL. In patients with nonresectable carcinoma, 9 of 10 patients tested were shown to have significantly strong LAS cell activity. However, TCGF-activated PBL from 10 normal healthy controls did not significantly suppress LAK cell activity.

To determine the phenotypic characterization of the LAK and LAS cell population, cytokine-activated PBL were analyzed by 2-color flow cytometry. The results are summarized in comparing the immunologic phenotype of PBL, rIL-2-activated PBL, and TCGF-activated PBL defined by monoclonal antibody labeled with distinct fluorochromes. There was no difference in the percentage of $CD8^+CD11^-$ cells remaining unchanged by PBL cultivated with rIL-2 between

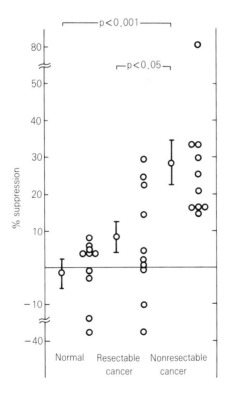

Fig 2 Suppressor cell function of TCGF-activated PBL from normal healthy controls and gastric cancer (resectable and nonresectable) patients. Percent suppression estimated by target:killer cells:suppressor cell source ratio, 1:10:40.

normal healthy controls and patients with resectable carcinoma. However, the rIL-2-activated PBL from patients with nonresectable carcinoma significantly decreased the percentage of $CD8^+CD11^-$ cells as compared with PBL (19.4 ± 1.9% vs 10.2 ± 2.5%, $p < 0.05$). The percentage of $CD8^+CD11^-$ cells was significantly increased by culture with TCGF in the 3 experimental groups. The percentage of $CD8^+$ cells coexpressing the $CD11^+$ antigen was dramatically decreased by culture with rIL-2 and TCGF. More significant was the increase in the percentage of $CD4^+Leu\ 8^-$ in rIL 2- and TCGF-activated PBL. The rIL-2- and TCGF-activated PBL from normal controls significantly decreased the percentage of $CD4^+Leu\ 8^+$ cells (31.1 ± 2.5% vs 13.9 ± 2.0% and 11.6 ± 2.3%, $p < 0.01$), but the percentage of $CD4^+Leu\ 8^+$ cells cultured with rIL-2 and TCGF from cancer patients remained unchanged compared with those of PBL. However, the percentage of $CD4^+Leu\ 8^+$ cells in rIL-2- and TCGF-activated PBL from gastric cancer patients was significantly increased compared with those from normal healthy controls (18.9 ± 1.3% and 23.9 ± 2.4% vs 13.9 ± 1.0%, $p < 0.05$; 25.0 ± 2.2% and 22.2 ± 3.8% vs 11.6 ± 2.3%, $p < 0.01$).

The percentage of $HLA\text{-}DR^+CD8^-$ cells in rIL-2-activated PBL was significantly increased in experimental groups as compared with those of PBL ($p < 0.001$), and the percentage of cells in TCGF-activated PBL remained unchanged in normal healthy controls and in patients with resectable carcinoma. The percentage of $HLA\text{-}DR^+CD8^-$ cells cultured with TCGF from patients with resectable carcinoma was significantly different from that of PBL from nonresectable carcinoma patients ($p < 0.01$). The percentage of $HLA\text{-}DR^+$ cells coexpressing cytotoxic/suppressor marker $CD8^+$ was markedly increased in TCGF-activated PBL from the 3 experimental groups compared with those of PBL and rIL-2-activated PBL ($p < 0.001$). Furthermore, TCGF-activated PBL from cancer patients significantly increased the percentage of $HLA\text{-}DR^+CD8^+$ cells compared with normal controls (41.1 ± 2.5% and 45.9 ± 2.6% vs 30.4 ± 3.9%, $p < 0.01$).

The percentage of $CD4^+HLA\text{-}DR^-$ cells in rIL-2-activated PBL remained unchanged compared with those of PBL, but the percentage of the cells in TCGF-activated PBL was significantly decreased compared with those of PBL. The percentage of $CD4^+HLA\text{-}DR^-$ cells in TCGF-activated PBL from patients with nonresectable carcinoma was significantly decreased compared with that of TCGF-activated PBL from normal controls ($p < 0.01$). The percentage of $CD4^+$ coexpressing $HLA\text{-}DR^+$ cells in rIL-2- and TCGF-activated PBL was significantly increased compared with that of PBL ($p < 0.001$). In addition, the percentage of $CD4^+HLA\text{-}DR^+$ in rIL-2- and TCGF-activated PBL from cancer patients was shown to increase compared with that of normal healthy controls ($p < 0.001$).

The percentage of $Leu\ 7^+CD16^-$ cells in the 3 experimental groups was increased by cultivation with rIL-2. However, the proportion of $Leu\ 7^+CD16^-$ cells in rIL-2-activated PBL was decreased according to the progression of tumor growth. The percentage of $Leu\ 7^+CD16^-$ cells in TCGF-activated PBL was significantly decreased compared with those of PBL ($p < 0.01$). Cell cultivation with rIL-2 or TCGF in each of the 3 groups did not change the percentage of $HLA\text{-}DR^+CD25^-$ cells. However, the percentages of $HLA\text{-}DR^+CD25^+$ cells in

Table 2 2-color flow cytometric analysis of PBL, rIL-2-activated PBL, and TCGF-activated PBL from normal healthy controls and gastric cancer (resectable and nonresectable) patients.

	Normal*			Cancer (resectable)*			Cancer (nonresectable)*		
	PBL	rIL-2	TCGF	PBL	rIL-2	TCGF	PBL	rIL-2	TCGF
CD8+CD11−	16.0 ± 0.9†	17.9 ± 2.5	58.6 ± 4.8	16.4 ± 1.6	15.5 ± 3.2	48.0 ± 6.5	19.4 ± 1.9	10.2 ± 2.5	51.6 ± 4.3
CD8+CD11+	6.8 ± 0.8	2.3 ± 0.5	1.2 ± 0.4	8.6 ± 1.1	1.5 ± 0.5	1.8 ± 0.7	7.0 ± 1.0	2.7 ± 1.5	1.7 ± 0.7
CD8−CD11+	12.3 ± 1.2	8.0 ± 1.9	0.1 ± 0.1	12.3 ± 1.2	6.3 ± 2.3	0.3 ± 0.2	12.9 ± 1.6	10.9 ± 2.5	0.4 ± 0.3
CD4+Leu8−	13.4 ± 2.2	51.4 ± 2.1	29.0 ± 3.0	17.8 ± 3.3	56.1 ± 3.8	25.1 ± 4.6	15.6 ± 3.8	46.0 ± 4.3	25.9 ± 5.1
CD4+Leu8+	31.1 ± 2.5	13.9 ± 1.0	11.6 ± 2.3	21.7 ± 3.5	18.9 ± 1.3	25.0 ± 2.2	25.7 ± 4.6	23.9 ± 2.4	22.2 ± 3.8
CD4−Leu8+	26.7 ± 2.0	2.0 ± 0.6	11.1 ± 2.9	15.4 ± 3.8	2.8 ± 0.9	13.8 ± 4.4	18.2 ± 4.1	3.4 ± 0.9	16.6 ± 3.1
HLA-DR+CD8−	21.2 ± 0.9	40.4 ± 5.4	20.3 ± 6.8	18.6 ± 1.1	33.1 ± 2.8	22.6 ± 2.0	20.2 ± 1.1	42.2 ± 3.9	14.4 ± 2.5
HLA-DR+CD8+	5.5 ± 0.8	8.2 ± 1.2	30.4 ± 3.9	5.9 ± 0.5	10.5 ± 2.4	41.1 ± 2.5	7.5 ± 1.9	9.7 ± 2.5	45.9 ± 2.6
HLA-DR−CD8+	15.3 ± 1.2	4.9 ± 1.3	19.7 ± 4.5	13.8 ± 1.0	5.1 ± 1.6	8.0 ± 2.0	13.6 ± 1.2	3.6 ± 0.6	11.1 ± 3.7
CD4+HLA-DR−	42.8 ± 1.9	48.2 ± 3.9	26.9 ± 3.4	45.5 ± 3.3	51.6 ± 4.0	20.7 ± 4.5	48.4 ± 2.7	39.5 ± 2.4	15.9 ± 3.8
CD4+HLA-DR+	3.2 ± 0.5	17.6 ± 1.6	13.7 ± 1.2	2.5 ± 0.4	21.4 ± 2.5	29.2 ± 4.9	3.5 ± 0.6	22.4 ± 2.3	26.5 ± 3.8
CD4−HLA-DR+	20.4 ± 2.4	11.5 ± 2.1	19.1 ± 2.3	16.1 ± 1.9	7.6 ± 1.9	24.9 ± 4.8	12.4 ± 0.9	16.2 ± 5.5	31.7 ± 3.5
Leu7+CD16−	7.7 ± 1.2	17.5 ± 2.3	2.3 ± 0.8	6.6 ± 1.2	11.5 ± 2.2	2.8 ± 0.8	7.1 ± 2.4	10.3 ± 2.3	3.5 ± 1.1
Leu7+CD16+	9.2 ± 1.8	1.5 ± 0.3	0.3 ± 0.1	8.8 ± 2.1	1.2 ± 0.3	0.6 ± 0.4	4.6 ± 3.0	2.1 ± 0.7	0.3 ± 0.1
Leu7−CD16+	3.7 ± 1.1	1.6 ± 0.6	0.3 ± 0.2	3.5 ± 0.5	1.7 ± 0.9	0.1 ± 0.1	2.5 ± 1.0	1.7 ± 0.7	0.5 ± 0.3
HLA-DR+CD25−	25.4 ± 1.3	26.0 ± 2.3	34.9 ± 4.8	24.9 ± 1.3	24.2 ± 3.9	29.2 ± 6.1	25.4 ± 1.7	18.7 ± 3.3	29.6 ± 4.8
HLA-DR+CD25+	1.0 ± 0.2	25.3 ± 3.8	18.0 ± 5.6	0.8 ± 0.1	21.9 ± 3.1	36.0 ± 7.1	0.7 ± 0.2	35.5 ± 4.9	39.0 ± 6.4
HLA-DR−CD25+	1.5 ± 0.3	5.7 ± 0.82	4.5 ± 1.5	0.9 ± 0.2	12.2 ± 2.4	5.6 ± 1.4	0.9 ± 0.2	14.6 ± 3.1	6.0 ± 2.1

*Each experimental group consisted of 10 patients.
†Each value represents mean percentage of positive cells ± SE.

rIL-2- and TCGF-activated PBL were significantly increased compared with those of PBL ($p < 0.001$ and $p < 0.01$, respectively). The most marked effect was the increased proportion of HLA-DR$^+$CD25$^+$ cells in rIL-2- and TCGF-activated PBL from patients with nonresectable carcinoma.

Figure 3A shows the overall survival rate curves of patients in the 2 treatment groups. Of the 98 patients in the chemotherapy group, 36 died, whereas 26 of 115 patients died in the immunochemotherapy group. The patients in the latter group lived significantly longer than those in the former group ($p < 0.05$). The effectiveness of immunochemotherapy in all patients was also analyzed by the histopathologic stages of carcinoma. The patient survival rate for each treatment group was compared for stage I plus II, and stage III plus IV. The survival rate in the 2 treatment groups was comparable for patients with stage I plus II (data not shown), because of an excellent 5-year survival rate of 95.4% at the time of the survival survey. Among the cases of histopathologic stage III plus IV, 34 of 53 patients died in the chemotherapy group and 26 of 61 patients died in the immunochemotherapy group (Fig 3B). A highly statistically significant prolongation of life span was observed with the combination treatment of tegafur and N-CWS (generalized Wilcoxon test, $P_0 = 0.0025$; log-rank test, $P_0 = 0.0019$, as shown in Fig 3B). Among all cases included for analysis, 5-year (1800 day) survival rates of 60.2% for the chemotherapy group and 73.2% for the immunochemotherapy group were noted. In stage III plus IV, 5-year (1800-day) survival rates of 28.8% for the former group and 52.4% for the latter group were observed. Consequently, 50% survival period in the chemotherapy group was only 722 days, whereas in the immunochemotherapy group, the 50% survival period was 1800 days or more, since it was better than 50% at the time of the survival survey (March 31, 1985).

Discussion

LAK cells were originally described by Grimm, Rosenberg, and their colleagues (12,13) as IL-2-activated effector cells that appeared to be clearly divergent from natural killer (NK) cells. NK-resistant and NK-susceptible target tumor cells were lysed by the LAK cells. We showed that LAK cells were generated by cultivation with rIL-2 in gastric cancer patients and the cells killed K562 and Daudi cells. In this study, we also analyzed the antigen expression of LAK effector cells by 2-color flow cytometry of lymphoid cell subpopulations after rIL-2 culture. The data indicated that CD4$^+$Leu 8$^-$, CD4$^+$HLA-DR$^+$, Leu 7$^+$CD16$^-$, and HLA-DR$^+$CD25$^+$ cell fractions were enriched in the LAK effector cells. Although phenotypic characterization of LAK cells has not been clarified, many investigators have reported that LAK cells have a marker, at least a CD8 or CD4 molecule (14–19). The LAK cells reported above expressed dominantly CD4$^+$Leu 8$^-$ but not CD8$^+$CD11$^-$ antigen. These results are in accordance with the data of Rayner et al (14), Fleischer et al (15), and Maggi et al (16).

LAK cell activity induced by rIL-2 decreased according to the progression of tumor growth (Table 1). However, the exogeneous addition of rIFN-γ could augment the lytic activity of LAK cells against both K562 and Daudi cells. The results suggested that LAK generation in PBL from cancer patients is mediated by rIL-2 in collaboration with IFN-γ produced in PBL cultures. The cell populations responsible for augmented LAK cell activity showed a phenotype of CD8$^+$ CD11$^-$ and Leu 7$^+$CD16$^-$ (data not shown). These results suggest that LAK cells might be heterogeneous with regard to phenotypic and functional characteristics.

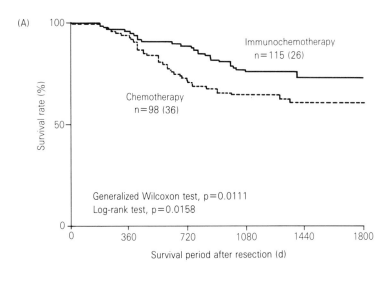

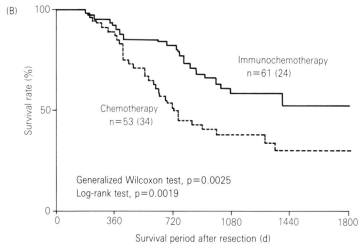

Fig 3 Survival rates of patients with surgical resection of gastrc carcinoma. A, All evaluable postoperative patients. B, Postoperative patients with stage III + IV gastric carcinoma. Numbers in parentheses are numbers of patients who died. Reprinted, with permission, from Koyama S, Ozaki A, Iwasaki Y, et al. (3).

The present study also showed the generation of $CD8^+CD11^-$ LAS cells in in vitro cultivation with TCGF from patients with gastric carcinoma. This suppression of cytotoxicity is exerted by directly blocking the activity of the LAK cells. This suppressive activity could not be accounted for by a minor crowding effect of the added TCGF-activated PBL or by the depletion of nutrients from culture medium by metabolizing TCGF-activated PBL, since TCGF-activated PBL from normal healthy controls did not significantly suppress the LAK cell activity (Fig 2). Our data presented here suggested that the potent suppressive effect of TCGF-activated PBL in patients with gastric carcinoma are due to suppressor cell properties of the cells themselves. The result is essentially in agreement with our previous work (7).

Our previous study showed that the functional human suppressor T cells that were expanded with TCGF revealed the characteristic phenotype of $CD8^+$ T cell-mediated suppression. The percentage of $CD8^+CD11^-$ cells believed to be killer T cells (20) was significantly increased by culture with TCGF in normal healthy controls and in patients with either resectable or nonresectable carcinoma, as compared with that of PBL ($16.9 \pm 0.9\%$ vs $58.6 \pm 4.8\%$; $16.4 \pm 1.6\%$ vs $48.0 \pm 6.5\%$; $19.4 \pm 1.9\%$ vs $51.6 \pm 4.3\%$, $p < 0.001$, respectively). The percentage of $CD8^+$ cells coexpressing the $CD11^+$ antigen, considered to be suppressor T cells (21,22), was dramatically decreased by culture with TCGF in the 3 experimental groups ($6.8 \pm 0.8\%$ vs $1.2 \pm 0.4\%$; $8.6 \pm 1.1\%$ vs $1.8 \pm 0.7\%$; $7.0 \pm 1.0\%$ vs $1.7 \pm 0.7\%$, $p < 0.01$, respectively). Thus TCGF resulted in preferential expansion of $CD8^+CD11^-$ cells and in unresponsiveness of $CD8^+CD11^+$ cells in both normal healthy controls and gastric cancer (resectable and nonresectable) patients. Taken together with functional and phenotypic analyses, the cell population responsible for LAS-effector T cells in our system is exclusively mediated by $CD8^+CD11^-$ cells but not by $CD8^+CD11^+$ cells. On the other hand, dominantly expressed $CD8^+CD11^-$ cells on TCGF-activated PBL from normal healthy controls did induce LAK-effector T cells. The functional diversity was therefore suggested to exist within the $CD8^+CD11^-$ cell population of TCGF-activated PBL.

TCGF-activated PBL in each group were shown to decrease the percentage of cells with the NK phenotype. The results suggested that neither LAS nor LAK cells activated with TCGF contained NK cells. It was shown that suppressor T cell growth was necessary for the facilitation of initial inducer T cell activation following antigenic stimulation (23). Indeed, TCGF-activated PBL from cancer patients showed a significantly increased proportion of suppressor-inducer T cell marker $CD4^+Leu 8^+$ as compared with those of cells in normal healthy controls (Table 2). Suppressor-inducer cells contained within the $CD4^+Leu 8^+$ subset might therefore be necessary for the proliferation of LAS cells contained within the $CD8^+CD11^-$ subset. The results described here agree with the conclusions reached by Bensussan et al (23).

The proportion of $HLA-DR^+CD8^+$ and $HLA-DR^+CD25^+$ cells in TCGF-activated PBL from cancer patients was increased compared with those of normal healthy controls (Table 2). This result suggests that the immune response to tumor cells (antigens) may be enhanced in cancer patients.

From the results described above, the apparent inability of TCGF-activated PBL from cancer patients to develop killer cell activity is not due to a total lack of immune response but rather to a dynamic process involving the activation of suppressor T cells and resulting in the suppression of antitumor immunity in cancer patients. Thus, in view of the suppression of the killer cell activity in cancer patients, functional recovery of the killer cell activity against tumor, by inactivation or elimination of circulating activated suppressor T cells, would be a prerequisite for a successful approach to the immunotherapy of cancer.

For these reasons, we selected for this study postoperative patients who had undergone gastrectomy for carcinoma. Patients with systemic metastasis of gastric carcinoma or for whom surgery was noncurative, as evaluated by macroscopic examination at operation, were not registered for this trial. We presented the results of a randomized, controlled study of tegafur with or without N-CWS in patients undergoing gastrectomy for gastric carcinoma. The overall survival rates for the immunochemotherapy group were significantly longer than those for the chemotherapy group ($p < 0.05$) (Fig 3A). According to the distribution stage of the disease, survival rates of patients with stage III + IV carcinoma in the immunochemotherapy group were statistically significantly better than those in the chemotherapy group ($p < 0.005$) (Fig 3B). In the analysis of survival rate based on the stage distribution of the disease, we combined patients with stage III and stage IV cancer. The number of stage III patients analyzed consisted of 39 in the chemotherapy group and 52 in the immunochemotherapy group. However, we had only a small number of eligible stage IV patients (14 in the chemotherapy group, and only 9 in the immunochemotherapy group), because we did not register patients with absolute noncurative operation, based on macroscopic examination. Thus, our patients with stage IV cancer closely corresponded to those with stage III, according to histopathologic evaluation. Therefore, we were able to investigate the combined survival rate of patients with stage III + IV carcinoma.

Background factors that may have influenced patient survival were analyzed, and it was noted that survival rates were not statistically influenced by bias from such background factors, as described previously in detail (3). No statistical differences were found in surgical curability, stage of distribution of cancer, or age and sex distribution between the chemotherapy and immunochemotherapy groups. Imanaga and Nakazato (24) reported that the 50% survival period for chemotherapy with mitomycin C in postoperative patients with stage III cancer was 2 years. In our study, the chemotherapy group with stage III + IV cancer consisted of 39 patients with stage III cancer, and 14 patients with stage IV cancer. It was shown that the survival rate of patients in our study was equivalent to that found by Imanaga and Nakazato (24), in spite of the inclusion of patients with advanced stage IV carcinoma. This clearly indicates that the significant effectiveness of N-CWS in the immunochemotherapy group presented here is not due to an inferior survival rate of patients in the chemotherapy group.

The mechanisms of cell-mediated antitumor activity of N-CWS have been described (25-27), and the accumulated experimental data have led to its clinical application in human cancer (2,3,6). Although the mode of action of N-CWS in human cancer systems is obscure, one of the authors showed increased proportions of CD4$^+$ and Leu 7$^+$ cells in postoperative gastric cancer patients treated 4 times with N-CWS (28). Thus, the administration of N-CWS may induce helper T cells and NK cells, which exert an antitumor effect against autochthonous tumors in patients. Indeed, we have demonstrated in this report that the CD4$^+$ Leu 8$^-$ cells generated by rIL-2 show lytic activity against tumor cells.

Acknowledgment

This study was supported in part by a grant-in-aid for Scientific Research (No. 62570307) from the Ministry of Education, Science and Culture, Japan.

References

1. Ochiai T, Sato H, Hayashi R, et al. Postoperative adjuvant immunotherapy of gastric cancer with BCG-cell wall skeleton. 3- to 6-year follow up of a randomized clinical trial. Cancer Immunol Immunother 1983;14:167–71.
2. Ochiai T, Sato H, Sato H, et al. Randomly controlled study of chemotherapy versus chemoimmunotherapy in postoperative gastric cancer patients. Cancer Res 1983;43:3001–7.
3. Koyama S, Ozaki A, Iwasaki Y, et al. Randomized controlled study of postoperative adjuvant immunochemotherapy with *Nocardia rubra* cell wall skeleton (N-CWS) and Tegafur for gastric carcinoma. Cancer Immunol Immunother 1986;22:148–54.
4. Azuma I, Taniyama T, Yamawaki M, et al. Adjuvant and antitumor activities of *Nocardia* cell-wall skeleton. Jpn J Cancer Res (Gann) 1976;67:733–6.
5. Azuma I, Yamawaki M, Yasumoto K, Yamamura Y. Antitumor activity of *Nocardia* cell wall skeleton preparations in transplantable tumors in syngeneic mice and patients with malignant pleurisy. Cancer Immunol Immunother 1978;4:95–100.
6. Yamamura Y, Ogura T, Sakatani M, et al. Randomized controlled study of adjuvant immunotherapy with *Nocardia rubra* cell wall skeleton for inoperable lung cancer. Cancer Res 1983;43:5575–9.
7. Koyama S, Fukao K, Fujimoto S. The generation of interleukin 2-dependent suppressor T-cells from patients with systemic metastasis of gastric carcinoma and the phenotypic characterization of the cells defined by monoclonal antibodies. Cancer 1985;56:2437–45.
8. Koyama S, Ebihara T, Fukao K, Osuga T. Two-color flow cytometric analyses of the peripheral blood lymphocytes (PBL) and lymphokine-activated PBL in gastric cancer patients. Jpn J Cancer Clin 1988;34:345–41. (In Japanese)
9. Koyama S, Fujimoto S, Tada T, Sakita T. Effect of Bacillus Calmette-Guérin cell wall skeleton on the induction of the cytotoxic and suppressor T cells against syngeneic tumor in the mouse. Int J Cancer 1981;27:819–35.
10. Koyama S, Yoshioka T, Sakita T. Suppression of cell-mediated antitumor immunity by complete Freund's adjuvant. Cancer Res 1982;42:3215–9.
11. Koyama S, Yoshioka T, Sakita T, Fujimoto S. Generation of T cell growth factor (TCGF)-dependent splenic lymphoid cell line with cell-mediated immunosuppressive reactivity against syngeneic murine tumor. Eur J Cancer Clin Oncol 1985;21:257–61.

12. Grimm EA, Mazumder A, Zhang HZ, Rosenberg SA. Lymphokine-activated killer cell phenomenon. Lysis of natural killer resistant fresh solid tumor cells by interleukin-2 activated autologous human peripheral blood lymphocytes. J Exp Med 1982;155:1823–41.

13. Rosenstein M, Yron I, Kaufmann Y. Rosenberg SA. Lymphokine-activated killer cells. Lysis fresh syngeneic NK–resistant murine tumor cells by lymphocytes cultured in IL 2. Cancer Res 1984;44:1946–53.

14. Rayner AA, Grimm EA, Lotze MT, et al. Lymphokine-activated killer (LAK) cell phenomenon. IV: Lysis by LAK cell clones of fresh human tumor cells from autologous and multiple allogeneic tumors. J Natl Cancer Inst 1985;75:67–75.

15. Fleischer B, Schrezenmeier H, Wangner H. Function of the CD4 and CD8 molecules on human cytotoxic T lymphocytes: regulation of T cell triggering. J Immunol 1986;136:1625–8.

16. Maggi E, Parronchi P, Prete GD, et al. Frequent T4-positive cells with cytolytic activity in spleens of patients with Hodgkin's disease (a clonal analysis). J Immunol 1986;136:1516–20.

17. Tilden AB, Itoh K, Balch CM. Human lymphokine-activated killer (LAK)cells: identificantion of two types of effector cells. J Immunol 1986;138:1068–73.

18. Hersey P, Bolhuis R. 'Nonspecific' MHC-unrestricted killer cells and their receptors. Immunol Today 1987;8:233–9.

19. Lanier LL, Phillips JH. Evidence for three types of human cytotoxic lymphocyte. Immunol Today 1986;7:132–4.

20. Clement LT, Dagg MK, Landy A. Characterization of human lymphocytes subpopulations: Alloreactive cytotoxic T-lymphocyte precursor and effector cells are phonotypically distinct from Leu 2$^+$ suppressor cells. J Clin Immunol 1984;4:394–402.

21. Landy A, Gartland GL, Clement LT. Characterization of a phenotypically distinct subpopulation of Leu 2$^+$ cells that suppresses T cell proliferative responses. J Immunol 1983;131:2757–61.

22. Clement LT, Grossi CE, Gartland GE. Morphologic and phenotypic feature of subpopulation of Leu 2$^+$ cells that suppresses B cell differentiation. J Immunol 1984;133:2461–8.

23. Bensussan A, Acuto O, Hassey RE, et al. T3-Ti receptor triggering of T8$^+$ suppressor T cells leads to unresponsiveness to interleukin 2. Nature 1984;311:565–7.

24. Imanaga H, Nakazato H. Results of surgery for gastric cancer and effect of adjuvant mitomycin C on cancer recurrence. World J Surg 1977;1:213–21.

25. Ito M, Iizuka H, Masuno T, et al. Killing of tumor cells in vitro by macrophages from mice given injections of squalene-treated cell wall skeleton of *Nocardia rubra*. Cancer Res 1981;41:2925–30.

26. Kawase I, Uemiya M, Yoshimoto T, et al. Effect of *Nocardia rubra* cell wall skeleton on T-cell mediated cytotoxicity in mice bearing syngeneic sarcoma. Cancer Res 1981;41:660–6.

27. Haraguchi S, Kurakata S, Matsuo T, Yoshida TO. Strain differences in the antitumor activity of an immunopotentiator, *Nocardia rubra* cell-wall skeleton, in B10 congenic and recombinant mice. Jpn J Cancer Res (Gann) 1985;76:400–13.

28. Koyama S, Fukao K, Sakita T. Cellular mechanisms of adjuvant effect of immunotherapy with *Nocardia rubra*-CWS on postoperative gastric cancer patients. Proc Jpn Cancer Assoc 1984;43:167. (In Japanese)

Randomized controlled study of chemoimmunotherapy for acute myelogenous leukemia with *Nocardia rubra* cell wall skeleton and irradiated allogeneic leukemic cells

Hiroyuki Nakamura,[1] Ryuzo Ohno,[2] Kazumasa Yamada,[2]* Nobuya Ogawa,[3] Tohru Masaoka[1]

[1]*Fifth Department of Internal Medicine, Center for Adult Diseases, Osaka,* [2]*First Department of Internal Medicine, Nagoya University School of Medicine, Nagoya, and* [3]*Department of Pharmacology, Ehime University School of Medicine, Ehime, Japan*

Introduction

Since acute myelogenous leukemia (AML) in complete remission is a minimal residual disease with a greatly reduced tumor burden, it is a suitable condition for testing potentially successful immunotherapy. As a result of several different immunotherapeutic trials, many groups have tried immunotherapy with BCG or its derivatives, and promising results have been reported (1–6). The effect of immunotherapy in AML has been controversial, however, since the most positive results have been obtained in uncontrolled, nonrandomized trials (7). *Nocardia rubra* cell wall skeleton (N-CWS) is a constituent of the cell wall subfractionated from *N. rubra*, which is taxonomically related to BCG. The antitumor activity induced by N-CWS has been shown to be more potent than the activity induced by BCG-CWS in many experimental systems (8). We have therefore conducted a randomized, controlled study of immunotherapy in adult AML to determine whether immunotherapy with N-CWS and irradiated allogeneic AML cells would prolong the duration of remission and the survival of patients with AML. This was a cooperative study at 2 institutions. Interim analyses of results at 6 and 66 months after entry into the trial have already appeared (9,10). We report here the follow-up results of this study, 9 years and 4 months after its start.

---

*Present address: Department of Internal Medicine, Nagoya University Branch Hospital, Nagoya, Japan.

Patients and methods

Seventy-three previously untreated patients with AML (FAB criteria: M1, M2, M4, and M5), aged 15 or older, and who had achieved their 1st complete remission at The Center for Adult Diseases, Osaka, or at Nagoya University Hospital, entered this study between December 1978 and December 1981. They were induced into complete remission either by DCMP 2-step therapy (11) or by BHAC-DMP therapy (12).

DCMP 2-step therapy consisted of: 10–14-day courses of cytarabine 80 mg/m² per day, 2-h intravenous infusion; 6-mercaptopurine 70 mg/m² per day orally; prednisolone 20 mg/m² per day, orally; and daunorubicin 25 mg/m² per day, intravenously, which was given on the 1st and the 2nd day, and every 2 to 4 days if required. The dose of cytarabine and the frequency of daunorubicin injection were adjusted so as to attain cell counts of less than 1500/mm³ for white cells and less than 15 000/mm³ for nucleated cells in bone marrow at the end of the 10–14-day treatment period. If leukemic cells remained in the bone marrow 3 to 7 days after the discontinuation of this 1st step of the therapy, the 2nd step of the therapy was administered, with relatively lower doses of cytarabine (40 mg/m² per day), 6-mercaptopurine (40 mg/m² per day), and prednisolone (20 mg/m² per day) for 3 to 7 days.

In BHAC-DMP therapy, the treatment schedule was almost the same as for DCMP 2-step therapy except that cytarabine was replaced by behenoylcytarabine (170 mg/m² per day, 2-h intravenous infusion), and the 2nd step was not included in the protocol.

After having achieved complete remission, the patients received 3 additional courses of consolidation therapy with the same drug combination (Fig 1). Cytarabine 80 mg/m² per day or behenoylcytarabine 170 mg/m² per day, 6-mercaptopurine 70 mg/m² per day, and prednisolone 20 mg/m² per day were given for 7 days, and daunorubicin 25 mg/m² per day was given on the 1st and last days.

After completion of consolidation therapy, the patients were divided into groups according to their types of leukemia (M1, M2, M4, or M5) and and then by age (15–49 years old, or 50 or older) and were randomized into either a maintenance chemotherapy-alone group or a maintenance chemotherapy plus immunotherapy group, by a block-randomization method assigned for each hospital (Fig 1). Maintenance chemotherapy consisted of 2 regimens given alternately every 5 weeks for a period of 2 years. One regimen was a 5-day course of the same DCMP (or BHAC-DMP) combination therapy as that used in the consolidation therapy. The other regimen consisted of vincristine 1.5 mg/m² per week for 2 weeks, cyclophosphamide 600 mg/m² per week for 2 weeks, 6-mercaptopurine 70 mg/m² per day for 2 weeks, and prednisolone 20 mg/m² per day for 2 weeks. Immunotherapy consisted of 400 μg of N-CWS, a squalene-treated freeze-dried form prepared by Fujisawa Pharmaceutical Co., Ltd. (Osaka, Japan), and 1×10^7 irradiated (1000 rad) allogeneic AML cells, given intradermally or subcutaneously, at 4 sites at the upper arms and thighs once a week, except when maintenance therapy was being given. Allogeneic AML cells had been ob-

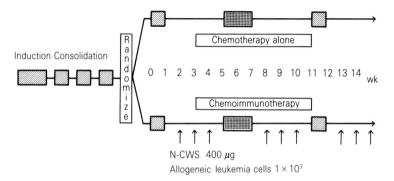

Fig 1 Study design. ▨ Behenoyl ara-C + daunorubicin + 6-mercaptopurine + pred-nisolone; ▦ vincristine + cyclophosphamide + 6-mercaptopurine + prednisolone. Reprinted, with permission, from Ohno R, Nakamura H, Kodera Y, et al (10).

tained from peripheral blood or bone marrow of patients with AML at diagnosis. The cells were separated with Ficoll-Hypaque (Sigma) density-gra-dient centrifugation, frozen in a programmed freezer, stored in liquid nitrogen, and thawed before use. The dose of N-CWS was decreased if the local skin reac-tions were intense. The patients in both groups were followed at outpatient clinics at 1–2-week intervals until termination of maintenance chemotherapy (2 years later) and at 2–4-week intervals until relapse. Immunotherapy was con-tinued as long as the patients were in remission, but only N-CWS was given after the maintenance chemotherapy was discontinued. The regimens for reinduction and maintenance therapy after relapse were not specified.

This study was controlled by a statistician (N. Ogawa), who had no affiliation to either hospital in which the study was carried out. The protocol defined that patients should be regarded as having dropped out if they relapsed within 1 month after the randomization, if they did not receive the consolidation and maintenance therapies defined by the protocol, or if patients in the chemoim-munotherapy group received less than 4 doses of immunotherapy. Actuarial remission duration and survival were calculated according to the Kaplan-Meier method. The generalized Wilcoxon test was used to compare duration of remis-sion and survival. Treatment cohorts were compared by the χ^2 test with Yates' correction. Remission duration was calculated from the date of complete remis-sion to relapse. Survival was computed from the date of diagnosis to death, since remission induction therapy was started within 1 week of diagnosis in all cases.

Results

From December 1978 to December 1981, a total of 73 adult patients with AML (M1, M2, M4, and M5) who had achieved complete remission were entered into the study (Table 1). Thirty-eight patients were randomized to the chemoim-

Table 1 Patient characteristics. Reprinted, with permission, from Ohno R, Nakamura H, Kodera Y, et al (10).

Characteristics*	Chemoimmunotherapy	Chemotherapy	Total
No. of patients			
Entered	38	35	73
Excluded	1	0	1
Dropped out	5	1	6
Evaluable patients	32	34	66
Age (y)			
15–49	25	24	49
50–63	7	10	17
Sex			
M:F	17:15	15:19	32:34
Type of leukemia			
Acute myeloblastic[†]	26	27	53
Acute myelomonocytic[‡] or			
monoblastic[§]	6	7	13
Remission induction therapy			
DCMP 2-step	7	14	21
BHAC-DMP	25	20	45

*There were no significant differences between each cohort by χ^2 test. FAB criteria: [†]M1, M2, [‡]M4, or [§]M5.

munotherapy group and 35 to the chemotherapy-alone group. One patient in the chemoimmunotherapy group was excluded from the evaluation because he was in his 2nd complete remission when registered. One patient from each group was regarded as having dropped out of the trial because each relapsed within 1 month after randomization. Three patients in the chemoimmunotherapy group were also regarded as having dropped out because they received no injection of N-CWS and allogeneic AML cells (2 cases) and only 1 injection (1 case), because of severe hepatitis. One patient in the chemoimmunotherapy group was also regarded as having dropped out because he received no consolidation therapy. Therefore, 32 patients (17 M, 15 F, median age 36.5) in the chemoimmunotherapy group and 34 patients (15 M, 19 F, median age 39.5) in the chemotherapy-alone group were evaluated. There were 26 acute myeloblastic leukemia (M1, M2) and 6 acute monocytic leukemia (M4, M5) in the chemoimmunotherapy group and 27 acute myeloblastic leukemia and 7 acute monocytic leukemia in the chemotherapy-alone group. Peroxidase staining of leukemic cells was positive in all cases. As remission induction therapy, 7 received DCMP 2-step and 25 BHAC-DMP in the chemoimmunotherapy group, and 14 DCMP 2-step and 20 BHAC-DMP in the chemotherapy-alone group. The interval from the date of complete remission to the date of randomization was 53 ± 55 days (mean ± SD) in the chemoimmunotherapy group and 43 ± 37 in the chemotherapy-alone group. There was no statistically significant difference between the above cohorts of both groups when compared by the χ^2 test. The reason why fewer patients received DCMP 2-step therapy in the chemoim-munotherapy group was that 4 of 11 patients in this cohort dropped out.

Remission and survival curves were compared by the generalized Wilcoxon test at 6, 66, and 112 months after patients' entry into the study. The interim analysis at 6 months after entry revealed a borderline beneficial effect of immunotherapy, as seen in remission duration (p=0.080) and survival time (p=0.098) (9). When the data were analyzed at 66 months after entry, immunotherapy showed a borderline beneficial effect in remission duration (p=0.080), but not in survival time (p=0.314) (10). At 112 months after entry, there was a borderline significant difference in remission duration (p=0.069) between the 2 groups (Fig 2), prolonging the 50% remission period by 120 days (440 versus 320 days), but no significant difference in survival time (p=0.238), although the 50% survival was 168 days longer in the chemoimmunotherapy group (757 versus 589 days) (Fig 3). At the time of writing, 8 patients (12.1%) are still alive, and 7 of those (10.6%) are alive without any relapse. Of these 7 relapse-free survivors, 5 were in the chemoimmunotherapy group.

Toxicity of N-CWS was acceptable. With longer use of N-CWS, no serious side effects were observed beyond those reported previously (10) (Table 2). About half the patients experienced some kind of side effect; fever was the most frequent, and local skin reactions, malaise after injection, and skin eruptions were also observed in some patients.

Discussion

Since a beneficial effect of immunotherapy with BCG was first reported for

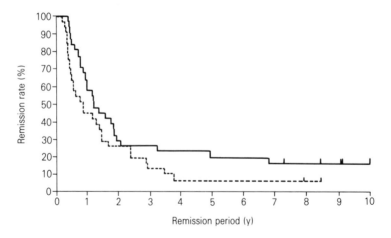

Fig 2 Remission duration analyzed at 9 years and 4 months after patient entry into study. Chemoimmunotherapy (– – – –), chemotherapy alone (———); p = 0.069.

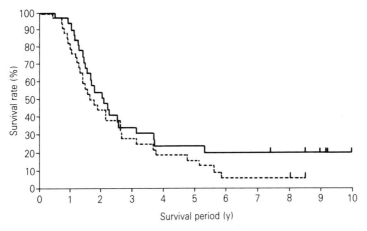

Fig 3 Survival length analyzed at 9 years and 4 months after patient entry into study. Chemoimmunotherapy (----), chemotherapy alone (——); p = 0.238.

Table 2 Side effects of immunotherapy with N-CWS and irradiated allogeneic AML cells. Reprinted, with permission, from Ohno R, Nakamura H, Kodera Y, et al (10).

Side effect*	No. of patients (%)	
Fever (°C)	14	(38.9)
37.0–37.9	5	(13.9)
38.0–38.9	5	(13.9)
39.0–39.9	3	(8.3)
≥ 40	1	(2.8)
Local skin reaction	10	(27.8)
Swelling	6	(16.7)
Abscess	2	(5.6)
Ulcer	2	(5.6)
Pain at injection site	2	(5.6)
Malaise	3	(8.3)
Eruption	2	(5.6)
Joint pain	1	(2.8)

*Side effects of the immunotherapy were analyzed 66 months after entry into the study (10).

childhood acute lymphoblastic leukemia by Mathé et al (1), several groups have described the therapeutic value of immunotherapy in the treatment of AML using BCG alone or in combination with irradiated leukemic cells (2–6). However, there has been considerable controversy about the effect of immunotherapy in AML, because most of the positive effects of earlier studies were not obtained in randomized controlled studies (7).

N-CWS is a component of the cell wall purified from *N. rubra*, which is taxonomically related to BCG. N-CWS was developed in Japan by Yamamura and Azuma, and its chemical structure, adjuvant activity, and antitumor activity have been extensively investigated in tumor-bearing animals (13–17). Yamamura et al reported a significantly prolonged survival after immunotherapy with N-CWS in patients with small cell carcinoma of the lung at stages III and IV and in patients with pleural effusion (18). Yasumoto et al also reported significantly prolonged remission for patients with operable lung cancer and prolonged survival in the curative operation group after immunotherapy with N-CWS (19). Significantly prolonged survival was reported by Ochiai et al for patients with noncuratively resected gastric cancer after immunotherapy with N-CWS (20), and the effectiveness of N-CWS as an adjuvant immunotherapeutic agent was also observed by Koyama et al in postoperative gastric cancer patients (21).

Our protocol in this clinical investigation was designed to be a cooperative, randomized, and controlled study, directed by an independent controller. The interim analysis, 6 months after patient entry into the study, indicated that immunotherapy with N-CWS and irradiated allogeneic AML cells improved the remission duration and the survival duration of adult AML, with a borderline significance (9). The analyses at 66 months (10) and 112 months after entry, however, showed borderline beneficial effects of the immunotherapy only in remission duration and not in survival time. Nevertheless, immunotherapy prolonged the 50% survival by 168 days (757 versus 589 days). There are currently 5 disease-free long-term survivors in the chemoimmunotherapy group, and 2 in the chemotherapy group. The side effects of N-CWS, such as fever and ulcer at injection sites, have been acceptable; even with longer use of N-CWS, they have been temporary and not serious.

References

1. Mathé G, Amiel JL, Schwarzenberg L, et al. Active immunotherapy for acute lymphoblastic leukemia. Lancet 1969;i:697–9.
2. Powles RL, Crowther D, Bateman CJT, et al. Immunotherapy for acute myelogenous leukemia. Br J Cancer 1973;28:365–76.
3. Gutterman JU, Hersh EM, Rodriguez V, et al. Chemoimmunotherapy of adult acute leukemia: prolongation of remission in myeloblastic leukemia with BCG. Lancet 1974;ii:1405–9.
4. Vogler WR, Chan YK. Prolonging remission in myeloblastic leukemia by Tice-strain bacillus Calmette-Guérin. Lancet 1974;ii:128–31.
5. Hamilton-Fairly G. Immunotherapy in the management of myelogenous leukemia. Arch Intern Med 1976;136:1406–8.
6. Ohno R, Ueda R, Imai K, et al. A clinical trial of cell wall skeleton of BCG in chemoimmunotherapy of acute leukemia. Jpn J Cancer Res (Gann) 1978;69:179–86.
7. Terry WD, Windhorst D, eds. Immunotherapy of cancer: present status of trials in man. New York: Raven Press;1978.
8. Yamamura Y, Yasumoto K, Ogura T, Azuma I. *Nocardia rubra*-cell wall skeleton in the therapy of animal and human cancer. In: EM Hersh, ed. Augmenting agents in

cancer therapy. New York: Raven Press;1981:71–90.

9. Nakamura H, Masaoka T, Ohno R, et al. A randomized controlled study of immunotherapy for acute myelogenous leukemia with *Nocardia rubra* cell-wall skeleton and irradiated allogeneic leukemia cells. Acta Haematol Jpn 1983;46:1087–92. (In Japanese)

10. Ohno R, Nakamura H, Kodera Y, et al. Randomized controlled study of chemoimmunotherapy of acute myelogenous leukemia (AML) in adults with *Nocardia rubra* cell-wall skeleton and irradiated allogeneic AML cells. Cancer 1986;57:1483–8.

11. Uzuka Y, Lion SK, Yamagata S. Treatment of acute leukemia using intermittent combination chemotherapy with daunomycin, cytosine arabinoside, 6-mercaptopurine and prednisolone: DCMP two-step therapy. Tohoku J Exp Med 1979; 118 (suppl):212–25.

12. Kato Y, Kawashima K, Ohno R, Yamada K. Treatment of adult nonlymphocytic leukemia with BHAC-DMP therapy. Acta Haematol Jpn 1983;46:1077–86. (In Japanese)

13. Azuma I, Taniyama T, Yamawaki M, et al. Adjuvant and antitumor activities of *Nocardia* cell-wall skeleton. Jpn J Cancer Res (Gann) 1976;67:733–6.

14. Azuma I, Yamawaki M, Yasumoto K, Yamamura Y. Antitumor activity of *Nocardia* cell wall skeleton preparations in transplantable tumors in syngeneic mice and patients with malignant pleurisy. Cancer Immunol Immunother 1978;4:95–100.

15. Ogura T, Namba M, Hirao F, et al. Association of macrophage activation with antitumor effect on rat syngeneic fibrosarcoma by *Nocardia rubra* cell wall skeleton. Cancer Res 1979;39:4706–12.

16. Ito M, Iizuka H, Masuno T, et al. Killing of tumor cells in vitro by macrophages from mice given injections of squalene-treated cell wall skeleton of *Nocardia rubra*. Cancer Res 1981;41:2925–30.

17. Kawase I, Uemiya M, Yoshimoto T, et al. Effect of *Nocardia rubra* cell wall skeleton on T-cell mediated cytotoxicity in mice bearing syngeneic sarcoma. Cancer Res 1981;41:660–6.

18. Yamamura Y, Ogura T, Sakatani M, et al. Randomized controlled study of adjuvant immunotherapy with *Nocardia rubra* cell wall skeleton for inoperable lung cancer. Cancer Res 1983;43:5575–9.

19. Yasumoto K, Yaita H, Ohta M, et al. Randomly controlled study of chemotherapy versus chemoimmunotherapy in postoperative lung cancer patients. Cancer Res 1985;45:1413–7.

20. Ochiai T, Sato H, Sato H, et al. Randomly controlled study of chemotherapy versus chemoimmunotherapy in postoperative gastric cancer patients. Cancer Res 1983;43:3001–7.

21. Koyama S, Ozaki A, Iwasaki Y, et al. Randomized controlled study of postoperative adjuvant immunochemotherapy with *Nocardia rubra* cell wall skeleton (N-CWS) and tegafur for gastric cancer. Cancer Immunol Immmunother 1986;22:148–54.

Clinical application of *Nocardia rubra* cell wall skeleton for acute nonlymphatic leukemia

Susumu Kishimoto,[1] Kazuo Yunoki,[2] Tsuyoshi Yamaguchi,[3] Michito Ichimaru,[3] Fumio Kawano,[4] Kiyoshi Takatsuki,[4] Kouichi Araki,[5] Yasumasa Suetomo,[6] Michihiro Takada,[6] Makoto Matsumoto,[7] Kouichiro Nishioka,[8] Shuji Hashimoto,[8] Nobuya Ogawa[9]

[1]*Third Department of Internal Medicine, Osaka University School of Medicine, Osaka,* [2]*Tarumizu City Medical Center, Tarumizu Central Hospital, Tarumizu,* [3]*Department of Hematology, Atomic Disease Institute, Nagasaki University School of Medicine, Nagasaki,* [4]*Second Department of Internal Medicine, Kumamoto University School of Medicine, Kumamoto,* [5]*Second Department of Internal Medicine, Ryukyu University School of Medicine, Okinawa,* [6]*Oita Memorial Hospital, Oita,* [7]*Institute of Cancer Research, Kagoshima University School of Medicine, Kagoshima,* [8]*Second Department of Internal Medicine, Kagoshima University School of Medicine, Kagoshima,* [9]*Department of Pharmacology, Ehime University School of Medicine, Ehime, Japan*

Introduction

The effectiveness of BCG in the treatment of acute lymphoblastic leukemia was first reported by Mathé et al (1). Azuma et al (2) later prepared BCG cell wall skeleton (BCG-CWS), composed of a mycolic acid-arabinogalactan-mucopeptide complex, as an active component of BCG. They also showed that BCG-CWS was less toxic than living BCG and that it was effective in prolonging the survival period of patients with leukemia and other malignant diseases. The clinical effectiveness of BCG-CWS has also been shown by Kishimoto et al (3) and Yamada et al (4), but these positive results were based mainly on comparative studies with historical controls. Azuma et al (5) reported that the cell wall skeleton of *Nocardia rubra* (N-CWS) could be advantageously used in place of BCG-CWS, and that it was more useful than BCG-CWS for the immunotherapy of human cancer.

Previous clinical studies have indicated that the clinical evaluation of immunotherapy should be conducted by a well-designed, randomized, controlled study in which the survival or the remission period is compared without reference to historical controls. In this study, therefore, the adjuvant activity of N-CWS on the maintenance chemotherapy of acute nonlymphatic leukemia (ANLL) was evaluated by a strictly randomized clinical trial in patients who had achieved complete remission after repeated courses of induction chemotherapy.

Patients and methods

Forty-one patients with ANLL who had achieved complete remission entered this trial between January 1979 and December 1981. The age of patients studied was limited to between 14 and 60 years. Cases associated with severe liver function disorders or severe infectious diseases at the point of complete remission were excluded from this trial. All patients were induced into complete remission mainly by either DCMP or DCVP therapy. DCMP therapy usually consisted of combined use of daunorubicin (25 mg/m^2 per day, iv on day 1), cytarabine (20 mg/m^2 per day iv on days 1 to 4), 6-mercaptopurine (80 mg/m^2 per day po on days 1 to 6), and prednisolone (60 mg/m^2 per day po on days 1 to 4). DCVP therapy consisted of daunorubicin (25 mg/m^2 per day iv on day 1), cyclophosphamide (300 mg/m^2 per day po on days 1 to 5), vincristine (1.5 mg/m^2 per day iv on day 1), and prednisolone (80 mg/m^2 per day po on days 1 to 5). After achieving complete remission, the patients received several additional courses of consolidation therapy with the same drug combination.

After completion of the consolidation therapy, the patients were randomized into either a maintenance chemotherapy only group or a maintenance chemotherapy plus immunotherapy group by a block-randomization method. Maintenance chemotherapy consisted of the same regimen as consolidation chemotherapy. The clinical effect was evaluated at the end of June 1982, and the cases surviving at that point were reevaluated in January 1984.

In the immunochemotherapy group, 200 to 300 μg of N-CWS was injected intradermally, the dose being divided into 4 sites at the upper arms and thighs, every 2 weeks for the first 5 times and then subsequently every 4 weeks. The dose of N-CWS was decreased discretionally if the local skin reactions caused by the injection were intense. In the patients showing a relapse, the immunotherapy was resumed after complete remission was reinduced by chemotherapy (Fig 1).

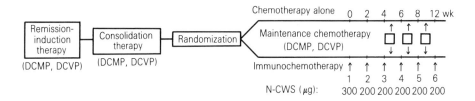

Fig 1　Protocol for randomization trial. For abbreviations, see text.

The investigators and the controller discussed whether each case was suitable for statistical analysis. The patients were regarded as having dropped out if they died within 60 days of registering, or if patients in the immounochemotherapy group received less than 5 days of immunotherapy.

The survival period after a defined diagnosis had been made and the 1st remission duration were calculated according to the Kaplan-Meier product-limit method. The generalized Wilcoxon test was used for comparing the durations of remission and survival. Treatment cohorts were compared by the χ^2 test; Yates' correction and Fisher's exact probability method were also used.

Results

Six of a total of 41 patients with ANLL (acute myelogenous leukemia [AML], acute monocytic leukemia [AMoL], and acute promyelocytic leukemia [APL]) who achieved complete remission were excluded from this study as unsuitable for statistical analysis. Seventeen were randomly assigned to the immunochemotherapy group (group N) and 18 to the chemotherapy alone group (group C). Group N consisted of 12 patients with AML, 2 with AMoL, and 3 with APL. Group C consisted of 14 patients with AML, 1 with AMoL, and 3 with APL. No statistical difference was found between the 2 groups in such background factors as disease constitution of ANLL, age, sex, and so on. There were 8 male and 9 female patients in group N, and 8 male and 10 female patients in group C, with a median age of 34.3 and 35.7 years, respectively. The numbers of treatments with N-CWS were 5 to 30 (median 14.2) and the total doses of N-CWS were 1100 to 8500 μg (median 3324 $\pm$ 2062 μg).

At the final evaluation period in this study (the 1st observation was at the end of June 1982), 6 patients in group N survived, and 4 of those were in the 1st period of remission. At the same time, 5 patients in group C survived, and 3 were in the 1st period of remission. At the 2nd observation (January 10, 1984), there were 4 surviving patients in group N and 3 in group C.

Figure 2 shows survival curves for all patients with ANLL, including AML, AMoL, and APL. These curves were calculated according to the Kaplan-Meier product-limit method. The 50% survival period was 811 days in group N and 416 days in group C, a significant difference (generalized Wilcoxon test, p < 0.05).

Notwithstanding the poor prognosis for APL, the survival period for APL is usually long after the induction of complete remission. If we therefore excluded the APL cases, the survival curve of 14 patients in group N could be compared with that of 15 patients in group C. As shown in Fig 3, the 50% survival period was 904 days for group N and 427 days for group C, a barely statistically significant difference (p < 0.1).

Next, we investigated the initial remission length. The remission duration curves of all ANLL patients, and of ANLL patients excluding those with APL, are shown in Figs 4 and 5, respectively. The 50% remission duration was 349 days for group N and 202 days for group C, a difference that was not statistically significant. The 50% remission duration for ANLL patients excluding those with

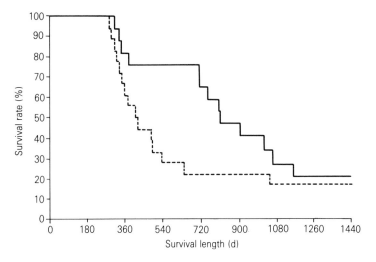

Fig 2 Survival curves of patients with ANLL (AML, AMoL, APL). The 50% survival period was 811 days in the immunochemotherapy group (—— group N), of 17 patients and 416 days in the chemotherapy alone group (---- group C) of 18 patients. $p < 0.05$ ($Z_0 = 1.988$).

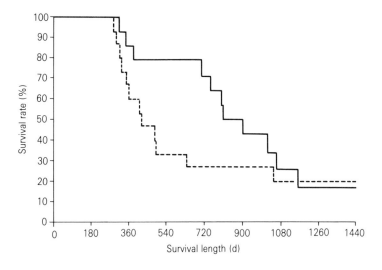

Fig 3 Survival curves of ANLL patients (excluding APL). The 50% survival period was 904 days in group N (—— 14 patients) and 427 days in group C (---- 15 patients). $p < 0.10$ ($Z_0 = 1.651$).

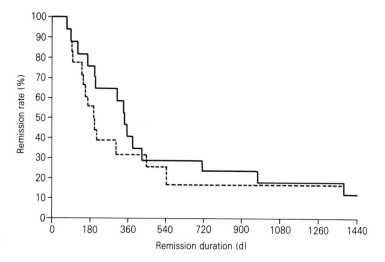

Fig 4 Remission duration curves for patients with ANLL (AML, AMoL, APL). The 50% remission duration was 349 days in group N (—— 17 patients) and 202 days in group C (---- 18 patients). NS ($Z_0 = 1.089$).

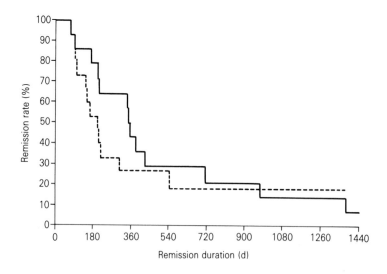

Fig 5 Remission duration curves for patients with ANLL (excluding APL). The 50% remission duration was 349 days in group N (—— 14 patients) and 202 days in group C (---- 15 patients). NS ($Z_0 = 1.250$).

APL was also not significantly different between the 2 groups (Figs 4 and 5).

In patients showing a relapse the reinduction of complete remission was investigated. In group N, 7 of 13 relapsed cases were reinduced into complete remission in less time than required for the initial induction of remission. On the other hand, in group C, only 2 of 14 relapsed cases were reinduced into complete remission. The difference in reinduction of complete remission between the 2 groups was significant (Fisher's exact probability method, $p < 0.05$).

Of 21 patients who received N-CWS, side effects were observed in 12 (57.1%): fever over 38°C several hours after the injection of N-CWS was noted in 3 cases (14.3%); local skin reactions were noted in 11 patients (52.4%), including local skin redness in 1 (4.8%), swelling in 3 (14.3%), induration in 3 (14.3%), abscess in 2 (9.5%), and ulceration in 2 (9.5%).

The patients surving at the end of June 1982 were reevaluated on January 10, 1984. Four of 6 patients in group N were still alive at this point. One AML and 1 APL patient were still in the initial period of remission, which was 4 to 5 years. Three of 5 patients in group C were still alive at this point. Two patients with AML were also in the initial period of remission, which was 3 to 4 years.

Discussion

In the chemotherapy of ANLL the intensive use of multidrug combinations has increased the complete remission rates (6,7). The increase in the remission rate, however, has only slightly improved the remission duration or the survival period for the patients.

Since active immunotherapy with BCG for acute leukemia was reported to be effective by Mathé et al (1), many investigators (8,9) have reported the usefulness of BCG for prolonging remission in AML. Azuma et al (2) prepared BCG-CWS as an active component of BCG and then reported that N-CWS could be used advantageously in place of BCG-CWS (5).

In this study, the effectiveness of N-CWS for ANLL was investigated in a cooperative, randomized, controlled study. After complete remission had been induced by chemotherapy and additional consolidation therapy, immunotherapy was given every 2 weeks for the first 5 doses and then every 4 weeks thereafter. Of the 41 patients with ANLL who entered this trial, 6 were excluded. The patients who entered the study were therefore 17 in group N and 18 in group C.

Statistical analysis 7 months after the closure of the study indicated that immunochemotherapy significantly improved the survival length of the patients with ANLL (including those with APL). There was a significant difference between the 2 groups in 50% survival period ($p < 0.05$). When APL cases were excluded from this study, however, little difference was observed between the 2 groups ($p < 0.1$).

The study on the initial remission duration showed no difference between group N and group C, whether the analysis was done for all cases of ANLL or for ANLL excluding APL. In relapsed cases, however, reinduction of complete remission seemed to be more easily achieved in group N than in group C (p < 0.05). Whittaker et al (9) also reported that immunotherapy with BCG contributed to the reinduction of complete remission in relapsed AML.

Nakamura et al (10) and Ohno et al (11) studied the effect of immunotherapy with N-CWS on the remission duration and survival period for adults with AML in a prospective, randomized, controlled study. During the 3-year period from December 1978 to December 1981, a total of 73 patients who had achieved complete remission entered the study. They reported that immunotherapy showed a borderline beneficial effect on remission duration and on survival period 6 months after study entry. When the data were analyzed 30 months after entry, however, there was a borderline significant difference in the remission duration but no significant difference in the survival duration. In our study, immunotherapy significantly increased survival duration but had no significant effect on remission duration. The significant prolongation of survival seemed to be mainly due to the increase of reinduction rate in group N.

Acknowledgment

The results of this study have already been published in Japan (12).

References

1. Mathé G, Amiel JL, Achwarzenberg L, et al. Active immunotherapy for acute lymphoblastic leukaemia. Lancet 1969;i:697-9.
2. Azuma I, Kishimoto S, Yamamura Y, Petit JF. Adjuvanticity of mycobacterial cell walls. Jpn J Microbiol 1971;15:193-7.
3. Kishimoto S, Araki K, Saito T. Immunotherapy with BCG or its derivatives in acute myelogenous leukemia. In: Yamamura Y, Kitagawa K, Azuma I, eds. Cancer immunotherapy and its immunological bases. Gann Monogr Cancer Res 1978;21:189-98.
4. Yamada K, Kawashima K, Morishima Y, et al. Chemoimmunotherapy of acute myelogenous leukemia in adults with BCG cell-wall skeleton. In: Yamamura Y, Kitagawa M, Azuma I, eds. Cancer immunotherapy and its immunological bases. Gann Monogr Cancer Res 1978;21:199-209.
5. Azuma I, Taniyama T, Yamawaki M, et al. Adjuvant and antitumor activities of *Nocardia* cell-wall skeletons. Jpn J Cancer Res (Gann) 1976;67:733-6.
6. Uzuka Y, Lion SK, Yamagata S. Treatment of adult acute leukemia using intermittent combination chemotherapy with daunomycin, cytosine arabinoside, 6-mercaptopurine and prednisolone: DCMP two step therapy. Tohoku J Exp Med 1979;118 (Suppl):212-25.
7. Peterson BA, Bloomfield CD, Bosl GJ, et al. Intensive five-drugs combination chemotherapy for adult acute nonlymphocytic leukemia. Cancer 1980;46:663-8.
8. Vogler WR, Chan YK. Prolonging remission in myeloblastic leukemia by Tice-strain bacillus Calmette-Guérin. Lancet 1974;ii:128-31.
9. Whittaker JA, Slater AJ. The immunotherapy of acute myelogenous leukemia using intravenous BCG. Br J Haematol 1977;35:263-73.
10. Nakamura H, Masaoka T, Ohno R, et al. A randomized controlled study of im-

munotherapy for acute myelogenous leukemia with *Nocardia rubra* cell-wall skeleton and irradiated allogeneic leukemia cells. Acta Haematol Jpn 1983;46:1086–92.

11. Ohno R, Nakamura H, Kodera Y, et al. Randomized controlled study of chemoimmunotherapy of acute myelogenous leukemia (AML) in adults with *Nocardia rubra* cell-wall skeleton and irradiated allogeneic AML cells. Cancer 1986;57:1483–8.

12. Kishimoto S, Yunoki K, Nishioka K, et al. Adjuvant activity of *Nocardia* cell-wall skeleton on maintenance chemotherapy of acute non-lymphatic leukemia. Acta Haematol Jpn 1983;46:1093–8. (In Japanese)

Adjuvant immunotherapy by *Nocardia rubra* cell wall skeleton for head and neck malignancies: a randomized, controlled study

Shun-ichi Sakai

Department of Otorhinolaryngology, Kagawa Medical School, Kagawa, Japan

Introduction

This paper describes a randomized, controlled clinical study, performed cooperatively by 8 Japanese clinics, to analyze the effect of adjuvant immunotherapy by the cell wall skeleton of *Nocardia rubra* (N-CWS). *N. rubra* is an actinomycete that exists in earth, is gram positive, Sauer resistant, and grows in aerobic culture. The cell wall skeleton is similar to that of *Mycobacterium* (BCG) spp and may be adopted as a substitute for BCG-CWS in immunotherapy for human malignancies.

In recent years, there have been many reports on immunotherapy for malignancies. It is, however, seldom that one finds a report describing a randomized, controlled study. It is especially doubtful whether immunotherapy for head and neck tumors, mostly squamous cell carcinoma, is effective.

Materials and methods

From the patients who visited our clinics from March 1980 to July 1982, 356 cases with head and neck carcinoma were selected by our protocol. They were divided by the envelope method into 2 groups: the 1st group was treated by immunotherapy with N-CWS, and the 2nd group received no immunotherapy. The basic treatment for both groups was combined surgery, irradiation, and chemotherapy, which was considered the best combination based our experience. The patients excluded from the study either had cancer that was too advanced to justify radical therapy or had macroscopically detectable tumor masses even after 3 months of treatment. N-CWS treatment consisted of induction and maintenance doses. The former comprised 4 successive weekly 500-μg doses administered intracutaneously into an upper arm, with 2 or 3 doses of 25 μg administered (preferably) directly into the tumor mass. The maintenance doses consisted of the same intracutaneous dose given monthly for 2 years.

242

The clinical course was observed until July 1984. We calculated the rate of recurrence-free patients and survivors by the Kaplan-Meier method. Differences between the groups were evaluated by the Wilcoxon test. A neutral controller checked the method and the results.

As Table 1 shows, results from 80 patients were not evaluated in the statistical tests, and 276 cases were analyzed. In studying the background factors, we found no significant differences between 132 N-CWS patients and 144 control patients (Table 2).

Results

The N-CWS group tended to show higher remission and survival rates than the control group, but no statistical significance was found (Fig 1). When the results were divided into 2 classes according to the clinical tumor stage, patients in stages I and II still showed no significant differences between the N-CWS group and the control group (Fig 2). For patients in stages III and IV, however, remission rates were still not significantly different, but the survival rates were significantly different ($p < 0.1$; Fig 3). Remission rates were 11% higher (nonsignificant) and the survival rates were 7% higher (significant) after N-CWS treatment.

The side effects of N-CWS treatment were slight fever, skin lesion at the injection site, abscess, or ulcer (Table 3). These temporary side effects occurred in only 33.3% of patients.

Discussion

Yamamura and coworkers (1–4) developed N-CWS as an immunotherapy for

Table 1 Reasons for patient exclusion.

Reason for exclusion	No. of N-CWS-treated patients	No. of control patients
Protocol violation	2	1
>76 years of age	5	3
Nonmalignancy	1	2
Double cancer	0	1
Metastatic cancer	0	1
Severe complication	1	1
Interruption of radical treatment	3	4
Residual tumor in 4 mo	20	21
Loss to follow-up within 4 mo	4	2
Other	5	3
Total	41	39

Table 2 Comparability of patients analyzed.

Background factor	No. of N-CWS patients*	No. of control patients†	Comparability test result
Sex			
Male	96	111	
Female	36	33	NS
Age (y)			
19–49	22	32	
50–59	42	47	
60–69	39	48	
70–75	29	17	NS
Primary site			
Maxilla	28	28	
Larynx	54	55	
Oral cavity	39	43	
Pharynx	11	18	NS
Neck metastasis			
Yes	37	36	
No	95	108	NS
Clinical stage			
I	31	35	
II	29	41	
III	44	46	
IV	28	22	NS
Surgery			
Yes	86	83	
No	46	61	NS
Radiotherapy			
Yes	94	111	
No	38	33	NS
Chemotherapy			
Yes	51	60	
No	81	84	NS

*Of a total of 132 patients.
†Of a total of 144 patients.
NS, no significant difference.

human malignancies. The immunity is not specific to the tumor, as has been shown experimentally. Clinical trials have been reported for postoperative gastric cancer patients by Ochiai et al (5), for inoperable lung cancer by Yamamura et al (6), for lung cancer by Yasumoto et al (7), and for head and neck malignancies by Sakai et al (8). Although our results from a randomized, controlled trial for head and neck carcinoma did not show significant differences,

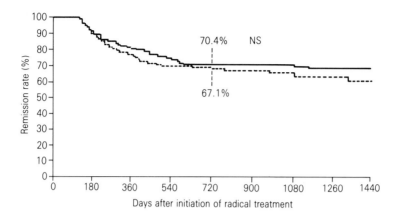

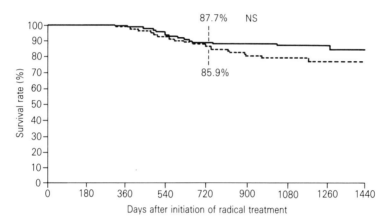

Fig 1 Comparison of remission and survival curves in all patients studied. —— N-CWS-treated patients (132 cases); ----- control patients (144 cases); no significant differences.

there was a tendency for the positive adjuvant immunotherapy to aid the ordinary radical treatment, especially in advanced cases at clinical stages III and IV. This result encourages us to continue with further trials. Even a 5% reduction in recurrence rate as a result of adjuvant immunotherapy can be considered an excellent result.

Acknowledgments

The author thanks his coworkers at the following 8 institutes: Department of

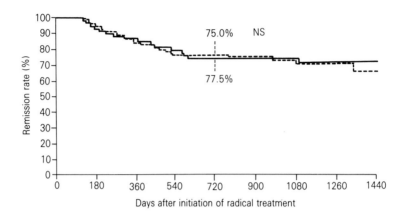

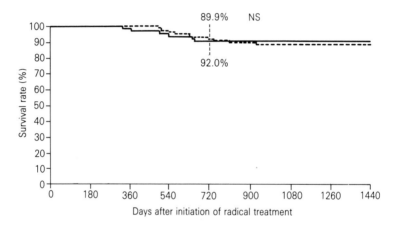

Fig 2 Comparison of remission and survival curves in stages I and II. ——— N-CWS-treated patients (60); ----- control patients (76); no significant differences.

Otolaryngology, Kagawa Medical School; Department of Otolaryngology, Medical Faculty of Osaka University; Department of Otolaryngology, Center for Adult Diseases, Osaka; Department of Otolaryngology, Nara Medical School; Department of Otolaryngology, Medical Faculty of Kagoshima University; Second Department of Oral Surgery, Dental Faculty of Osaka University; First Department of Oral Surgery, Osaka Dental School; and First Department of Oral Surgery, Dental Faculty of Hiroshima University.

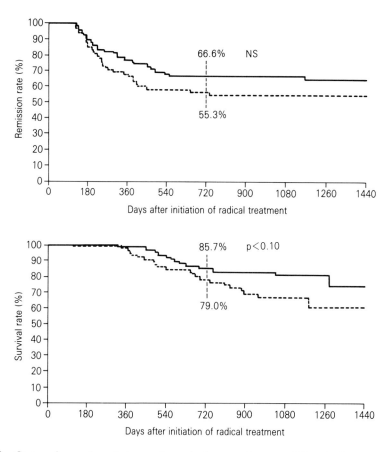

Fig 3 Comparison of remission and survival curves in stages III and IV. —— N-CWS-treated patients (72); ----- control patients (68); upper curves, significant difference between the 2 curves; lower curves, p<0.1 (*Z* = 1.765).

Table 3 Side effects of N-CWS treatment.*

Side effect	No. of patients
Local ulcer	55
Fever (>38°C)	27
(<38°C)	14
Chill	3
Malaise	2
Eruption	2
Pain	2
Arthralgia	1
Lymphadenopathy	1

*Of 188 patients treated with N-CWS, 72 (33.3%) showed side effects.

References

1. Sone S, Filder IJ. In situ activation of tumoricidal properties in rat alveolar macrophages and rejection of experimental lung metastases by intravenous injections of *Nocardia rubra* cell wall skeleton. Cancer Immunol Immunother 1982;12:203-9.
2. Saijo N, Ozako A, Beppu Y, et al. In vivo and in vitro effects of *Nocardia rubra* cell wall skeleton on natural killer activity in mice. Jpn J Cancer Res (Gann) 1983;74:137-42.
3. Yamamura Y, Ogura T, Hirao F, et al. Phase I study with cell wall skeleton of *Nocardia rubra*. Cancer Treat Rep 1981;65:707-9.
4. Yamamura Y, Yasumoto K, Ogura T, Azuma I. *Nocardia rubra*-cell wall skeleton in the therapy of animal and human cancer. In: EM Hersh, ed. Augmenting agents in cancer therapy. New York: Raven Press; 1981:71-90.
5. Ochiai T, Sato H, Sato H, et al. Randomly controlled study of chemotherapy versus chemoimmunotherapy in postoperative gastric cancer patients. Cancer Res 1983;43:3001-7.
6. Yamamura Y, Ogura T, Sakatani M, et al. Randomized controlled study of adjuvant immunotherapy with *Nocardia rubra* cell wall skeleton for inoperable lung cancer. Cancer Res 1983;43:5575-9.
7. Yasumoto K, Yamamura Y. Randomized clinical trial of nonspecific immunotherapy with cell wall skeleton of *Nocardia rubra*. Biomed Pharmacother 1984;38:48-54.
8. Sakai S. Adjuvante Immuntherapie bei Kopf- und Halstumoren; Eine randomisierte kontrollierte Studie. HNO 1986;11:109-14.

Preliminary results of a trial with *Nocardia rubra* cell wall skeleton for the prevention of respiratory tract cancer in a high-risk group

Yukio Nishimoto,[1] Michio Yamakido,[2] Shinichi Ishioka[2]

[1]*Hiroshima Hospital of West Japan Railway Company,* [2]*Department of Internal Medicine, Hiroshima University School of Medicine, Hiroshima, Japan*

Introduction

A poison gas factory was established by the Japanese army in 1929 on the small island of Okunojima, located in the Inland Sea of Japan. The initial products of the factory were hydrocyanic acid and phosgene. In 1933, the factory started to produce mustard gas and lewisite, for which the peak production year was 1937. The factory was in operation until the end of World War II, in 1945, when it was closed by the order of the Allied Command, and the poison gases stored at the factory were disposed of.

Since 1952, we have been conducting clinical and pathological studies on lung cancer among former workers at the Okunojima poison gas factory (1). Wada et al in 1968 (2) reported a high incidence of respiratory neoplasia among former poison gas workers.

In 1956, Collins (3) reported a method for estimating the growth rate of a tumor and time of development of lung cancer, in which tumors are measured on chest X-ray films. We used this method in a study on a poison gas worker who had been engaged in mustard gas production in a poison gas factory and developed lung cancer. The areas of the tumor in 5 chest X-ray films were plotted on a semilogarithmic graph, and a line between the 5 points was extrapolated. The line suggested that tumor cells divided once in 5.5 months, and lung cancer developed around March 1941 (Fig 1). This patient worked at the poison gas factory between November 1940 and September 1945, so cancer seems to have developed 6 months after the start of employment. The latent period of the cancer was very long (13 years, 10 months), although this estimation is based on the assumption that cancer cells divide at regular intervals. We report the effects of *Nocardia rubra* cell wall skeleton (N-CWS), which was administered during this latent

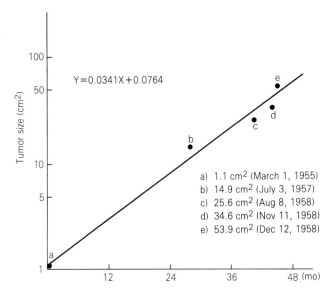

Fig 1 Increase in tumor size in a patient employed at the poison gas factory between November 1940 and September 1945. His work involved mustard gas production, and he died on April 14, 1959.

period to modify immune function, in delaying the development of clinical manifestation of and preventing lung cancer.

Subjects and methods

The former poison gas workers were divided into 3 groups according to their type of work in the factory. Group A consisted of workers engaged directly in the production of poison gases such as mustard gas and lewisite. Group B consisted of workers who had come in contact with these gases. Group C consisted of those engaged in production of other gases or who were working in medical and/or administrative sectors. A dose of 200 μg of N-CWS was administered to male poison gas workers and controls matched for background factors such as sex, age, type of work at the poison gas factory, duration of work, and Brinkman index, and the results were compared between the 2 groups. Tables 1 and 2 show the background factors in the N-CWS group in the 2nd trial, which started in April 1984. Most of subjects belonged to groups A and B, the high-risk groups for respiratory tract cancer epidemiologically. Natural killer (NK) cell activity against K-562 dervived from chronic myelogenous leukemia was determined by the ^{51}Cr-release assay method. Serum interferon was assayed by the cytopathic effect (CPE) inhibition and dye uptake method using FL cells and Sindbis virus (4). For statistical analysis, the χ^2 test, generalized Wilcoxon test, generalized Savage test, and Z-test were used.

Table 1 Duration and type of work of subjects in N-CWS group in 2nd trial (from April 1984).

Duration of work (y)	Type of work			Total
	A	B	C	
<0.5	2	4	3	9
0.5–5	59	43	18	120
>5	24	19	3	46
Total	85	66	24	175

Table 2 Age of subjects and type of work in N-CWS group in 2nd trial (from April 1984).

Age (y)	Type of work			Total
	A	B	C	
50–59	6	5	1	12
60–69	41	25	12	78
70–79	30	28	10	68
80+	8	8	1	17
Total	85	66	24	175

Results

1st trial

Table 3 shows the results of the 1st trial, carried out between April 1977 and April 1982. In this trial, N-CWS 200 μg sc was administered to 187 male poison gas workers once every 3 months. Clinical and immunologic examinations were performed, and the results compared with those of controls matched for background factors such as sex, age, type of work at the poison gas factory, and duration of work. Cancer developed in 12 workers in the N-CWS-treated group and 13 in the control group. Respiratory cancer, which often develops in poison gas workers, occurred in 5 of the N-CWS-treated subjects and 4 of the control group. There was no difference in the incidence of all cancers or respiratory cancer between the 2 groups.

Changes in immunologic parameters

During the 1st trial, a basic study was carried out on immunopotentiation by N-CWS in poison gas workers. Figure 2 (5) shows the time course of NK cell activity before and after percutaneous injection of N-CWS 200 μg. NK cell activity increased significantly 2 weeks after injection and returned to preadministration

Table 3 Development of malignant tumors at the 1st trial* (April 1977–November 1982).

Malignant tumor	N-CWS group	Control group	χ^2 test
Respiratory tract			
Lung	4 ⎫ 5	3 ⎫ 4	NS
Larynx	1 ⎭	1 ⎭	
Digestive system			
Esophagus	1 ⎫	0 ⎫	
Stomach	3 ⎪ 6	8 ⎪ 9	NS
Colon	1 ⎪	1 ⎪	
Pancreas	1 ⎭	0 ⎭	
Others			
CML	1 1	0 0	NS
Total	12	13	NS

*N-CWS group, 187 cases with sc injection of N-CWS 200 μg every 3 months; control group, 187 cases without treatment.

(Target cell, K-562)

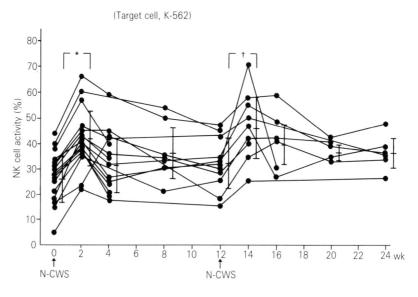

Fig 2 Changes in NK cell activity after N-CWS injection. N-CWS 200 μg was injected into poison gas workers and NK cell activity against K-562 was measured before and after N-CWS administration.*p<0.001; †p<0.05. Reprinted, with permission, from Yamakido M, Ishioka S, Onari K, et al (5).

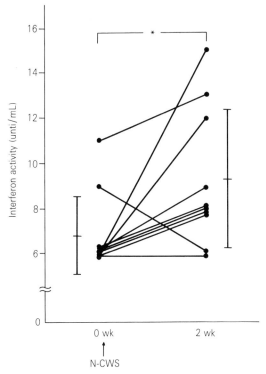

Fig 3 Changes in interferon activity after N-CWS injection. *p < 0.05. Reprinted, with permission, from Yamakido M, Ishioka S, Onari K, et al (5).

levels after 4 weeks. Readministration after 12 weeks produced similar results. The ADCC and monocyte-mediated cytostatic activity increased 2 weeks after administration, as with NK cell activity, and tended to return to the preadministration level after 4 weeks (data not shown).

Figure 3 (5) shows changes in interferon activity after sc injection of N-CWS 200 μg. A significant increase was also observed 2 weeks after administration.

The data obtained during the 1st trial show a peak of various immunoparameters 2 weeks after N-CWS administration and a return to the preadministration level after 1 month. These findings suggest that the interval of N-CWS administration (once every 3 months) is not adequate to maintain an immunopotentiated state.

2nd trial

In the 2nd trial, started in April 1984, 200 μg of N-CWS was administered sc once a month. During the period between April 1984 and February 1988, malignant tumors were clinically demonstrated in 7 of the 175 workers in the N-CWS-treated group and in 14 of the control subjects. The incidence tended to be lower in the treated group. Among respiratory malignant tumors, small cell lung cancer was detected in 1 of the N-CWS group subjects, and lung cancer and laryngeal

Table 4 Development of malignant tumors at the 2nd trial* (April 1984–February 1988).

Malignant tumor	N-CWS group		Control group		χ^2 test
Respiratory tract					
Lung	1 ⎫ 1		2 ⎫ 4		NS
Larynx	0 ⎭		2 ⎭		
Digestive system					
Esophagus	0 ⎫		1 ⎫		
Stomach	1 ⎪		3 ⎪		
Colon	0 ⎬ 4		2 ⎬ 7		NS
Liver	1 ⎪		0 ⎪		
Bile duct	2 ⎭		1 ⎭		
Others					
Prostate	0 ⎫		1 ⎫		
Kidney	1 ⎪		0 ⎪		
Skin	0 ⎬ 2		1 ⎬ 3		NS
Lymphoma	1 ⎪		0 ⎪		
Bladder	0 ⎭		1 ⎭		
Total	7		14		$p < 0.1$

*N-CWS group, 175 cases with sc injection of N-CWS 200 μg each month; control group, 175 cases without treatment.

Table 5 Number of malignant tumors in 2nd trial.

Group	With malignant tumor	Without malignant tumor	Total
N-CWS group	7(1)*	168	175
Control group	14(4)	161	175
Total	21(5)	329	350

$\chi_c^2 = 1.824$ (p<0.1).
*Number of respiratory tract cancers in parentheses.

cancer were each detected in 2 subjects (total 4) in the control group. Cancer of the digestive tract was observed in 4 subjects in the N-CWS group and 7 in the control group (Table 4).

The number of workers who developed cancer during the 2nd trial in the N-CWS-treated group and in the control group were analyzed by the χ^2 test. As shown in Table 5, the number of workers who developed cancer tended to be lower in the N-CWS-treated group.

	N-CWS group		Control group	
April 1984			←Prostate	(A; 74 y)
	←Common bile duct	(B; 81 y)	←Lung	(B; 88 y)
			←Stomach	(A; 80 y)
April 1985	←Bile duct	(C; 68 y)	←Stomach	(B; 66 y)
			←Colon	(B; 79 y)
			←Larynx	(A; 78 y)
April 1986	←Malignant lymphoma	(A; 65 y)	←Esophagus	(A; 75 y)
	←Stomach	(A; 72 y)		
			←Lung	(A; 84 y)
			←Skin	(A; 75 y)
April 1987	←Liver	(A; 72 y)	←Bile duct	(B; 77 y)
	←Lung	(A; 81 y)	←Larynx	(A; 70 y)
	←Kidney	(B; 78 y)	←Stomach	(A; 71 y)
			←Bladder	(A; 79 y)
			←Colon	(B; 81 y)

Fig 4 The time of detection of malignant tumors in N-CWS and control groups (April 1984–February 1988).

Figure 4 shows the time of detection of cancer after the start of the 2nd trial. In the control group, during the 1st year of the period, 3 cases were detected, 1 of which was lung cancer. During the following year, 4 cases were detected, 1 of which was cancer of the larynx and, during the subsequent period, 7 cases were detected, including 1 lung cancer and 1 laryngeal cancer. Thus, in the control group a constant number of cancer cases have been detected each year. In the N-CWS group during the 1st year, 2 cases were detected, during the next year, 1 case, and during the 3rd year, 4 cases, 1 of which was lung cancer.

When compared to the control group, malignant tumors were detected in the N-CWS group after the 2nd year following the start of N-CWS administration.

The curves shown in Fig 5 represent the number of workers with cancer in the N-CWS-treated and control groups. The generalized Wilcoxon and Savage tests revealed no statistical difference between the 2 curves.

Standard errors of the incidence of cancer were obtained from the curves of the stage of occurrence of cancer in workers, using the Greenwood approximation formula based on the survival rates calculated by the Cutler-Ederer method (Fig 6). Differences in the incidence of cancer were evaluated between the N-CWS-treated and control groups during 4 periods, ie, during the 1st, 2nd, and 3rd years following the start of the 2nd trial and after the 3rd year. No difference was observed at the 1st, 2nd, and 3rd years. However, the incidence tended to be lower in the treated group after the 3rd year, providing hope for the prognosis.

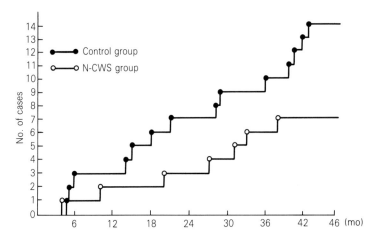

Fig 5 Occurrence of malignant tumors in N-CWS and control groups (April 1984–February 1988). No statistical difference between the N-CWS and control groups was detected using the generalized Wilcoxon test (Breslow, p=0.1465) and generalized Savage test (Mantel-Cox, p=0.1452).

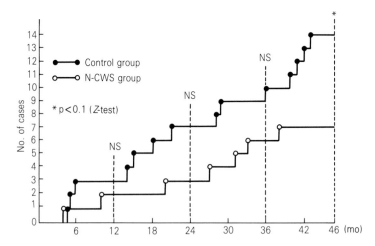

Fig 6 Standard errors of the incidence of cancer obtained from the curves of the stage of occurrence of cancer in workers, using the Greenwood approximation formula, based on survival rates calculated by the Culter-Ederer method (Z-test) (April 1984–February 1988). No difference was observed at the 1st, 2nd, and 3rd years, although the incidence tended to be lower in the treated group after the 3rd year.

Table 6 Side effects observed with administration of N-CWS.

Side effect	No. of cases (%)	No. of dropouts
Fever	20 (11.4)	1
Skin reaction	17 (9.7)	1
Skin ulcer	4 (2.3)	1
Headache	2 (1.1)	0
General tiredness	1 (0.6)	0

Adverse effects of N-CWS

The adverse effects of N-CWS administration observed during the 2nd trial are shown in Table 6. Slight fever was the most frequently observed adverse effect (20 workers, 11%) followed, in order, by skin reactions, such as redness, swelling, and suppuration at the site of injection (17 workers), skin ulcer at the site of injection (3), and headache (2). No abnormality in liver function was observed in any worker. The administration of N-CWS was discontinued in 3 workers (1.7%) because of side effects (fever, skin reaction, and skin ulcer, each in 1 worker).

Discussion

Epidemiological analysis of the period between 1952 and 1981 revealed that the incidence of respiratory malignant tumors in poison gas workers was 3.9 times higher than that in the general population of Japan (6). In particular, the incidence was markedly higher in workers who engaged in mustard gas (Yperite) production for 6 months or more. The results suggest that cancer of the respiratory tract was induced by mustard gas. Since 1977, with the aim of preventing or delaying the development of lung cancer in these workers by strengthening their immunologic surveillance system, administration of N-CWS has been carried out.

N-CWS was developed by Azuma et al (7), and animal experiments conducted by Hirao et al (8) have shown that it prevents carcinogenesis. Immunologic abnormalities such as depressed mitogen response and T cell subset abnormalities have been reported in poison gas workers (9,10).

We have not found any reports of methods of cancer prevention for a group at high risk of cancer. There are limited possibilities for a method of cancer prevention which could be used for nontumor-bearing or for latent-period cases. We cannot use radiation or chemotherapeutic agents that may adversely effect immune function or cause malignant neoplasia. In this paper, we have proposed a method for possible cancer prevention using a biological response modifier, N-CWS. In the 1st trial, N-CWS was administered once every 3 months and we found no difference between the N-CWS and control groups. The immunologic findings, however, suggested that the intervals between N-CWS administration (once every 3 months) were too long to maintain the immunopotentiated state. Therefore, in the 2nd trial, initiated in April 1984, N-CWS was administered once per month, after which the number of workers who developed cancer was lower in the N-CWS-treated group (7 workers) than in the control group (14). Malignant tumors in the respiratory tract, which are characteristic tumors in poison gas workers, developed in 1 of the treated group but in 4 of the controls. These results suggest the efficacy of N-CWS in preventing cancer.

Statistical analysis by the χ^2 test showed that the number of workers who developed cancer was lower in the N-CWS-treated group than in the control group.

Standard errors of the incidence of cancer were obtained from the curves of the stage of occurrence of cancer in workers, using the Greenwood approximation formula based on survival rates calculated by the Cutler-Ederer method. Although no difference was observed for the 1st, 2nd, and 3rd years, the incidence of cancer was lower in the treated group after the 3rd year, giving rise to hope for the future of this treatment.

N-CWS, a biological response modifier, has been reported to induce transient fever, and swelling, pain, suppuration, and skin ulcer at the site of injection (11, 12). In our trial, when these side effects were severe, the dose of N-CWS was reduced to 200, 100, or 50 μg, but administration was continued. During the 2nd trial of N-CWS administration once per month, dropouts were fewer than expected, ie, only 3 due to side effects, demonstrating the safety of N-CWS. No severe side effects of N-CWS have been reported in cancer patients. In our trial, minor fever on the day of administration, and skin reactions at the site of injection, such as redness and pain, were each observed in about 10% of the workers. When these side effects appeared, we reduced the dosage and, in some cases, the interval of administration was changed to 3 months. At least until now, no correlation between the reduction of the dosage and cancer development has been observed.

We can therefore conclude that immunologic prevention of cancer is theoretically valid, but the clinical effects should be carefully evaluated. In future, we would like to continue this clinical study and obtain more accurate data on the immunologic prevention of cancer by consecutive administration of N-CWS.

References

1. Wada S, Nishimoto Y, Miyanishi M, et al. Review of Okunojima poison gas factory regarding occupational environment. Hiroshima J Med Sci 1962;11:75–80.
2. Wada S, Miyanishi M, Nishimoto Y, et al. Mustard gas as a cause of respiratory neoplasia in man. Lancet 1968;i:1161–3.
3. Collins VP, Loeffler RK, Tivey H. Observations on growth rates of human tumors. Am J Roentgenol Radium Ther Nucl Med 1956;76:988–1000.
4. Kohase M, Kohno S, Saito S. Quality control of human interferon preparations.

Tampakushitsu Kakusan Koso [Protein, Nucleic Acid and Enzyme] 1981;12:355-63. (In Japanese)

5. Yamakido M, Ishioka S, Onari K, et al. Changes in natural killer cell, antibody-dependent cell-mediated cytotoxicity and interferon activities with administration of *Nocardia rubra* cell wall skeleton to subjects with high risk of lung cancer. Jpn J Cancer Res (Gann) 1983;74:896-901.

6. Nishimoto Y, Yamakido M, Ishioka S, et al. Epidemiological studies on lung cancer in Japanese mustard gas workers. Proceedings of the international symposium of the Princess Takamatsu Cancer Research Fund 1988:95-101.

7. Azuma I, Yamawaki M, Yasumoto K, Yamamura Y. Antitumor activity of *Nocardia rubra* cell-wall skeleton preparations in transplantable tumors in syngeneic mice and patients with malignant pleurisy. Cancer Immunol Immunother 1978;4:95-100.

8. Hirao F, Sakatani M, Nishikawa H, et al. Effect of *Nocardia rubra* cell-wall skeleton on the induction of lung cancer and amyloidosis by 3-methyl cholanthrene in rabbits. Jpn J Cancer Res (Gann) 1980;71:398-401.

9. Yamakido M, Yanagida J, Ishioka S, et al. Immune functions of former poison gas workers. I: Mitogenic response of lymphocytes and serum factors. Hiroshima J Med Sci 1986;35:117-26.

10. Yamakido M, Yanagida J, Ishioka S, et al. Immune functions of former poison gas workers. II: Lymphocyte subsets and interleukin 2 production. Hiroshima J Med Sci 1986;35:127-34.

11. Yamamura Y, Ogura T, Sakatani M, et al. Randomized controlled study of adjuvant immunotherapy with *Nocardia rubra* cell wall skeleton for inoperable lung cancer. Cancer Res 1983;43:5575-9.

12. Yasumoto K, Yaita H, Ohta M, et al. Randomly controlled study of chemotherapy versus chemoimmunotherapy in postoperative lung cancer patients. Cancer Res 1985;45:1413-7.

Author index

Subject index